# Neurosurgery and Global Health

Isabelle M. Germano

**Editor**

# Neurosurgery and Global Health

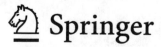 Springer

*Editor*
Isabelle M. Germano
Department of Neurosurgery
Icahn School of Medicine at Mount Sinai
New York, NY, USA

ISBN 978-3-030-86658-7          ISBN 978-3-030-86656-3    (eBook)
https://doi.org/10.1007/978-3-030-86656-3

This Springer imprint is published by the registered company Springer Nature Switzerland AG
The registered company address is: Gewerbestrasse 11, 6330 Cham, Switzerland

*In memory of all neurosurgeons worldwide who dedicated and sacrificed their lives while caring for their patients during the COVID-19 pandemic.*

# Preface

My passion for and dedication to neurosurgery education throughout my career have given me the opportunity to meet with many dedicated and brilliant neurosurgeons around the world. This was accentuated during the past 4 years when I served as the chair of the Education and Training Committee for the World Federation of Neurosurgical Societies (WFNS), a nonprofit, non-governmental organization representing 119 national neurosurgical societies worldwide. During this journey, I recognized that the similarities of our neurosurgical experiences were far greater than the differences. Regardless of the geographical context, the common goal of the neurosurgeons I was working with was to better understand our field and, by so doing, to better serve our patients. Scientific curiosity, deep dedication, incredible work ethics, entrepreneurship, and creativity were common traits among neurosurgeons around the world, and not the exception. Finally, I sensed a common theme that transcended geographical boundaries: the desire to collaborate and exchange ideas and experiences.

To continue the journey we started in the field, while setting up training course and lectures, I envisioned creating a project that would bring us together and perhaps could build a foundation for future collaboration, not just among ourselves but with all the trainees we have in common. Therefore, I decided to create this book with more than 150 authors spanning all 5 continents. I encouraged the lead author of each chapter to find collaborators from each of the five continents. This had a doubly positive net effect. First, the chapter is seen and rendered through multiple lenses and therefore most likely to be more representative of reality. Second, the opportunity to write together started or fostered continued collaborative efforts.

The book opens with an excursive on the role of neurosurgery in worldwide health care. This chapter touches on disparities and proposes strategies and opportunities to overcome them. The history of neurosurgery is then briefly reviewed. The many areas pioneered and developed by neurosurgeons are extraordinary. The overarching theme over the years was to develop new, more effective high-end solutions for complex diseases and to provide access to neurosurgical services for all patients.

In developing the structure for this book, I had in mind the needs of several groups of readers. The first group was those readers who question why neurosurgery should be part of global health. For that group, We created chapters to provide a concise descriptive account of what neurosurgery is all about. In so doing, it became evident that it was not going to be an easy task. Neurosurgery has expanded to cover many sub-specialties. Additionally, it touches on other fields like disaster response, ethics, quality, and safety of care.

The second group of readers to whom I have striven to cater are those who are already familiar with the multifaceted aspects of neurosurgery but have a desire to learn how future neurosurgeons are trained around the world. Current literature on this topic is scant.

My third audience was those neurosurgeons who, like myself, focused on the art and the science of medicine during medical school. Many have mastered technical expertise, pushed the boundaries of discovery, and developed new treatment paradigms. Yet, many were not given the tools to integrate the art and science with the economic forces influencing our work. Hence, I designed the third part of the book to highlight some of the economic aspects of neurosurgery.

This book was written when the COVID-19 pandemic first started. Without a doubt, the pandemic has caused tremendous disruption in global neurosurgery. Yet I believe it has also caused us to unite as a global community and to harness collective efforts for positive changes. Many of the lessons learned during this time have contributed to our resilience and preparedness for the future; some of the changes might even have pushed our neurosurgery boundaries to places where we wouldn't have been without it.

New York, NY, USA                                                          Isabelle M. Germano

# Contents

# Contributors

**John R. Adler Jr.** Department of Neurosurgery, Stanford University, Stanford, CA, USA

**Mehmet Osman Akçakaya** Neurosurgical Department, Florence Nightingale Hospital, Demiroglu Bilim University, Istanbul, Turkey

**Rime Al Baroudi** Department of Neurosurgery, International Cheikh Zaid Hospital, Abulcassis University of Health Sciences, Rabat, Morocco

**Abdulrahman Al-Shudifat** Neurosurgery Department, Faculty of Medicine, University of Jordan, Amman, Jordan

**Oscar L. Alves** Neurosurgery Department, Centro Hospitalar de Gaia/Espinho, Vila Nova de Gaia, Portugal

Neurosurgery Department, Hospital Lusiadas Porto, Porto, Portugal

**Ahmed Ammar** Department of Neurosurgery, King Fahd University Hospital, Al Khobar, Saudi Arabia

**Russell J. Andrews** World Federation of Neurosurgical Societies, Nyon, Switzerland

Nanotechnology & Smart Systems, NASA Ames Research Center, Moffett Field, CA, USA

**Lilyana Angelov** Neurological Surgery, Cleveland Clinic Lerner College of Medicine of Case Western Reserve University, Section of Spinal Radiosurgery and Director of BBTC's Primary CNS Lymphoma Program, Brain Tumor and Neuro-Oncology Center, Cleveland Clinic, Cleveland, OH, USA

**Ahmed Ansari** Department of Neurosurgery, Jawahar Lal Nehru Medical College, Aligarh Muslim University, Aligarh, Uttar Pradesh, India

**Luis Ernesto Ricaurte Arcos** University of Medical Sciences, Habana, Cuba

**Miguel A. Arraez** Department of Neurosurgery, Malaga University, Malaga, Spain

**Souad Bakhti** Neurosurgery Department, Neurosurgery Algiers Medical School University, Algiers, Algeria

**Ronnie E. Baticulon** Division of Neurosurgery, University of the Philippines – Philippine General Hospital, Manila, Philippines

**Suchanda Bhattacharjee** Nizams Institute of Medical Sciences (NIMS), Hyderabad, India

**Lucia Bederson** Icahn School of Medicine at Mount Sinai, New York, NY, USA

**Maria M. Bederson** Carl Illinois College of Medicine, Champaign, IL, USA

**Mark Bernstein** Division of Neurosurgery, Toronto Western Hospital, University of Toronto, Toronto, ON, Canada

**Indira Devi Bhagavatula** National Institute of Health Research Global Health Research Group on Neurotrauma, University of Cambridge, Cambridge, UK

National Institute of Mental Health & Neuro Science, Bangalore, India

**Dhananjaya I. Bhat** Neurosurgery, RV ASTER, Bengaluru, India

**Alexandre Jose Bourcier** David Geffen School of Medicine, The University of California, Los Angeles, CA, USA

**David P. Bray** Department of Neurosurgery, Emory University School of Medicine, Atlanta, GA, USA

**Marike L. D. Broekman** Department of Neurosurgery, Leiden University Medical Center, Leiden, The Netherlands

Department of Neurosurgery, Haaglanden Medical Center, The Hague, The Netherlands

**Richard W. Byrne** Department of Neurosurgery, Rush Medical College, Rush University Department of Neurosurgery, Chicago, IL, USA

**Alexandre C. Carpentier** Chief Neurosurgery Department, Pitie Salpetriere Hospital, Sorbonne University, Founder CarThera Inc., Paris, France

**Marco Cenzato** Neurosurgical Department, Grande Ospedale Metropolitano Niguarda, Milano, Italy

**Meena N. Cherian** Emergency & Surgical Care Program, Geneva Foundation for Medical Education & Research (GFMER), Geneva, Switzerland

**Jebet Beverly Cheserem** National Institute of Health Research Global Health Research Group on Neurotrauma, University of Cambridge, Cambridge, UK

Aga Khan University Hospital, Nairobi, Kenya

**David Clark** National Institute of Health Research Global Health Research Group on Neurotrauma, University of Cambridge, Cambridge, UK

University of Cambridge, Cambridge, UK

**Nigel Crisp**  Independent Member, House of Lords, London, UK
All-Party Parliamentary Group on Global Health, London, UK

**Aneela Darbar**  Aga Khan University Hospital, Karachi, Pakistan

**Rosaline de Koning**  Medical Sciences Department, University of Oxford, Oxford, UK

**B. Indira Devi**  National Institute of Mental Health and Neurosciences, Bengaluru, India

**Katharine Drummond**  Department of Neurosurgery, The Royal Melbourne Hospital, Parkville, VIC, Australia
Department of Surgery, University of Melbourne, Parkville, VIC, Australia

**Najia El Abbadi**  Department of Neurosurgery, International Cheikh Zaid Hospital, Abulcassis University of Health Sciences, Rabat, Morocco

**Abdesslam El Khamlichi**  Hôpital des Spécialités, ONO Service de Neurochirurgie BP 6444 Rabat-Instituts, Rabat, Morocco

**Anthony Figaji**  National Institute of Health Research Global Health Research Group on Neurotrauma, University of Cambridge, Cambridge, UK
University of Cape Town, Cape Town, South Africa

**Di Meco Francesco**  Department of Neurosurgery, Fondazione IRCCS Istituto Neurologico Carlo Besta, Milan, Italy

**Anthony T. Fuller**  Department of Neurosurgery, Duke University, Durham, NC, USA

**Isabelle M. Germano**  Department of Neurosurgery, Icahn School of Medicine at Mount Sinai, New York City, NY, USA
Department of Neurosurgery, Icahn School Medicine at Mount Sinai and Department of Economics, NYU Stern School of Business, NYU, New York City, NY, USA

**André Grotenhuis**  Radboud University Center Nijmegen Medical Center, Nijmegen, The Netherlands

**S. William A. Gunn**  Emergency Humanitarian Operations, World Health Organization, Rolle, Switzerland
International Association for Humanitarian Medicine, Rolle, Switzerland

**Michael M. Haglund**  Duke Department of Neurosurgery, SIngHealth Duke-NUS Global Health Institute, Duke Health, Duke University, Durham, NC, USA

**Mojgan Hodaie**  Division of Neurosurgery, Toronto Western Hospital, University of Toronto, Toronto, ON, Canada

**Stephen Honeybul**  Department of Neurosurgery at Royal Perth Hospital Neurological Surgery, Perth, WA, Australia

**Peter Hutchinson** National Institute of Health Research Global Health Research Group on Neurotrauma, University of Cambridge, Cambridge, UK

University of Cambridge, Cambridge, UK

**Walter D. Johnson** Department of Neurosurgery and School of Public Health, Loma Linda, CA, USA

Center for Global Surgery, Loma Linda University, Loma Linda, CA, USA

Former Lead, Emergency and Essential Surgical Care Programme, World Health Organization, Geneva, Switzerland

**Marianne Juhler** Department of Clinical Medicine, Rigshospitalet – Neurocentret, Copenhagen, Denmark

**Kalango Kalangu** University of Zimbabwe, College of Health Sciences, Department of Neurosurgery, Harare, Zimbabwe

**Aristotelis Kalyvas** Division of Neurosurgery, Toronto Western Hospital, University of Toronto, Toronto, ON, Canada

**Ulrick Sidney Kanmounye** Research Department, Association of Future African Neurosurgeons, Yaounde, Cameroon

**Claire Karekezi** Rwanda Military Hospital, Kigali, Rwanda

**Yoko Kato** Department of Neurosurgery, Fugita Health University, Bantane Hospital, Nagoya, Aichi, Japan

**Andrew Kaye** Department of Neurosurgery, Hadassah University Hospital, Ein Karem, Kyriat Hadassah, Jerusalem, Israel

**Yves Jordan Kenfack** University of Texas Southwestern Medical School, Dallas, TX, USA

**Annette Kennedy** International Council of Nurses, Geneva, Switzerland

**Talat Kırış** Neurosurgery Department, American Hospital and Koc University, Istanbul, Turkey

**Satoshi Kuroda** Department of Neurosurgery, University of Toyama, Graduate School of Medicine and Pharmaceutical Sciences, Toyama, Japan

**John Laidlaw** Department of Neurosurgery, The Royal Melbourne Hospital, Parkville, VIC, Australia

**Guiseppe Lanzino** Department of Neurological Surgery, Mayo Clinic, Rochester, MN, USA

**Rifat Latifi** Department of Surgery, Westchester Medical Center, Valhalla, NY, USA

New York Medical College School of Medicine, Valhalla, NY, USA

**Laura Lippa** Department of Neurosurgery, Ospedali Riuniti, Livorno, Italy

**Wirginia Maixner** Royal Children's Hospital Melbourne, Parkville, VIC, Australia

**Emmanuel M. Makasa** University Hospitals, Lusaka, Zambia

Wits-SADC Regional Collaboration Centre for Surgical Healthcare, University of the Witwatersrand, Johannesburg, Republic of South Africa

Former Health Counsellor at the Permanent Mission of the Republic of Zambia to the United Nations in Geneva and Vienna, Johannesburg, Republic of South Africa

**Marcos Maldaun** Society of Neuro-Oncology Latin America (SNOLA), Sao Paulo, Brazil

**Marcos Masini** School of Medicine Faciplac, Brasília, Brazil

Hospital Lago Sul, Brasília, Brazil

**Heidi McAlpine** Department of Neurosurgery, The Royal Melbourne Hospital, Parkville, VIC, Australia

**Edward Mee** Department of Neurosurgery, Auckland City Hospital, Grafton, Auckland, New Zealand

**Martina Messing-Jünger** Pediatric Neurosurgeon, Head of neurosurgery, Chefärztin der Abteilung Neurochirurgie, Zentrum für Kinderchirurgie, -orthopädie und -neurochirurgie, Sankt Augustin, Germany

**Sergio Moreno-Jiménez** Instituto Nacional de Neurología y Neurocirugía, Mexico City, Mexico

**Stephan A. Munich** Department of Neurosurgery, Rush Medical College, Rush University Department of Neurosurgery, Chicago, IL, USA

**Edjah K. Nduom** Department of Neurosurgery, Emory University, Atlanta, GA, USA

**Bárbara Nettel-Rueda** Department of Neurosurgery, Hospital de Especialidades, Centro Médico Nacional Siglo XXI, IMSS, Mexico City, Mexico

**Federico Nicolosi** Humanitas Research Hospital, Rozzano, Milan, Italy

**Jeff Ntalaja** Hopital Ngaliema, Kinshasa, Democratic Republic of Congo

**Eylem Ocal** Pediatric Neurosurgeon, Little Rock, AR, USA

**Setthasorn Zhi Yang Ooi** Centre for Medical Education (C4ME), Cardiff University School of Medicine, Cardiff, UK

**Nelson M. Oyesiku** Department of Neurosurgery, Emory University School of Medicine, Atlanta, GA, USA

**Susan C. Pannullo** Department of Neurological Surgery, New York-Presbyterian Hospital and Weill Cornell Medicine, New York, NY, USA

**Diana Marcela Sánchez Parra** NIHR Global Health Research Group on Neurotrauma, Universidad de Cambridge, Cambridge, UK

Neurotrauma and Global Neurosurgery Fellowship Program, Meditech Foundation, Cali, Colombia

**Leonidas M. Quintana** World Federation of Neurosurgical Societies, Nyon, Switzerland

Valparaiso University School of Medicine, Valparaiso, Chile

**Mahmood Qureshi** Yaya Centre, Nairobi, Kenya

**Alejandra Rabadán** Department of Neurosurgery, Faculty of Medicine, Buenos Aires University, Buenos Aires, Argentina

**Paolo Raimondo** UpSurgeOn, Milan, Italy

**Faith C. Robertson** Department of Neurosurgery, Leiden University Medical Center, Leiden, The Netherlands

Department of Neurosurgery, Massachusetts General Hospital and Harvard Medical School, Boston, MA, USA

**Scott Robertson** Neurosurgery Department, Laredo Medical Center, University of the Incarnate Word School of Osteopathic Medicine, Laredo, TX, USA

**Jeffrey V. Rosenfeld** Monash University, Melbourne, VIC, Australia

Alfred Hospital, Melbourne, VIC, Australia

**Gail Rosseau** Department of Neurosurgery, George Washington University School of Medicine and Health Sciences, Washington, DC, USA

**Andrés M. Rubiano** Neuroscience Institute, INUB-MEDITECH Research Group, Universidad El Bosque, Bogotá, Colombia

Neurological Surgery Service, Vallesalud Clinic, Cali, Colombia

NIHR Global Health Research Group on Neurotrauma, Universidad de Cambridge, Cambridge, UK

**Francesco Sala** Department of Neuroscience, Biomedicine and Movement Sciences, Section of Neurosurgery, University of Verona, Verona, Italy

**Madjid Samii** International Neuroscience Institute, Hannover, Germany

**Lorraine Sebopelo** Faculty of Medicine, University of Botswana, Gaborone, Botswana

**Franco Servadei** Department of Biomedical Sciences, Humanitas University, Milan, Italy

Department of Neurosurgery, Humanitas Clinical and Research Center – IRCCS, Milan, Italy

**Salman Sharif** WFNS Spine Committee, Izmir, Turkey

Liaquat National Hospital & Medical College, Karachi, Pakistan

**Rajeev Sharma** Department of Neurosurgery, AIIMS, New Delhi, India

**Teresa Somma** Department of Neurosciences and Reproductive and Odontostomatological Sciences, Division of Neurosurgery, Università degli Studi di Napoli Federico II, Naples, Italy

**Giannantonio Spena** HospitalNeurosurgery, Policlinico San Matteo Foundation, Pavia, Italy

**Cameron Stewart** Faculty of Law, Sydney, NSW, Australia

**Katarzyna Świątkowska-Wróblewska** Szpital Świętego Wojciecha, Poznań, Poland

**Souhil Tliba** Bejaia University Hospital Center, Bejaia University, Research Laboratory "Biological Engineering of Cancers", Bejaia, Algeria

**Kurt Yaeger** Department of Neurosurgery, Icahn School of Medicine at Mount Sinai, New York City, NY, USA

**Fumio Yamaguchi** Nippon Medical School, Department of Neurosurgery for Community Health, Tokyo, Japan

**Ismail Zaed** Department of Biomedical Sciences, Humanitas University, Milan, Italy

Department of Neurosurgery, Humanitas Clinical and Research Center – IRCCS, Milan, Italy

**Nelci Zanon** Pediatric Neurosurgeon, Department of Neurology and Neurosuregery, Federal University of São Paulo, São Paulo, Brazil

**Mehmet Zileli** Ege University, Izmir, Turkey

WFNS Spine Committee, Izmir, Turkey

**Yvan Zolo** Faculty of Health Sciences, University of Buea, Buea, Cameroon

**Rodrigo Ramos Zúñiga** Department of Neurosciences, Translational Institute of Neuroscience, University Center of Health Sciences, University of Guadalajara, Guadalajara, Mexico

**Edie Zusman** NorthBay Medical Center, Fairfield, CA, USA

# Part I
# The Role of Neurosurgery in Global Health

Isabelle M. Germano

Global health has been defined as the area of study, research, and practice that places a priority on improving health by prevention and clinical care and achieving equity in health for all people worldwide. The concept of global health is one that includes all involved, as opposed to the term "international health" which usually excludes one's own country, is less inclusive, and possibly adds a connotation of paternalism/colonialism. The main focus of global health has evolved over the years to include not just infectious diseases, such as influenza, tuberculosis, yellow fever, cholera, AIDS, and more recently Covid-19, but to include chronic diseases or conditions such as obesity and diabetes that have become prominent global health issues as well. Additionally, global health is taking into account issues that transcend borders such as climate change, urbanization, health equity, social justice, and income disparity, to mention a few. Global health also focuses on "public health" issues, defined as the actions a community takes to ensure that members of that community can remain healthy (prevention). A few examples of public health-related projects include vaccination programs, fluoridation of drinking water, improved family planning, reduction in the rate of occupational injury, and greater motor vehicle safety.

Why should global health matter to everyone, everywhere? For some, improving health globally is just *"the right thing to do."* For others, improving global health is important because it *potentially* leads to *incredible worldwide economic growth.* Vaccination is a prime example of this. Before the Covid-19 pandemic, between 2010 and 2015, vaccines prevented at least 10 million deaths worldwide. The more people who receive vaccinations, the less likely a disease will spread. As a global community, if our neighbors do not have what they need to prevent and treat diseases, it puts everyone at greater risk. The opposite is also true; when everyone can access health care, we are all better able to combat diseases, which in turn increases worldwide productivity.

Neurosurgery is among the youngest of the surgical disciplines. Although evidence of skull trepanation dates back to over two million years ago [1, 2], it is not until the late nineteenth century, when anesthesia, antisepsis, and hemostasis became available, that our field expanded. It continues to expand. Recent technological advances rapidly progress, to the point that inoperable tumors and pathologies once thought to be incurable are successfully managed and corrected by neurosurgeons. Neurosurgery is considered a tertiary care specialty, meaning that patients being treated require a high level of care that is dependent on highly specialized physicians and equipment. In turn, this typically implies a higher financial cost to the hospital/ institution where the neurosurgery procedures occur and higher cost to the patient receiving the care/their insurance intermediary. This assumption is only partially true, as many basic neurosurgical procedures are life-saving procedures and do not depend on equipment more sophisticated than some of the other surgeries. Recognizing the importance of neurosurgery within the basics of global health has propelled neurosurgery to become an active voice in global health in recent years.

In 2015, the Lancet Commission on Global Surgery provided global needs-based evidence pushing global surgery into the field of global health [3, 4]. In this seminal article, the dire need for global surgery is reviewed, showing the vast inequities present in global access to safe, affordable quality surgery. This called for a global response. Since then, projects and interventions have continued to expand and flourish, with many innovative and impactful approaches developed worldwide, some of which include neurosurgery. The focus of neurosurgery within global health is that of prioritizing improving the health outcomes and achieving health equity worldwide for all people who are affected by neurosurgical conditions or have a need for neurosurgical care.

This Part of the book provides a thorough understanding of the role of neurosurgery in global health in each of the subspecialties. Over 27 million people are estimated to sustain traumatic brain injury (TBI) every year. Chapter 3 highlights specific issues faced in low-resource settings and proposes strategies on how this can be resolved, including an exciting new methodology to improve care for patients suffering from TBI.

Chapter 4 highlights the importance of pediatric neurosurgery in providing services to the children of the world. Current projections show that the global population will be 8 billion by 2025 and the next billion global inhabitants will still be children by then. Over 90% of them will be born in low and intermediate income (LMIC). Better quality neurosurgical care to pediatric patients can be provided through the rapid advances in technology and surgical techniques.

The burden of cerebrovascular diseases (CVD) continues to rise in LMIC. Eighty percent of all CVD-related deaths occur in LMIC, yet the amount of global health spending on noncommunicable disease prevention and treatment remains disproportionately low when compared to the global burden of these diseases. Chapter 5 reviews how the field of cerebral vascular neurosurgery has evolved over recent years to position neurosurgery as a key player for the care of CVD.

Over the past decade, neurosurgical oncology has made strides on each of the five continents. With an aging population and worldwide increased quality of healthcare delivery and resources, the burden of oncological diseases, including those affecting the brain and spine, is projected to increase over the next two decades. Chapter 6 develops concepts of the epidemiology of brain tumors and the current cross-collaboration of national and international neurosurgical organizations focusing on these diseases to improve the field.

Whereas the vast majority of spine disorders do not require surgical intervention, surgical intervention, when indicated, can prevent lifelong disability. Patient selection is a key element in this field in ensuring a successful neurosurgical outcome. Chapter 7 reviews the role of spine neurosurgeons worldwide to create education for patients and physicians aimed at improving outcomes for patients with spine disorders.

Disability caused by tremor, epilepsy, depression, and central pain accounts for more worldwide disability than cancer, heart disease, or HIV-related disorders. Functional neurosurgeons address these important neurological diseases using precision surgery and novel technologies to restore network disorders. Chapter 8 reviews the past and present of this multifaceted subspecialty within neurosurgery and provides exciting views on its future directions.

Both natural and man-made mass casualty events, known as disasters, result in hundreds of thousands of deaths each year. Neurosurgery can play an important role in the humanitarian response to mass casualty disasters. Chapter 9 reviews the critical role of neurosurgeons in disaster response. This is primarily focused on head and spine trauma; however, it expands to other aspects as well.

Poorly coordinated efforts in healthcare delivery and medical errors contribute to increased patient mortality, decreased patient satisfaction, and increased cost in all medical fields including neurosurgery. With its complex nature, neurosurgery is deeply associated with a very slim margin for error and a very high potential for life adverse events. Chapter 10 reviews the key facts on safety and their impact on medical care within neurosurgery, including future opportunities to further enhance quality and safety of neurosurgery patients worldwide.

Medical ethics is a fundamental element at the core of our daily medical practice, regardless of our specialty and/or where we practice in the world. Chapter 11 highlights some of the ethical considerations common to all neurosurgeons worldwide. These include the concept of mental capacity, and the fine line between innovation, clinical research, conflict of interest and the many other gray areas present in the bioethical landscape.

Over the past century, neurosurgery has made significant progress in each of the subspecialties that today allow us to provide care for a broader number of neurological disorders worldwide. Chapter 12 reviews efforts necessary to further raise the standard of neurosurgical care across the globe. These include not only volunteerism, but also creating sustainable, self-sufficient, neurosurgical global infrastructures.

In conclusion, our field spans an incredibly wide range of techniques and technologies focused on caring for an expanding number of patients with neurological and other disorders currently accounting for a large burden of global diseases. Neurosurgeons remain passionate about their work. We envision that the increased desire to collaborate and to build infrastructure to care for patients with neurological disorders will result in improved care worldwide.

# References

1. Dart R. The predatory incremental technique of Australopithecus. Am J Phys Anthropol. 1949;7:1–38.
2. Andrushko VA, Verano JW. Prehistoric trepanation in the Cuzco region of Peru: a view into an ancient Andean practice. Am J Phys Anthropol. 2008;137(1):4–13. https://doi.org/10.1002/ajpa.20836. PMID 18386793.
3. Meara JG, Leather AJ, Hagander L, Alkire BC, Alonso N, Ameh EA. Global surgery 2030: evidence and solutions for achieving health, welfare, and economic development. Lancet. 2015;386:569–624.
4. Burroughs PM, Bloomfield GS. Cardiovascular disease research and the development agenda in low- and middle-income countries. Glob Heart. 2015;10(1):71–3.

# Chapter 1
# The Role of Neurosurgery in Worldwide Health Care and Its Disparities: An Overview

**Franco Servadei and Ismail Zaed**

## Abbreviations

| | |
|---|---|
| HIC | High-income country |
| ICP | Intracranial pressure |
| LMIC | Low- or middle-income country |
| RCT | Randomized clinical trial |
| RTA | Road traffic accidents |
| SCI | Spinal cord injury |
| TBI | Traumatic brain injury |
| WFNS | World Federation of Neurosurgical Societies |

Neurosurgery is a relatively new branch of surgery that became an independent specialty in the large majority of countries only after World War II. Despite being a specialty field within surgery that cares for a relatively small percentage of patients, neurosurgery plays an important role globally in reducing the overall burden of diseases. This is particularly true in countries with limited resources, also known as low-and middle-income countries (LMICs).

Neurosurgery is increasingly important in global health because, *when both neurosurgical and anesthesiology services are available*, a significant number of common conditions can be effectively treated or eliminated by neurosurgical interventions (Table 1.1). For example, traumatic brain injury (TBI) has been

F. Servadei (✉) · I. Zaed
Department of Biomedical Sciences, Humanitas University, Milan, Italy

Department of Neurosurgery, Humanitas Clinical and Research Center – IRCCS, Milan, Italy

© The Author(s), under exclusive license to Springer Nature Switzerland AG 2022     5
I. M. Germano (ed.), *Neurosurgery and Global Health*,
https://doi.org/10.1007/978-3-030-86656-3_1

**Table 1.1** The impact of neurosurgical interventions on health care

| Neurosurgical intervention | Health-care impact |
| --- | --- |
| Traumatic brain injury (TBI) | TBI is the first cause of death and disability in multi-trauma patient |
| Spinal cord injury (SCI) | SCI remains the first cause of long-term disability in the young population |
| Pediatric neurosurgery | In 40 African countries where over 50% of the population is below the age of 20 years, many curable diseases in children are related to our specialty |
| Brain tumors | A large part of intracranial tumors are benign and can be cured by surgery |
| Cerebrovascular (CV) diseases | CV diseases remain a top cause of death worldwide and can be treated minimally invasively |
| Movement/psychiatric disorders and epilepsy | They are increasingly recognized as major causes of death and disability worldwide and can be treated minimally invasively |
| Degenerative spine conditions | They are increasingly recognized as major causes of disability worldwide and can be treated by neurosurgeons |

reported to be the primary cause of death and disability in any multi-trauma patient. Spinal cord injuries (SCIs) remain the first cause of long-term disability in the young population, significantly impacting the national workforce. Spinal cord tumors and most of the other spine degenerative diseases are cared for by neurosurgeons all over the world. A large proportion of intracranial tumors are benign and can be cured with an appropriate surgical treatment. Finally, it is important to note that in 40 African countries, where over 50% of the population is below the age of 20 years [1], many curable diseases in children such as hydrocephalus, spina bifida, and myelomeningocele are successfully treated by neurosurgeons.

Neurosurgery has recently benefited from a general technological improvement that increased the armamentarium of neurosurgical options for the treatment of diseases. One example is the use of endoscopy for skull base tumors and stereotactic radiosurgery. Another is vascular neurosurgery that has made enormous scientific and technological progress; in collaboration with endovascular physicians, interventions are minimally invasive and provide successful outcomes. Functional neurosurgery has expanded its boundaries to play a primary role in the treatment of what were once considered to be classical "neurological" and "psychiatric" diseases, such as extrapyramidal disorders and obsessive-compulsive disorder.

According to a recent study about the neurosurgical workforce around the globe, there are currently around 50,000 neurosurgeons in the workforce. Their distribution among the world population is not homogeneous. In the majority of high-income countries (HICs), such as the USA, Canada, Australia, Japan, and Western European countries, the current ratio is 1 neurosurgeon per 100,000 inhabitants. However, in other parts of the world, particularly in Africa and Southeast Asia, there is a drastic lack of neurosurgical workforce, which results in the absence of urgently needed neurosurgical procedures [2]. Recent data show that globally approximately 5 billion people lack access to surgical care of any kind, leading to an estimated 16.9 million deaths annually that could potentially have been avoided [1]. These disparities are particularly concentrated in LMICs, where nine out of ten people cannot access even the most basic surgical care [1].

Modern medicine is based on high-quality papers that generate evidence-based guidelines for everyday clinical activities. In this context, randomized clinical trials (RCTs) are critically important, since they provide the highest level of scientific evidence in clinical settings. Unfortunately, less than 9% of all RCTs in neurosurgery were performed in LMICs [3]. The situation is self-explanatory when RCTs focused on neurotrauma are considered. There are currently two published RCTs on the topic of cranial decompression. In the DECRA study, all of the patients were from HICs [4]. Similarly, in the RESCUE ICP study, about 91% of patients were from HICs [5]. Yet, the majority of TBI occur in LMICs, not in HICs, raising the question that such RCTs are not representative of and/or applicable to the global burden of TBI disease. There is disparity between countries with a high burden of TBI and those in which most of the research is conducted [6]. In the two RCTs mentioned above, the improvement in clinical outcomes observed in the surgical patients between 6 and 12 months after injury [4, 5] is most likely due to improvement in perioperative management of long-term complications. These include hydrocephalus, cranioplasty, sepsis, and a longer period of intensive rehabilitation. How many countries in the world have the appropriate infrastructure and/or the financial means to afford this?

Furthermore, these and other RCTs have generated evidence-based guidelines [7] which cannot be applied in many countries because of the absence of available resources. As an alternate approach, there is another process that can allow the so-called practical suggestions such as the consensus conference method. In this case, we can include in the process of consensus even non-class I or II papers coming from areas of the world where trauma is an endemic disease. We can also include experts from Africa, Southeast Asia, and Central America [8].

If we examine the publication input from LMICs, we can see how less than 5% of published papers in the neurosurgical literature come from these countries [9]. More specifically, in traumatic brain injury (TBI), almost 80% of published papers come from the USA and Europe [6], and similar data are reported in spinal cord injury [10]. In the same papers, it is reported that there is an inverse relationship between publications and the incidence of both head and spine trauma. This results in a paradoxical scenario, where we have very few scientific publications from the countries in which trauma is an endemic disease, whereas in countries where the incidence of trauma is decreasing, we have most of the published papers. This scientific gap is also increased by the important clinical differences in patient cohorts: whereas, in the "Western" countries such as Europe, the mean age of patients is over 60 years and the main cause of trauma is falls at home [11], in LMIC, patients are much younger, and the main cause of TBI is road traffic accidents (RTA) [12]. This difference is also reflected by the frequency and the diversity of post-traumatic hematomas: in Europe and the USA, patients experience mostly brain contusions and chronic subdural hematomas, whereas in LMICs, they typically sustain acute epidural and subdural hematomas. Besides all these differences, it should be pointed out that the large majority of state-of-the-art monitoring devices, like microdialysis, pO2, and intracranial pressure (ICP), are not easily accessible in those countries. Given all these documented differences, how can we believe that the same suggestions for management can be applied everywhere?

Is it possible to improve this situation and decrease these disparities? Yes, but it will take concerted efforts consistently made on a number of fronts. First, we know it is possible to improve the number of neurosurgeons in areas with a limited workforce because of success we have already witnessed in some LMICs. Through a passion for training engendered by the World Federation of Neurosurgical Societies (WFNS) initiatives and by the increasing number of training programs in many universities, the number of neurosurgeons in sub-Saharan Africa increased five times over 18 years (79 in 1998, 369 in 2016), and the ratio decreased from one neurosurgeon/eight million (1998) to one neurosurgeon/two million (2018) [13].

In order to improve access and decrease disparities, we must also meet the equipment needs of LMIC neurosurgeons. Recent surveys [14, 15] have shown that there is a clear lack of diagnostic devices and surgical instruments (microscope, endoscope, neuro-navigation) in most parts of Africa and Southeast Asia. For example, MRI is available in only 30 to 60% of hospitals. A recent paper demonstrated that the delivery of surgical instruments in these countries is effective and improves patient outcomes [16]. We clearly have to improve this experience and can do so by dramatically increasing donations of instruments even from non-profit organizations.

In order to reduce disparities, we must also increase the number of publications in countries with limited facilities. A recent survey showed that one of the top priorities for young neurosurgeons in LMICs is clinical research and publications [17]. There are many examples of collaborations resulting in clinical research and surgical help between Western universities and LMIC institutions in neurosurgery. The list includes Tanzania and Cornell University, USA [18]; Uganda and Duke University, USA [19]; Cambodia and Harvard University, USA [20]; Indonesia and Humanitas University, Italy, and Cambridge University, UK [9]; and Zanzibar and Valencia University, Spain [21]. The good news is that these represent only very few examples of a large number of "twin" institutions' collaborations. In addition, the recently completed RESCUE-ASDH (*R*andomised *Evaluation* of *S*urgery with *C*raniectomy for patients *U*ndergoing *E*vacuation of *A*cute *S*ub*D*ural *H*aematoma) study [22] included LMIC centers in its randomized clinical studies. Even more important, neurosurgeons from these countries (including India, Malaysia, and Hong Kong) were included in well-organized consensus conferences which resulted in important practical recommendations recently done by the University of Cambridge and by the WFNS [8].

It is also critical that we explore and maximize the use of low-cost devices for advanced surgical approaches in countries with limited resources. The Malawi and the Chhabra shunts developed for the treatment of hydrocephalus are two examples of low-cost devices. Dr. Benjamin Warf has reported the success of endoscopic third ventriculostomy in Ugandan children with hydrocephalus, limiting the usage of the ventriculoperitoneal shunt [23, 24]. Even awake surgery for brain tumors has been shown to be feasible in poor-resource settings [25] as well as endoscopic approaches both for hydrocephalus and skull base tumors [26].

The arrival of the worldwide COVID-19 pandemic has severely stressed global health-care delivery and has starkly demonstrated the public health inequities that we all knew existed but often have largely ignored. It has sparked an unprecedented need to share information worldwide. This need to collaborate and share information, and even equipment, is critically important in neurosurgery.

The COVID-19 pandemic has shown globally how far we were from reality at the outset. The first mistake made by every single country and continent is that we all believed "We are different." We told ourselves "China is far away. COVID-19 will never cross oceans, we will protect ourselves; we are clever and prepared enough." WRONG! We told ourselves "The Italians have bad patient care and the population is old; therefore our mortality (in Spain, France, Belgium, UK) will never be like them." WRONG again: the mortality has been similar, if not higher. We said "We (in the USA, Brazil, Sweden) do not need to lock down; we are more clever. We will wait for mass immunization." WRONG! As we learned more about SARS-CoV-2, the pandemic experts in these countries all changed their minds. We told ourselves that the second wave will never arrive. Our current global situation shows how wrong we were about that assumption! Despite the development and distribution of vaccines, we remain in serious trouble worldwide, thanks in large part to individuals' resistance to common sense prevention methods such as masks and social distancing, to the development of viral variants, to governments lessening restrictions, and to general "COVID fatigue."

We also mistakenly told ourselves that neurosurgery will be preserved at any time, that we are indispensible for a large number of patients. Again we were WRONG. Our experience in Italy is such that in the most affected areas, like the city of Bergamo, for several weeks, neurosurgery was shut down and all neurosurgeons were sent to provide general care to COVID-19 patients [27].

Therefore, we have quickly reorganized patient evaluation and care to preserve at least some emergency activity [28]. The same situation happened in many other countries where the neurosurgical units were simply swept away by the COVID-19 tsunami. Surgical indications changed greatly overall. As an example, most of our non-tumoral and non-traumatic spine surgery disappeared from our operating lists, and even tumor surgery was re-formatted in this period [28, 29].

But we believe there are also positive messages from this disaster. We realized that we are NOT a separate body. Instead we are reminded we are doctors before becoming neurosurgeons. We learned how to deal with oxygen masks, how to intubate patients, and how to treat them properly. We showed that we are also able to quickly reorganize our services to provide neurosurgical emergency care with humility and a spirit of service in these difficult times [27]. We also found many ways of communicating without large or small meetings. We activated and became adept with webinars, teleconferences, etc. One positive effect was that many young neurosurgeons who could never travel to other continents for congresses are now exposed to the best possible teaching [29, 30]. We can and must continue to use these innovative communication methods to improve neurosurgery information access worldwide.

In conclusion, neurosurgery is a life-saving branch of surgery and an important part of neurosciences. To reach efficacy on a worldwide basis, we need strategies to reduce disparities between countries with more and countries with fewer resources. The COVID pandemic has taught us how to collaborate and how to find common solutions to a tremendous task. If we use the lessons learned, we can continue to make global progress to ensure increased access to safe and effective neurosurgery interventions in LMICs.

**Acknowledgments**  None.

**Disclosure of Potential Conflict of Interest**  The authors report no conflict of interest concerning the materials or methods used in this study or the findings specified in this paper.

**Funding**  The authors declare that the article content was composed in the absence of any commercial or financial relationships that could be construed as a potential conflict of interest.

# References

1. (a) Department of Economic and Social Affairs Population Dynamics of United Nations. (2020, 7 November) The 2019 Revision of World Population Prospects. Retrieved from: https://population.un.org/wpp/. (b) Mear JG, Greenberg SLM. The lancet commission on global surgery global surgery 2030: evidence and solutions for achieving health, welfare and economic development. Surgery. 2015;157:834–5. (c) Meara JG, Greenberg SLM. Global surgery as an equal partner in health: no longer the neglected stepchild. Lancet Glob Health. 2015;3(Suppl 2):S1–2.
2. Dewan MC, Rattani A, Fieggen G, Arraez MA, Servadei F, Boop FA, Johnson WD, Warf BC, Park KB. We would like to thank the following individuals for their dedication and contribution to identifying the global neurosurgical deficit. Collaborators are listed in alphabetical order: global neurosurgery: the current capacity and deficit in the provision of essential neurosurgical care. Executive summary of the global neurosurgery initiative at the program in global surgery and social change. J Neurosurg. 2018;1:1–10. https://doi.org/10.3171/2017.11. JNS171500. PMID: 29701548.
3. Griswold DP, Khan AA, Chao TE, Clark DJ, Budohoski K, Devi BI, Azad TD, Grant GA, Trivedi RA, Rubiano AM, Johnson WD, Park KB, Broekman M, Servadei F, Hutchinson PJ, Kolias AG. Neurosurgical randomized trials in low- and middle-income countries. Neurosurgery. 2020;87(3):476–83. https://doi.org/10.1093/neuros/nyaa049. PMID: 32171011; PMCID: PMC7426187.
4. Cooper DJ, Rosenfeld JV, Murray L, Arabi YM, Davies AR, Ponsford J, Seppelt I, Reilly P, Wiegers E, Wolfe R, DECRA Trial Investigators and the Australian and New Zealand Intensive Care Society Clinical Trials Group. Patient outcomes at twelve months after early decompressive craniectomy for diffuse traumatic brain injury in the randomized DECRA clinical trial. J Neurotrauma. 2020;37(5):810–6. https://doi.org/10.1089/neu.2019.6869. PMID: 32027212; PMCID: PMC7071071.
5. Hutchinson PJ, Kolias AG, Timofeev IS, Corteen EA, Czosnyka M, Timothy J, Anderson I, Bulters DO, Belli A, Eynon CA, Wadley J, Mendelow AD, Mitchell PM, Wilson MH, Critchley G, Sahuquillo J, Unterberg A, Servadei F, Teasdale GM, Pickard JD, Menon DK, Murray GD, Kirkpatrick PJ, RESCUEicp Trial Collaborators. Trial of decompressive Craniectomy for traumatic intracranial hypertension. N Engl J Med. 2016;375(12):1119–30. https://doi.org/10.1056/NEJMoa1605215. PMID: 27602507.

6. Tropeano MP, Spaggiari R, Ileyassoff H, Park KB, Kolias AG, Hutchinson PJ, Servadei F. A comparison of publication to TBI burden ratio of low- and middle-income countries versus high-income countries: how can we improve worldwide care of TBI? Neurosurg Focus. 2019;47(5):E5. https://doi.org/10.3171/2019.8.FOCUS19507. PMID: 31675715.
7. Hawryluk GWJ, Rubiano AM, Totten AM, O'Reilly C, Ullman JS, Bratton SL, Chesnut R, Harris OA, Kissoon N, Shutter L, Tasker RC, Vavilala MS, Wilberger J, Wright DW, Lumba-Brown A, Ghajar J. Guidelines for the management of severe traumatic brain injury: 2020 update of the decompressive craniectomy recommendations. Neurosurgery. 2020;87(3):427–34. https://doi.org/10.1093/neuros/nyaa278. PMID: 32761068; PMCID: PMC7426189.
8. Hutchinson PJ, Kolias AG, Tajsic T, Adeleye A, Aklilu AT, Apriawan T, Bajamal AH, Barthélemy EJ, Devi BI, Bhat D, Bulters D, Chesnut R, Citerio G, Cooper DJ, Czosnyka M, Edem I, El-Ghandour NMF, Figaji A, Fountas KN, Gallagher C, Hawryluk GWJ, Iaccarino C, Joseph M, Khan T, Laeke T, Levchenko O, Liu B, Liu W, Maas A, Manley GT, Manson P, Mazzeo AT, Menon DK, Michael DB, Muehlschlegel S, Okonkwo DO, Park KB, Rosenfeld JV, Rosseau G, Rubiano AM, Shabani HK, Stocchetti N, Timmons SD, Timofeev I, Uff C, Ullman JS, Valadka A, Waran V, Wells A, Wilson MH, Servadei F. Consensus statement from the international consensus meeting on the role of decompressive craniectomy in the management of traumatic brain injury: consensus statement. Acta Neurochir. 2019;161(7):1261–74. https://doi.org/10.1007/s00701-019-03936-y. PMID: 31134383; PMCID: PMC6581926.
9. Servadei F, Tropeano MP, Spaggiari R, Cannizzaro D, Al Fauzi A, Bajamal AH, Khan T, Kolias AG, Hutchinson PJ. Footprint of reports from low- and low- to middle-income countries in the neurosurgical data: a study from 2015 to 2017. World Neurosurg. 2019;130:e822–30. https://doi.org/10.1016/j.wneu.2019.06.230.
10. Tropeano MP, Spaggiari R, Ileyassoff H, Mabunda DJD, Anania CD, Costa F, Fornari M, Sharif S, Zileli M, Park KB, Servadei F. Traumatic spine injury: which discrepancy between the research output and the actual burden of the disease? World Neurosurg. 2020;142:e117–25. https://doi.org/10.1016/j.wneu.2020.06.131.
11. Roozenbeek B, Maas AI, Menon DK. Changing patterns in the epidemiology of traumatic brain injury. Nat Rev Neurol. 2013;9(4):231–6. https://doi.org/10.1038/nrneurol.2013.22.
12. Smart LR, Mangat HS, Issarow B, McClelland P, Mayaya G, Kanumba E, Gerber LM, Wu X, Peck RN, Ngayomela I, Fakhar M, Stieg PE, Härtl R. Severe traumatic brain injury at a tertiary referral center in Tanzania: epidemiology and adherence to brain trauma foundation guidelines. World Neurosurg. 2017;105:238–48. https://doi.org/10.1016/j.wneu.2017.05.101. PMID: 28559070; PMCID: PMC5575962.
13. Servadei F, Rossini Z, Nicolosi F, Morselli C, Park KB. The role of neurosurgery in countries with limited facilities: facts and challenges. World Neurosurg. 2018;112:315–21. https://doi.org/10.1016/j.wneu.2018.01.047.
14. Gnanakumar S, Abou El Ela Bourquin B, Robertson FC, Solla DJF, Karekezi C, Vaughan K, Garcia RM, Hassani FD, Alamri A, Höhne J, Mentri N, Stienen M, Laeke T, Moscote-Salazar LR, Al-Ahmari AN, Al-Jehani H, Nicolosi F, Samprón N, Adelson PD, Servadei F, Esene IN, Al-Habib A, Kolias AG, World Federation of Neurosurgical Societies Young Neurosurgeons Committee. The world federation of neurosurgical societies young neurosurgeons survey (part I): demographics, resources, and education. World Neurosurg. 2020;8:100083. https://doi.org/10.1016/j.wnsx.2020.100083. PMID: 33103109; PMCID: PMC7573644.
15. Karekezi C, El Khamlichi A, El Ouahabi A, El Abbadi N, Ahokpossi SA, Ahanogbe KMH, Berete I, Bouya SM, Coulibaly O, Dao I, Djoubairou BO, Doleagbenou AAK, Egu KP, Ekouele Mbaki HB, Kinata-Bambino SB, Habibou LM, Mousse AN, Ngamasata T, Ntalaja J, Onen J, Quenum K, Seylan D, Sogoba Y, Servadei F, Germano IM. The impact of African-trained neurosurgeons on sub-Saharan Africa. Neurosurg Focus. 2020;48(3):E4. https://doi.org/10.3171/2019.12.FOCUS19853. PMID: 32114560.
16. Venturini S, Park KB. Evaluating the effectiveness and the impact of donated neurosurgical equipment on neurosurgical units in low- and middle-income countries: the world federation of neurosurgical societies experience. World Neurosurg. 2018;109:98–109. https://doi.org/10.1016/j.wneu.2017.09.117. PMID: 28962958.

17. Robertson FC, Gnanakumar S, Karekezi C, Vaughan K, Garcia RM, Abou El Ela Bourquin B, Derkaoui Hassani F, Alamri A, Mentri N, Höhne J, Laeke T, Al-Jehani H, Moscote-Salazar LR, Al-Ahmari AN, Samprón N, Stienen MN, Nicolosi F, Fontoura Solla DJ, Adelson PD, Servadei F, Al-Habib A, Esene I, Kolias AG, WFNS Young Neurosurgeons Committee. The world federation of neurosurgical societies young neurosurgeons survey (part II): barriers to professional development and service delivery in neurosurgery. World Neurosurg. 2020;8:100084. https://doi.org/10.1016/j.wnsx.2020.100084. PMID: 33103110; PMCID: PMC7573643.

18. Lessing NL, Zuckerman SL, Lazaro A, Leech AA, Leidinger A, Rutabasibwa N, Shabani HK, Mangat HS, Härtl R. Cost-effectiveness of operating on traumatic spinal injuries in low-middle income countries: a preliminary report from a major east african referral center. Global Spine J. 2020;17:2192568220944888. https://doi.org/10.1177/2192568220944888. PMID: 32799677.

19. Adil SM, Elahi C, Gramer R, Spears C, Fuller A, Haglund M, Dunn T. Predicting the individual treatment effect of neurosurgery for TBI patients in the low resource setting: a machine learning approach in Uganda. J Neurotrauma. 2020;38(7):928–39. https://doi.org/10.1089/neu.2020.7262. PMID: 33054545.

20. Makhni MC, Vatan NM, Park PJ, Kabeer ZA, Cerpa M, Choi JH, Lombardi JM, Hong S, Kim Y, Lenke LG, Lehman R, Vycheth I, Park KB. Path to prevention of spinal trauma in a low- to middle-income country: a single-center study in Phnom Penh, Cambodia. J Am Acad Orthop Surg Glob Res Rev. 2019;3(10):e1900080. https://doi.org/10.5435/JAAOSGlobal-D-19-00080. PMID: 31773077; PMCID: PMC6855502.

21. Leidinger A, Piquer J, Kim EE, Nahonda H, Qureshi MM, Young PH. Experience in the early surgical management of myelomeningocele in Zanzibar. World Neurosurg. 2019;121:e493–9. https://doi.org/10.1016/j.wneu.2018.09.145. PMID: 30268549.

22. RESCUE-ASDH. Randomised evaluation of surgery with craniectomy for patients undergoing evacuation of acute subdural haematoma 2020. Retrieved from: http://www.rescueasdh.org

23. Adeloye A. Use of the Malawi shunt in the treatment of obstructive hydrocephalus in children. East Afr Med J. 1997;74(4):263–6. PMID: 9299832.

24. Warf BC. Comparison of 1-year outcomes for the Chhabra and Codman-Hakim Micro Precision shunt systems in Uganda: a prospective study in 195 children. J Neurosurg. 2005;102(4 Suppl):358–62. https://doi.org/10.3171/ped.2005.102.4.0358. PMID: 15926385.

25. Howe KL, Zhou G, July J, Totimeh T, Dakurah T, Malomo AO, Mahmud MR, Ismail NJ, Bernstein MA. Teaching and sustainably implementing awake craniotomy in resource-poor settings. World Neurosurg. 2013;80(6):e171–4. https://doi.org/10.1016/j.wneu.2013.07.003. PMID: 23871816.

26. Uche EO, Okorie E, Emejulu J, Ajuzieogu O, Uche NJ. Challenges and outcome of cranial neuroendoscopic surgery in a resource constrained developing African country. Niger J Clin Pract. 2016;19(6):811–5. https://doi.org/10.4103/1119-3077.183236. PMID: 27811456.

27. Cenzato M, DiMeco F, Fontanella M, Locatelli D, Servadei F. Editorial. Neurosurgery in the storm of COVID-19: suggestions from the Lombardy region, Italy (ex malo bonum). J Neurosurg. 2020:1–2. https://doi.org/10.3171/2020.3.JNS20960. PMID: 32276261; PMCID: PMC7161162.

28. Burke JF, Chan AK, Mummaneni V, Chou D, Lobo EP, Berger MS, Theodosopoulos PV, Mummaneni PV. Letter: the coronavirus disease 2019 global pandemic: a neurosurgical treatment algorithm. Neurosurgery. 2020;87(1):E50–6. https://doi.org/10.1093/neuros/nyaa116. PMID: 32242901; PMCID: PMC7184344.

29. Burks JD, Luther EM, Govindarajan V, Shah AH, Levi AD, Komotar RJ. Early changes to neurosurgery resident training during the COVID-19 pandemic at a large U.S. Academic Medical Center. World Neurosurg. 2020;144:e926–33. https://doi.org/10.1016/j.wneu.2020.09.125. PMID: 32992058; PMCID: PMC7521299.

30. Zaed I, Tinterri B. Letter to the editor: how is COVID-19 going to affect education in neurosurgery? A step toward a new era of educational training. World Neurosurg. 2020;140:481–3. https://doi.org/10.1016/j.wneu.2020.06.032. PMID: 32535051; PMCID: PMC7289099.

# Chapter 2
# Historical Perspective: The History of Neurosurgery

Madjid Samii

Neurosurgery made a fascinating advancement in the last century. Its historical development, however, was somewhat slower than that of other surgical specialties due to the complexity of the central nervous system. Initial attempts to treat brain disease surgically have been related to high morbidity and mortality. Only the better understanding of brain structure and function localization and the introduction of antisepsis, anesthesia, and hemostasis at the end of the nineteenth century led to increased interest and rapid advancement in the field. The other line of development of neurosurgery was to distribute the acquired knowledge and make this highly specialized care available to all patients around the world.

Many prominent surgeons contributed to this advancement despite the initial rather frustrating results. Victor Horsley is considered the founder of modern neurological surgery. Fedor Krause was the first to study human cerebral cortex in detail and developed new operative approaches. Harvey Cushing – considered as the "father of modern neurosurgery" – contributed both with the introduction of new techniques and approaches, such as the application of silver clip and suction, but also laid the conceptual basis of neuro-oncology. The progress of neurosurgery was dependent to a large extent on and was influenced by the discoveries in allied fields [1]. The discovery of the X-rays by Wilhelm Roentgen in 1895 had a major impact in medicine. In 1901, Oppenheim applied the new technique to the skull (cranial rentgenology), and in 1918, Walter Dandy introduced the air ventriculography. The cerebral angiography, introduced by Moniz in the 1920s, allowed for more precise diagnosis and preoperative visualization of the pathological lesions in the brain, which was a prerequisite for more accurate planning of surgeries that did not rely anymore only on the symptoms of the patient. Still, the information from these studies only indirectly presented the brain tumors or lesions.

M. Samii (✉)
International Neuroscience Institute, Hannover, Germany
e-mail: samii@ini-hannover.de; sekretariat.samii@ini-hannover.de

© The Author(s), under exclusive license to Springer Nature Switzerland AG 2022
I. M. Germano (ed.), *Neurosurgery and Global Health*,
https://doi.org/10.1007/978-3-030-86656-3_2

The modern era in neurosurgery began with the establishing of micro-neurosurgery and the introduction of more elaborate imaging tools. Microsurgical instruments and techniques and the operating microscope were introduced in the late 1950s and 1960s by a relatively small group of pioneering neurosurgeons. Jacobson and Donaghy were the first to use it in the lab and recommended it for use in the operating theater. Theodore Kurze (1957) is considered the first neurosurgeon to use the microscope in the operating room. W. House observed H. Wullstein in Germany operating otosclerosis with a microscope and later utilized the microsurgical techniques to approach acoustic neurinomas. Due to the efforts and contributions of L. Malis, G. Yasargil, C. Drake, M. Samii, and others in the 1960s, micro-neurosurgery became the standard of care in modern neurosurgery in the following decade. Many operative procedures already described or even abandoned previously were reviewed or modified with the help of microsurgery. Exemplary is the rediscovery of transsphenoidal surgery for pituitary adenomas that was almost completely abandoned by neurosurgeons after Cushing due to the deep, dark, and frequently blood-filled surgical field. It experienced a rebirth after the introduction of the surgical microscope [2].

Peripheral nerve surgery profited tremendously from the application of operating microscope and in itself stimulated the refining and acceptance of microsurgery.

The microsurgical revolution was enhanced greatly by the introduction of imaging methods that directly presented the brain lesions and the normal cranial and brain structures: the CT scan in 1972 by G. Hounsfield and the MRI by PC Lauterbur in the 1980s.

All these achievements decreased surgical morbidity and allowed for a paradigm change in neurosurgery. Neurosurgery did not aim simply on life preservation and prolongation anymore but rather on preservation of neurological functions. Surgeries became possible even in difficult and functionally important brain areas. The improved knowledge of microanatomy and the utilization of microsurgical technique allowed approaching and removing safely even deep-seated tumors via natural spaces or "anatomical corridors." Tumors in areas considered inaccessible or "no man's land" in the past could be accessed and removed. Radical and safe removal of complex tumors, such as acoustic neurinomas and skull base meningiomas, became feasible with low morbidity, almost no mortality, and good functional outcome. The progress of neuro-anesthesia and neuro-intensive care, as well as of neuro-rehabilitation, was the basis for optimizing the outcome of surgeries and severe brain trauma.

The progress in neurosciences and technology influenced directly and quickly many areas of neurosurgery. Glioma surgery profited from the introduction in the clinical practice of brain mapping methods allowing for individualized approach to each patient, considering the tumor location and particular brain organization. Brain mapping techniques are based either on electrophysiological methods that are applied during surgery or on preoperative and intraoperative imaging methods. Modern neuroimaging allows for precise diagnosis of the tumor, including its metabolic and molecular characteristics. On the other hand, it demonstrates the structure and organization of the surrounding normal brain, including the functional eloquent cortical areas (functional MRI) and its connecting fibers (DTI-based tractography). Neuronavigation became a routinely used tool, which allows for precise planning of surgery and implementing this plan during surgery, minimizing the risk to eloquent structures. The implementation of intraoperative imaging technology reduced the morbidity and increased the effectiveness of the surgeries even further.

A characteristic feature of neurosurgery is its close and open collaboration with related medical specialties, thus promoting the advancement and creation of new concepts and methods of treatment. Exemplary for that is the history of skull base surgery since the 1970s. The lesions of the skull base have been an area of interest to several surgical disciplines, each developing its own management forms and concepts but also limitations. The novel idea of skull base surgery was the interdisciplinary cooperation in order to overcome the limitations of the existing disciplines (M Samii, W Draf: *Surgery* of the *Skull Base: An Interdisciplinary Approach*) [3].

The search of safer therapeutic methods that would further decrease the morbidity and the close cooperation between neurosurgery and neuroimaging led to the origin of neuro-endovascular surgery or interventional neuroradiology. This catheter-based technique for endovascular diagnosis and treatment is now the most commonly practiced therapeutic approach for many vascular conditions affecting the brain and spinal cord, such as aneurysms and AVMs, as well as highly vascularized tumors (e.g., glomus jugulare tumors) [4].

Despite these major advances, some tumors cannot be healed by surgery alone. In the 1960s, Lars Leksell developed the Gamma Knife to treat intracranial lesions in a noninvasive fashion, creating the field of stereotactic radiosurgery [5]. Radiosurgery is a treatment method based on the delivery of high doses of radiation, stereotactically directed to an intracranial region of interest. It is utilized with increasing frequency around the world to treat "nonsurgical" tumors or tumor remnants, such as cavernous sinus meningiomas, or in case radical surgery for some tumor is not possible.

The refinement of stereotactic methods, in particular the precise access to deep brain regions, formed the basis of functional neurosurgery, which is among the most significant advances in neurosurgery. It expanded the role of neurosurgery for management of diseases that have not been traditionally considered as "neurosurgical." The initial destructive techniques have been supplemented by stimulation methods (implantation of stimulating electrodes in the target area). The pioneers of this new development were Siegfried and Benabid [6, 7]. Deep brain stimulation is effective in the treatment of Parkinson's disease, as well as other movement disorders – essential tremor and dystonia – obsessive-compulsive disorders, chronic pain, and epilepsy. Meanwhile, it has been applied in approximately 160,000 patients around the world. Its potential role in the management of other psychiatric conditions, such as addictions or Alzheimer disease, is under investigation [8].

Spine surgery developed parallel to that of brain surgery and profited enormously from the introduction of the new imaging methods – CT and MRI – that allowed precise diagnosis and correlation of the findings to the patient's symptoms. Thus, spinal and spinal cord procedures could be individually targeted to the needs of each patient, avoiding unnecessary extensive surgeries. Spinal fixation techniques were developed in the early twentieth century and revolutionized the care of millions of patients with unstable traumatic or other lesions causing instability. Their management previously was centered on prolonged immobilization using bed rest, traction, and bracing and was frequently ineffective. New techniques for spinal stabilization and instrumentation; the elaboration of new approaches, allowing safe access to every part of the spine; and the introduction of minimally invasive techniques transformed spine surgery [9, 10]. With the introduction of MRI in spine pathologies and of microsurgical techniques, the management of intramedullary tumors has been revolutionized. Multilevel laminectomies causing postoperative spinal deformity were replaced by the laminotomy technique, which prevents such complications.

Characteristic feature of neurosurgery is that it deals with some conditions that very frequently affect people all over the world, such as neurotrauma, but also with some rare and complex diseases. Modern neurosurgery was developed and could be practiced initially only in highly specialized medical centers in some developed countries, which limited the access of the patient. Major challenge has been how to open the access to modern neurosurgical care worldwide. Crucial in this regard over the past century was the foundation of neurosurgical organizations around the world and their close cooperation. Few countries founded the WFNS in 1955, the first president was Jefferson, and the first WFNS Congress was held in 1957 in Brussels (Congress president – Prof. A. Walder). WFNS initiated world congresses every 4 years in order to gather together neurosurgeons for scientific exchange. Since the 1970s, WFNS started organizing neurosurgical training courses in less developed countries. The WFNS Foundation was founded in 1998 with the goal to strengthen the education (founder and first president, M. Samii). The support of the foundation allowed neurosurgical training of many young doctors. Parallel to that, the WFNS organized a broad educational program, which was supported by many neurosurgeons, members of the education committee, to further spread the knowledge.

On the other hand, instrumental for this development was the individual dedication of some outstanding neurosurgeons who throughout their career personally travelled and trained neurosurgeons from all parts of the world. In the 1990s, there were only 500 neurosurgeons practicing in whole Africa (1 neurosurgeon for 1,350,000 inhabitants overall and 1 neurosurgeon for 6,368,000 inhabitants in sub-Saharan Africa, compared to 1/121,000 in Europe and 1/81,000 in North America) [11]. Despite all attempts and positive trends, the sub-Saharan region continues to suffer from a lack of both qualified personnel and well-equipped neurosurgical facilities.

The Project "Africa 100" was planned in order to educate rapidly and without bureaucracy young doctors from countries with few or without neurosurgeons. The past experience has showed that almost all neurosurgeons after their training remained in Europe or America due to lack of infrastructure in their home countries. Therefore, the Project Africa 100 decided to organize the education in North Africa in order to prevent brain drain but also to assure a brain gain for Africa. The pioneer work for the education was in Rabat under the guidance of El Khamlichi. Meanwhile, many young doctors completed their training in Rabat and started to work back in their countries. Despite all attempts and positive trends, the sub-Saharan region continues to suffer from a lack of both qualified personnel and well-equipped neurosurgical facilities. Hence, it remains a big challenge for global NS to pursue reaching a minimum of NS standards in all countries in the world.

These two trends' challenges – to develop new more effective high-end solutions for complex diseases and to provide access to good neurosurgical service for all patients – will certainly continue to define the future of our specialty.

# References

1. Ellis H. Harvey Cushing: father of modern neurosurgery. Br J Hosp Med (Lond). 2014;75(10):597.
2. Martins C, Rhoton AL. Encyclopedia of the neurological sciences. Academic Press; 2003.
3. Samii M, Draf W. Surgery of the skull base. An interdisciplinary approach. Springer Verlag; 1989.
4. Riina HA. Neuroendovascular surgery. J Neurosurg. 2019;131(6):1690–701.
5. Lasak JM, Gorecki JP. The history of stereotactic radiosurgery and radiotherapy. Otolaryngol Clin N Am. 2009;42(4):593–9.
6. Benabid AL, Pollak P, Gao D, Hoffmann D, Limousin P, Gay E, Payen I, Benazzouz A. Chronic electrical stimulation of the ventralis intermedius nucleus of the thalamus as a treatment of movement disorders. J Neurosurg. 1996;84:203–14.
7. Siegfried J, Lippitz B. Chronic electrical stimulation of the VL-VPL complex and of the pallidum in the treatment of movement disorders: personal experience since 1982. Stereotact Funct Neurosurg. 1994;62:71–5.
8. Lozano AM, Lipsman N, Bergman H, et al. Deep brain stimulation: current challenges and future directions. Nat Rev Neurol. 2019;15(3):148–60.
9. Kumar Kakarla U, Chang SW. History and advances in spinal neurosurgery. J Neurosurg Spine. 2019;31(6):775–85.
10. Walker CT, Kakarla UK, Chang SW, Sonntag VKH. History and advances in spinal neurosurgery. J Neurosurg Spine. 2019;31(6):775–85.
11. El Khamlichi A. African neurosurgery part II: current state and future prospects. Surg Neurol. 1998;49(3):342–7. El-Fiki M. African neurosurgery, the 21st-century challenge. World Neurosurg. 2010;73(4):254–8.

# Chapter 3
# The Role of Neurosurgery in Global Health Head Trauma

David Clark, Jebet Beverly Cheserem, Indira Devi Bhagavatula, Anthony Figaji, and Peter Hutchinson

## Brief Historical Background

Evidence of head trauma has been discovered in South Africa in skulls of *Australopithecus africanus*, a hominid precursor to *Homo sapiens*, from as far back as over 2 million years ago [1]. Trepanation during life (the earliest forerunner of modern craniotomies performed by neurosurgeons as well as perhaps the oldest medical procedure) has been discovered in skeletons dating back to around 7000 BC [2], although the largest and most extensively studied group of trephined

D. Clark · P. Hutchinson (✉)
National Institute of Health Research Global Health Research Group on Neurotrauma, University of Cambridge, Cambridge, UK

University of Cambridge, Cambridge, UK
e-mail: dj.clark@cantab.net; pjah2@cam.ac.uk

J. B. Cheserem
National Institute of Health Research Global Health Research Group on Neurotrauma, University of Cambridge, Cambridge, UK

Aga Khan University Hospital, Nairobi, Kenya

I. D. Bhagavatula
National Institute of Health Research Global Health Research Group on Neurotrauma, University of Cambridge, Cambridge, UK

National Institute of Mental Health & Neuro Science, Bangalore, India

A. Figaji
National Institute of Health Research Global Health Research Group on Neurotrauma, University of Cambridge, Cambridge, UK

University of Cape Town, Cape Town, South Africa
e-mail: anthony.figaji@uct.ac.za

© The Author(s), under exclusive license to Springer Nature Switzerland AG 2022
I. M. Germano (ed.), *Neurosurgery and Global Health*,
https://doi.org/10.1007/978-3-030-86656-3_3

19

skulls from any period in any region comes from Peru and Bolivia [3]. Anthropologists postulate that many of the trepanations from this region in South America were performed to treat head trauma, based on the frequency of adjacent skull fractures, male specimens and left-sided injuries (presumably from right-handed assailants) [4]. Mortality following these procedures was surprisingly low and appeared to decrease over time suggesting successive generations of these early surgeons were able to improve their practice considerably, with long-term survival rates reaching 78% by the time of the Incas [4]. The earliest written evidence of head injuries can be found in the Edwin Smith Papyrus, an ancient Egyptian surgical treatise thought to have been originally written around 3000 BC, which describes 48 patient presentations, of which 27 relate to different types of head injury [5]. In ancient Greece, Hippocrates (460–370 BC) – widely considered the "father of medicine" – also published his own treatise on the management of head injuries [6]. From these early pioneers to recent times, gradual progress in the understanding, diagnosis and management of head trauma has occurred over the centuries.

Significant advances in the management of head injury were made in the twentieth century, particularly for those patients with the most severe injuries. A systematic review of the case fatality of severe traumatic brain injury (TBI) [defined as Glasgow Coma Scale (GCS) 3–8] between 1885 and 2010 indicated that the most significant decrease in mortality was observed between 1970 and 1990 [7]. The authors attribute this dramatic drop to the introduction of intracranial pressure (ICP) monitoring and CT scanning. The measurement of ICP was first performed by Guillaume and Janny in 1951 [8], but it was the work of Nils Lundberg in 1960 that set the groundwork for the development of modern-day continuous monitoring of ICP at the bedside [9]. The development of CT scanning in 1971 [10], for which Hounsfield, a British electrical engineer, and Cormack, a South African physicist, were awarded the 1979 Nobel Prize, rapidly went on to revolutionise TBI care. The CT scan superseded existing modalities for making acute treatment decisions for traumatic intracranial pathology including skull radiographs, ventriculography and angiography [11, 12] as well as the practise of exploratory surgery for patients in whom transtentorial herniation was suspected [12]. The description of the original 14-point Glasgow Coma Scale (GCS) by Jennett and Teasdale in 1974 (updated to its modern-day, 15-point format in 1976) was another milestone in the management of head trauma. The GCS brought consistency to the recording of conscious levels in TBI between assessments and clinicians and is now used by neurosurgeons worldwide in both clinical practice and research [13, 14]. Similarly, the Glasgow Outcome Scale (GOS) was created in 1975 as a means of assessing overall functional outcome following TBI [15]. Following these monumental efforts to better understand the pathophysiology and natural history of traumatic intracranial injuries, the final few decades of the twentieth century were characterised by increasing recognition of the importance of preventing secondary brain injury in the treatment of severe TBI, including seminal studies on the deleterious effects of hypoxia [16, 17] and hypotension [16, 17] as well as the benefit conferred by prompt evacuation of intracranial extra-axial haematomas to reduce ICP [18–20].

## Traumatic Brain Injury (TBI): Current Status

The Global Burden of Disease study recently estimated that 27 million new TBI cases occurred in 2016 [21]. Although reliable data on the total number of deaths due to TBI worldwide is not available, evidence from autopsy studies suggests TBI is likely to account for many of the estimated five million deaths that occur due to injuries worldwide annually [22–24]. Approximately 90% of these trauma-related deaths are thought to occur in low- and middle-income countries (LMICs) [22]. Moreover, a post hoc analysis of the Corticosteroid Randomisation After Significant Head Injury (CRASH) trial found that mortality following severe TBI, the patient subpopulation with the worst prognosis, was higher in LMICs than high-income countries [25]. Similarly, a systematic review by Georgoff et al. showed that between 1975 and 2010, the case fatality ratio of severe TBI in the literature was higher in developing nations and, although survival was improving across the globe, it was doing so at a slower rate in developing nations [26]. It has been estimated that 21–38% of the burden of disease due to all injury globally (1–2 million fatalities each year and 52 million disability-adjusted life years) could be averted if the mortality following all trauma in LMICs was similar to that in high-income countries [27, 28]. In this section, we will discuss the progress that has been made in reducing the burden of disease due to TBI worldwide across the entire spectrum of interventions from prevention through to pre-hospital and in-hospital care and finally rehabilitation. Table 3.1 lists examples of key strategies that have been implemented to reduce burden of disease due to TBI for each phase of care.

**Table 3.1** Key strategies implemented to reduce the TBI disease burden

| Current status: what was accomplished until present | |
| --- | --- |
| Phase of care | Examples |
| Prevention | Helmet legislation for motorcycles and bicycles<br>ThinkFirst programme |
| Pre-hospital care | Training lay first responders |
| Neuroimaging | Increasing the number and upkeep of CT scanners |
| Critical care | Guidelines for severe TBI tailored to resources available (including monitoring and medications) |
| Surgery | Training neurosurgeons and delegating emergency neurotrauma procedures to appropriately trained general surgeons |
| Rehabilitation | Sharing of tasks with primary healthcare personnel and families |

## Prevention

The neurosurgical community has had a significant role to play in the recognition of the importance of the primary prevention of head trauma. Hugh Cairns, a British military neurosurgeon, observed that over 2000 motorcyclists and pillion passengers were killed in Britain in the first 21 months of World War II, that the majority of these deaths were due to head injuries and that wearing a helmet seemed to reduce the severity of injuries sustained [29]. On the basis of this evidence, Cairns submitted a report to the Director-General of the Army Medical Services and the Military Personnel Research Committee of the Medical Research Council and persuaded the Army to make wearing helmets mandatory while riding motorcycles in 1941. A dramatic fall in motorcycle-related deaths amongst army personnel was subsequently observed, leading Cairns to propose that helmets should also be adopted by civilian motorcyclists to reduce fatalities [30].

Since then, the use of helmets has become widespread in many regions and evidence from systematic reviews in recent decades indicates that helmets reduce head injuries [31, 32] and deaths in motorcyclists [32]. Moreover, helmeted cyclists have a lower risk of intracranial injury [33]. Evidence from population-based studies indicates that implementation of motorcycle helmet laws is associated with a reduction in deaths due to head injuries [34, 35] and, conversely, repealing these laws is associated with an increase in deaths [35]. Similarly, helmets have been shown to reduce head injuries in bicyclists [31], and bicycle helmet legislation prevents head injuries in bicyclists [36].

Efforts to prevent head injuries in motorcyclists are particularly important in LMIC. The 2013 WHO Global Status Report on Road Safety reports that one third of all road traffic deaths in the South-East Asian and Western Pacific regions involve motorcyclists and head injuries account for up to 88% of fatalities in motorcyclists in some LMICs [37]. Ninety countries, comprising 77% of the world's population, have a comprehensive helmet law, but only one third of countries rate enforcement of helmet laws as good [38]. Nevertheless, evidence exists to suggest correctly implemented and enforced helmet legislation can be effective at preventing head injuries in LMIC. In Vietnam, a review of all road traffic injury patients with head injuries admitted to 20 hospitals 3 months before and after the introduction of a compulsory helmet law nationally observed a 16% reduction in the risk of road traffic head injuries [39].

The primary prevention of head trauma is broader than the promotion of helmet usage only. In response to concerns about the national burden of disease due to TBI and traumatic spinal cord injury (tSCI), the American Association of Neurological Surgeons (AANS) and the Congress of Neurological Surgeons (CNS) created the National Head and Spinal Cord Injury Prevention Program in 1986 [40]. The programme was subsequently renamed the ThinkFirst National Injury Prevention Foundation and aims to prevent neurotrauma in young people due to road traffic accidents, violence and falls through a mixture of educational primary prevention programmes delivered by chapters in the United States and internationally [41].

These programmes explain the causes and effects of neurotrauma as well as its prevention and are delivered by injury prevention educators alongside individuals who have previously experienced a TBI or tSCI. Evaluations of the interventions have shown that participants' self-reported knowledge improves after attendance, and one study even demonstrated a decrease in the proportion of paediatric trauma admissions involving head and spine injuries after the delivery of the ThinkFirst programme [41].

## Pre-Hospital Care

A systematic review published in 2012 by Henry et al. indicated a 25% decreased risk of dying from trauma in areas with pre-hospital trauma systems compared to those without [42]. Pre-hospital hypoxia and hypotension are both poor prognostic indicators in severe TBI [16], and the introduction of effective pre-hospital care has been associated with better odds of a favourable outcome for these patients [43]. However, only 59 out of 195 countries (30%) have ambulance services with the capacity to transfer at least 75% of seriously injured patients to hospital [37]. Similarly, a survey of pre-hospital care in 13 LMICs found that a significant proportion of medical emergencies were transported to hospital by a commercial vehicle (such as a taxi or minibus) or private vehicle rather than emergency medical services [44]. A different survey of hospitals in LMICs caring for paediatric severe TBI patients found significant limitations in capacity to provide essential supportive care in the pre-hospital period, including airway support (62%), oxygen saturation monitoring (79%), oxygen administration (79%) and blood pressure measurement (50%) [45]. The high burden of disease due to trauma in LMICs coupled with a scarcity of pre-hospital resources has led to the development of innovative, cost-effective solutions to improve outcomes. For example, a 5-year prospective study in North Iraq and Cambodia found that training lay first responders in pre-hospital trauma care resulted in a reduction in trauma deaths in those regions from 40% to 14.9% during the study period [46]. Relatedly, the International Committee of the Red Cross's experience in conflict zones is that many patients with survivable head injuries die because of inadequate control of the airway during transfer from the scene of injury to the place of definitive care [47]. As such, the organisation's policy was reformed such that tracheotomies were performed in frontline field hospitals prior to evacuation – this straightforward change in care resulted in mortality being halved.

## Neuroimaging

Despite the significant benefits that access to CT scanning is recognised to offer in acute TBI care [7, 11, 12], the Baseline Country Survey on Medical Devices by the WHO conducted in 2013 indicated only 14% of the low-income countries included in the survey had at least one CT scanner per million people [48]. A prospective TBI registry in a tertiary hospital in rural Tanzania found that 95% of severe TBI patients needed but did not receive a head CT acutely [49]. To compound the problem, competencies in diagnostic procedures that were used to guide head injury management in the pre-CT era, such as ventriculography and angiography, are no longer generally considered essential requirements for trainees in neurosurgery, radiology or neurology anywhere in the world. Exploratory burr holes are occasionally still carried out in certain low-resource settings [50, 51], but their use is restricted to patients with appropriate clinical signs in extremis. Improving access to emergency CT scanning to diagnose traumatic intracranial injuries is likely to improve the outcome of TBI considerably in low-resource settings.

## Surgery

A significant number of patients require surgical care for TBI – a recent population-based study in Taiwan found 7.4 per 100,000 persons received surgical treatment for TBI in 2010 [52]. Moreover, Dewan et al. estimate that 45% of patients with an indication for an essential neurosurgical operation worldwide have TBI [53]. The burden is particularly great in LMICs, where it is estimated that approximately 4.5 million TBI cases need operative management every year [54]. Because of this demand, the World Bank's Disease Control Priorities report includes operative management for traumatic brain injury as one of the 44 surgical procedures considered essential to be available on an emergency basis to all worldwide [55, 56]. Despite this, access to neurosurgery remains extremely poor in some parts of the world – Punchak et al. estimated only 25% of the population in sub-Saharan Africa have access to neurosurgical care within a 2-h time window [57]. This is particularly worrisome for the care of TBI patients, where the relationship between time to surgery and outcome in patients with intracranial extra-axial haematomas is now well established [18–20]. This lack of access can at least partially be explained by the deficiency in trained neurosurgeons in those regions with the highest burden of disease. It has been estimated that 1 neurosurgeon performing TBI cases only is required per 212,000 people in LMICs [54]. However, a recent survey of neurosurgical capacity in sub-Saharan Africa found a significant deficit in trained neurosurgeons in the region – Ethiopia reported 1 neurosurgeon per 13,800,000 people [58]. Another survey conducted in 2016 and 2017 found that 33 countries worldwide had no neurosurgeon [59].

The shortage of trained neurosurgeons in areas with a high burden of TBI has led many countries to delegate aspects of the provision of neurosurgical care to non-neurosurgeons, such as general surgeons. In a recent survey of neurosurgical providers in LMICs, 43% indicated that non-neurosurgeons were involved in delivering neurosurgical care in some capacity in their country [60]. The procedures most frequently performed by non-neurosurgeons were burr holes and craniotomy for haematoma evacuation, the indication for both of which is usually head trauma. Reports from the literature indicate that delegation of neurosurgical care to general surgeons can be safe and effective [61, 62]. In Darwin, a remote and rural region of Australia, emergency neurosurgery has previously been provided by general surgeons – a 5-year retrospective review of their practice found that trauma was the most common indication and outcomes were comparable to urban neurosurgical centres when accounting for case mix [61]. Similarly, a study in the Philippines comparing emergency neurosurgery (mostly for head trauma) provided by consultant neurosurgeons and general surgical residents found no difference in mortality between the two groups [62]. As such, it is reasonable to conclude that delegation of emergency neurosurgery to non-neurosurgeons can be safe and appropriate in certain circumstances where there is a need due to geography or lack of resources. However, it is important to state here that the provision of care by non-neurosurgeons should not be seen as a definitive replacement in the long term and acknowledge the added value that specialist neurosurgical care offers in TBI. A retrospective review of the US and UK Combat Trauma Registries from Iraq and Afghanistan found that the presence of a deployed military neurosurgeon was associated with increased odds of survival in casualties with moderate or severe TBI [63]. As such, efforts to train neurosurgeons in areas where there is a deficit are also crucial.

## Neurocritical Care

The management of severe TBI in high-income countries (HICs) is often based on clinical practice guidelines, the most widely used of which is the Guidelines for the Management of Severe TBI published by the Brain Trauma Foundation (BTF) which focuses on the prevention of secondary brain injury [64]. However, the application of such guidelines is often not feasible in low-resource settings due to a lack of resources. A registry study in a neurosurgical unit in Tanzania found that adherence to the BTF guidelines for the treatment of severe TBI patients was not possible – none of the severe TBI patients in the study received continuous arterial blood pressure monitoring or ICP monitoring and just over a third received hyperosmolar therapy [64]. Furthermore, a survey of 247 hospitals in 68 LMICs found significant deficits in resources available for the monitoring of paediatric severe TBI, including ability to conduct invasive blood pressure monitoring (61%), central venous pressure monitoring (55%), serial CT scanning (41%) and ICP monitoring (22%) [45]. Major limitations in providing treatment were also identified, such as access to mannitol (88%), hypertonic saline (79%), fresh frozen plasma to treat coagulopathy (68%) and external ventricular drainage (14%). To tackle this, the Beyond One Option for Treatment of Traumatic Brain Injury: A Stratified Protocol (BOOTStraP) was developed in Colombia and provides a collection of clinical practice guidelines for all TBI tailored to the resources that are available [65] although its efficacy has yet to be formally assessed.

ICP monitoring remains the cornerstone of the management of severe TBI in high-income countries, but the evidence to support its use is observational [66, 67]. Due to the established role of ICP monitoring in clinical practice in most HICs, a clinical trial investigating ICP monitoring has never been considered feasible due to a lack of equipoise. However, ICP monitoring is not routinely available in many LMICs due to prohibitive cost and lack of available equipment. As such, such an environment was considered a reasonable setting to scrutinise the usefulness of ICP monitoring. The investigators of the Benchmark Evidence from South American Trials: Treatment of Intracranial Pressure (BEST:TRIP) trial set out to compare care guided by ICP monitoring to that guided by imaging and clinical examination (ICE) alone in six intensive care units in Bolivia and Ecuador [68]. Controversially, they concluded that "care focused on maintaining monitored intracranial pressure at 20 mm Hg or less was not shown to be superior to care based on imaging and clinical examination". However, the publication of the findings from BEST:TRIP and their interpretation prompted considerable debate in the literature, and some have interpreted the trial as indicating that ICP monitoring has no role in low-resource settings. A consensus-based interpretation was published by the authors [69], and one of the statements included was that the findings from the trial should be "applied cautiously to regions with much different treatment milieu". It is therefore possible that ICP monitoring has a role in certain low-resource settings if the environment is carefully considered and implemented thoughtfully. For example, a single-centre retrospective cohort study from Kerala in India found that ICP monitoring of severe TBI patients with diffuse brain injury was associated with a decreased need for neuroprotective management, radiation exposure and length of ICU stay [69]. Nevertheless, ICP monitoring is unlikely to be available in many settings in LMIC for years to come, and inexpensive and more readily available alternatives are currently being evaluated such as optic nerve sheath diameter on bedside ultrasonography [70].

Finally, the ability to prognosticate has long been recognised to be extremely important in planning management of TBI patients [71], and this is even more true in low-resource settings where treating when withdrawal would be more appropriate could result in a large volume of scarce resources being wasted. Despite this, an international survey in 2007 of doctors treating head injury found that only 37% agreed they could accurately assess prognosis [72]. Another study comparing the prognostication ability of Ugandan neurosurgical providers with the CRASH risk calculator found that those surveyed were consistently overoptimistic about the long-term prospects of TBI patients [73]. Interestingly, exposure to the predictions made by the calculator resulted in the clinicians in this cohort adjusting their opinions on the prognosis of patients to be less favourable. Advances in machine learning have brought about renewed interest in the utility of prognostic models for TBI in clinical practice and several of such models have recently been developed specifically for use in LMICs using local data sets [74, 75].

## Rehabilitation

Rehabilitation is an important part of TBI care, but resources are extremely limited in the majority of countries globally. Access to rehabilitation medicine is essentially non-existent in many LMICs. A 2009 review found that sub-Saharan Africa had no specialists in rehabilitation medicine [76]. The deficit in human resources is similar for allied healthcare professionals essential for neurorehabilitation. Physiotherapists are probably the most plentiful allied healthcare professionals involved in providing rehabilitation care worldwide, but there are many regions where access is extremely limited. For example, the WHO's Global Health Workforce Statistics indicate that 30 member countries have less than 10 physiotherapists nationwide [77]. Similarly, a 2020 survey of the member countries of the World Federation of Occupational Therapists found the number of occupational therapists worldwide ranged from 220 per 100,000 in Denmark to 0.01 per 100,000 in Tanzania [78]. Finally, the WHO *Mental Health Atlas 2017* reports there are 0.88 psychologists per 100,000 people globally, ranging from 9.04 per 100,000 in high-income countries to 0.05 per 100,000 in low-income countries [79] – even fewer are likely to have the specialist skills in neuropsychology that are required to effectively care for brain-injured patients. In recognition of this mismatch between demand and supply, the WHO distributes a manual entitled "Rehabilitation for Persons with Traumatic Brain Injuries" which is specifically aimed at mid-level rehabilitation workers and primary healthcare personnel [80]. The manual contains information on the effects of brain injuries as well as guides on how to relearn functional skills even when specialised rehabilitation equipment is not available. Task shifting and task sharing of rehabilitation of TBI patients to community health practitioners and families represents an exciting potential avenue for improving care in low-resource settings.

## Future Opportunities and Unmet Needs

Although significant progress has already been made, the examples in the previous section have made clear there are a number of avenues in which the burden of disease from TBI could be reduced globally. The first step in solving any problem is comprehensively describing it (Table 3.1). Despite this, the Commission on *Traumatic brain injury: integrated approaches to improve prevention, clinical care, and research* published in *The Lancet Neurology* in November 2017 highlighted a lack of high-quality, epidemiological data for TBI globally, particularly in LMICs [81]. Recent international collaborative studies, such as CENTER-TBI in Europe [82] and TRACK-TBI in the United States [83], have sought to try and address this. However, both studies mostly collected data on patients in high-income countries. The Global Neurotrauma Outcomes Study, an ongoing international, prospective, observational cohort study comparing outcomes following emergency surgery for TBI across different levels of human development, is one such effort to try and close this knowledge gap [84] While multicentre studies comparing practice and outcomes between countries are useful, population-based studies in individual countries are also required to truly understand the problem and such data from LMICs is currently essentially non-existent [81]. Interventional studies run specifically in LMICs are also lacking. A bibliometric review of neurosurgical randomised controlled trials (RCTs) found that only nine RCTs in neurotrauma with samples from

LMICs only had been published between 2003 and 2016. Moreover, significant between-hospital and between-country variation in outcomes and quality of care has been observed following TBI in HIC [85, 86]. Given the diversity of cultures and health systems in LMICs, it is likely that such heterogeneity also exists in TBI case mix, care and outcomes in this group of nations, and initiatives to reduce the burden of disease due to TBI through research or policy should take this into consideration. Furthermore, improvements in data capture technology mean more information about TBI patients is now routinely available than ever before. Combined with advances in statistical methodology, this data has the potential to revolutionise patient care through precision medicine approaches [81]. However, it is important that such efforts include data on TBI patients from LMICs so as not to further exacerbate the existing knowledge gap. Finally, it is clear that a holistic approach across the entire health system (including prevention, pre-hospital care, surgery, intensive care and rehabilitation) is likely required to truly address the complexity of improving care for TBI across the world [87].

# References

1. Dart R. The predatory incremental technique of Australopithecus. Am J Phys Anthropol. 1949;7:1–38.
2. Lillie MC. Cranial surgery dates back to Mesolithic. Nature. 1998;391(6670):854.
3. Verano JW, Finger S. Chapter 1: ancient trepanation. Handb Clin Neurol. 2010;95:3–14.
4. Verano J. Trepanation in prehistoric South America: geographic and temporal trends over 2000 years. In: Trepanation: history, discovery, theory. Leiden: Swets & Zeitlinger; 2003. p. 223–36.
5. Breasted J. The Edwin smith surgical papyrus. Chicago: University of Chicago press; 1930.
6. Panourias IG, Skiadas PK, Sakas DE, Marketos SG. Hippocrates: a pioneer in the treatment of head injuries. Neurosurgery. 2005;57(1):181–9; discussion 9.
7. Stein SC, Georgoff P, Meghan S, Mizra K, Sonnad SS. 150 years of treating severe traumatic brain injury: a systematic review of progress in mortality. J Neurotrauma. 2010;27(7):1343–53.
8. Guillaume J, Janny P. Continuous intracranial manometry; importance of the method and first results. Rev Neurol (Paris). 1951;84(2):131–42.
9. Lundberg N. Continuous recording and control of ventricular fluid pressure in neurosurgical practice. Acta Psychiatr Scand Suppl. 1960;36(149):1–193.
10. Hounsfield GN. Computerized transverse axial scanning (tomography). 1. Description of system. Br J Radiol. 1973;46(552):1016–22.
11. Zimmerman RA, Bilaniuk LT, Gennarelli T, Bruce D, Dolinskas C, Uzzell B. Cranial computed tomography in diagnosis and management of acute head trauma. AJR Am J Roentgenol. 1978;131(1):27–34.
12. Ambrose J, Gooding MR, Uttley D. E.M.I. scan in the management of head injuries. Lancet. 1976;1(7964):847–8.
13. Teasdale G, Jennett B. Assessment of coma and impaired consciousness. A practical scale. Lancet. 1974;2(7872):81–4.
14. Teasdale G, Jennett B. Assessment and prognosis of coma after head injury. Acta Neurochir. 1976;34(1-4):45–55.
15. Jennett B, Bond M. Assessment of outcome after severe brain damage. Lancet. 1975;1(7905):480–4.

16. Chesnut RM, Marshall LF, Klauber MR, Blunt BA, Baldwin N, Eisenberg HM, et al. The role of secondary brain injury in determining outcome from severe head injury. J Trauma. 1993;34(2):216–22.
17. Miller JD, Sweet RC, Narayan R, Becker DP. Early insults to the injured brain. JAMA. 1978;240(5):439–42.
18. Seelig JM, Becker DP, Miller JD, Greenberg RP, Ward JD, Choi SC. Traumatic acute subdural hematoma: major mortality reduction in comatose patients treated within four hours. N Engl J Med. 1981;304(25):1511–8.
19. Mendelow AD, Gillingham FJ. Extradural haematoma: effect of delayed treatment. Br Med J. 1979;2(6182):134.
20. Haselsberger K, Pucher R, Auer LM. Prognosis after acute subdural or epidural haemorrhage. Acta Neurochir. 1988;90(3-4):111–6.
21. Collaborators GTBIaSCI. Global, regional, and national burden of traumatic brain injury and spinal cord injury, 1990–2016: a systematic analysis for the Global Burden of Disease Study 2016. Lancet Neurol. 2019;18(1):56–87.
22. WHO. Injuries and violence: the facts. Geneva: WHO; 2014.
23. Saidi H, Oduor J. Trauma deaths outside the hospital: uncovering the typology in Kenyan capital. J Forensic Legal Med. 2013;20(6):570–4.
24. Pfeifer R, Schick S, Holzmann C, Graw M, Teuben M, Pape HC. Analysis of injury and mortality patterns in deceased patients with road traffic injuries: an autopsy study. World J Surg. 2017;41(12):3111–9.
25. De Silva MJ, Roberts I, Perel P, Edwards P, Kenward MG, Fernandes J, et al. Patient outcome after traumatic brain injury in high-, middle- and low-income countries: analysis of data on 8927 patients in 46 countries. Int J Epidemiol. 2009;38(2):452–8.
26. Georgoff P, Meghan S, Mirza K, Stein SC. Geographic variation in outcomes from severe traumatic brain injury. World Neurosurg. 2010;74(2-3):331–45.
27. Mock C, Joshipura M, Arreola-Risa C, Quansah R. An estimate of the number of lives that could be saved through improvements in trauma care globally. World J Surg. 2012;36(5):959–63.
28. Higashi H, Barendregt JJ, Kassebaum NJ, Weiser TG, Bickler SW, Vos T. Burden of injuries avertable by a basic surgical package in low- and middle-income regions: a systematic analysis from the Global Burden of Disease 2010 Study. World J Surg. 2015;39(1):1–9.
29. Cairns H. Head injuries in motor-cyclists. The importance of the crash helmet. Br Med J. 1941;2(4213):465–71.
30. Cairns H. Crash helmets. Br Med J. 1946;2(4470):322–3.
31. Thompson DC, Rivara FP, Thompson R. Helmets for preventing head and facial injuries in bicyclists. Cochrane Database Syst Rev. 2000;(2):CD001855.
32. Liu BC, Ivers R, Norton R, Boufous S, Blows S, Lo SK. Helmets for preventing injury in motorcycle riders. Cochrane Database Syst Rev. 2008;(1):CD004333.
33. Forbes AE, Schutzer-Weissmann J, Menassa DA, Wilson MH. Head injury patterns in helmetcd and non-helmeted cyclists admitted to a London Major Trauma Centre with serious head injury. PLoS One. 2017;12(9):e0185367.
34. Tsai MC, Hemenway D. Effect of the mandatory helmet law in Taiwan. Inj Prev. 1999;5(4):290–1.
35. Sosin DM, Sacks JJ, Holmgreen P. Head injury--associated deaths from motorcycle crashes. Relationship to helmet-use laws. JAMA. 1990;264(18):2395–9.
36. Macpherson A, Spinks A. Bicycle helmet legislation for the uptake of helmet use and prevention of head injuries. Cochrane Database Syst Rev. 2008;(3):CD005401.
37. WHO. Global status report on road safety. Geneva: WHO; 2013.
38. Banstola A, Mytton J. Cost-effectiveness of interventions to prevent road traffic injuries in low- and middle-income countries: a literature review. Traffic Inj Prev. 2017;18(4):357–62.
39. Passmore J, Tu NT, Luong MA, Chinh ND, Nam NP. Impact of mandatory motorcycle helmet wearing legislation on head injuries in Viet Nam: results of a preliminary analysis. Traffic Inj Prev. 2010;11(2):202–6.

40. Rosenberg RI, Zirkle DL, Neuwelt EA. Program self-evaluation: the evolution of an injury prevention foundation. J Neurosurg. 2005;102(5):847–9.
41. Youngers EH, Zundel K, Gerhardstein D, Martínez M, Bertrán C, Proctor MR, et al. Comprehensive review of the ThinkFirst injury prevention programs: a 30-year success story for organized neurosurgery. Neurosurgery. 2017;81(3):416–21.
42. Henry JA, Reingold AL. Prehospital trauma systems reduce mortality in developing countries: a systematic review and meta-analysis. J Trauma Acute Care Surg. 2012;73(1):261–8.
43. Rudehill A, Bellander BM, Weitzberg E, Bredbacka S, Backheden M, Gordon E. Outcome of traumatic brain injuries in 1,508 patients: impact of prehospital care. J Neurotrauma. 2002;19(7):855–68.
44. Nielsen K, Mock C, Joshipura M, Rubiano AM, Zakariah A, Rivara F. Assessment of the status of prehospital care in 13 low- and middle-income countries. Prehosp Emerg Care. 2012;16(3):381–9.
45. Wooldridge G, Hansmann A, Aziz O, O'Brien N. Survey of resources available to implement severe pediatric traumatic brain injury management guidelines in low and middle-income countries. Childs Nerv Syst. 2020;36(11):2647–55.
46. Husum H, Gilbert M, Wisborg T, Van Heng Y, Murad M. Rural prehospital trauma systems improve trauma outcome in low-income countries: a prospective study from North Iraq and Cambodia. J Trauma. 2003;54(6):1188–96.
47. Giannou C, Baldan M. War surgery: working with limited resources in armed conflict and other situations of violence, vol. 1. https://www.icrc.org/eng/assets/files/other/icrc-002-0973. pdf:. ICRC; 2009.
48. WHO. Global atlas of medical devices. Geneva: WHO; 2017.
49. Zimmerman A, Fox S, Griffin R, Nelp T, Thomaz EBAF, Mvungi M, et al. An analysis of emergency care delays experienced by traumatic brain injury patients presenting to a regional referral hospital in a low-income country. PLoS One. 2020;15(10):e0240528.
50. Eaton J, Hanif AB, Mulima G, Kajombo C, Charles A. Outcomes following exploratory burr holes for traumatic brain injury in a resource poor setting. World Neurosurg. 2017;105:257–64.
51. Fatigba HO, Allodé AS, Savi de Tové KM, Mensah ED, Hodonou AM, Padonou J. The exploratory burr hole: indication and results at one departmental hospital of benin. ISRN Surg. 2013;2013:453907.
52. Shi HY, Hwang SL, Lee IC, Chen IT, Lee KT, Lin CL. Trends and outcome predictors after traumatic brain injury surgery: a nationwide population-based study in Taiwan. J Neurosurg. 2014;121(6):1323–30.
53. Dewan MC, Rattani A, Fieggen G, Arraez MA, Servadei F, Boop FA, et al. Global neurosurgery: the current capacity and deficit in the provision of essential neurosurgical care. Executive summary of the global neurosurgery initiative at the program in global surgery and social change. J Neurosurg. 2018:1–10. https://doi.org/10.3171/2017.11.JNS171500.
54. Corley J, Lepard J, Barthélemy E, Ashby JL, Park KB. Essential neurosurgical workforce needed to address Neurotrauma in low- and middle-income countries. World Neurosurg. 2019;123:295–9.
55. Botman M, Meester RJ, Voorhoeve R, Mothes H, Henry JA, Cotton MH, et al. The Amsterdam declaration on essential surgical care. World J Surg. 2015;39(6):1335–40.
56. Mock CN, Donkor P, Gawande A, Jamison DT, Kruk ME, Debas HT, et al. Essential surgery: key messages from disease control priorities, 3rd edition. Lancet. 2015;385(9983):2209–19.
57. Punchak M, Mukhopadhyay S, Sachdev S, Hung YC, Peeters S, Rattani A, et al. Neurosurgical care: availability and access in low-income and middle-income countries. World Neurosurg. 2018;112:e240–e54.
58. Sader E, Yee P, Hodaie M. Assessing barriers to neurosurgical care in sub-Saharan Africa: the role of resources and infrastructure. World Neurosurg. 2017;98:682–8, e3.
59. Mukhopadhyay S, Punchak M, Rattani A, Hung YC, Dahm J, Faruque S, et al. The global neurosurgical workforce: a mixed-methods assessment of density and growth. J Neurosurg. 2019:1–7. https://doi.org/10.3171/2018.10.JNS171723.

60. Robertson FC, Esene IN, Kolias AG, Kamalo P, Fieggen G, Gormley WB, et al. Task-shifting and task-sharing in neurosurgery: an international survey of current practices in low- and middle-income countries. World Neurosurg. 2020;6:100059.
61. Luck T, Treacy PJ, Mathieson M, Sandilands J, Weidlich S, Read D. Emergency neurosurgery in Darwin: still the generalist surgeons' responsibility. ANZ J Surg. 2015;85(9):610–4.
62. Robertson FC, Briones R, Mekary RA, Baticulon RE, Jimenez MA, Leather AJM, et al. Task-sharing for emergency neurosurgery: a retrospective cohort study in the Philippines. World Neurosurg. 2020;6:100058.
63. Breeze J, Bowley DM, Harrisson SE, Dye J, Neal C, Bell RS, et al. Survival after traumatic brain injury improves with deployment of neurosurgeons: a comparison of US and UK military treatment facilities during the Iraq and Afghanistan conflicts. J Neurol Neurosurg Psychiatry. 2020;91(4):359–65.
64. Smart LR, Mangat HS, Issarow B, McClelland P, Mayaya G, Kanumba E, et al. Severe traumatic brain injury at a tertiary referral center in Tanzania: epidemiology and adherence to brain trauma foundation guidelines. World Neurosurg. 2017;105:238–48.
65. Rubiano AM, Vera DS, Montenegro JH, Carney N, Clavijo A, Carreño JN, et al. Recommendations of the Colombian consensus committee for the management of traumatic brain injury in prehospital, emergency department, surgery, and intensive care (Beyond One Option for Treatment of Traumatic Brain Injury: A Stratified Protocol [BOOTStraP]). J Neurosci Rural Pract. 2020;11(1):7–22.
66. Miller JD, Becker DP, Ward JD, Sullivan HG, Adams WE, Rosner MJ. Significance of intracranial hypertension in severe head injury. J Neurosurg. 1977;47(4):503–16.
67. Miller JD, Butterworth JF, Gudeman SK, Faulkner JE, Choi SC, Selhorst JB, et al. Further experience in the management of severe head injury. J Neurosurg. 1981;54(3):289–99.
68. Chesnut RM, Temkin N, Carney N, Dikmen S, Rondina C, Videtta W, et al. A trial of intracranial-pressure monitoring in traumatic brain injury. N Engl J Med. 2012;367(26):2471–81.
69. Vora TK, Karunakaran S, Kumar A, Chiluka A, Srinivasan H, Parmar K, et al. Intracranial pressure monitoring in diffuse brain injury-why the developing world needs it more? Acta Neurochir. 2018;160(6):1291–9.
70. Lee SH, Kim HS, Yun SJ. Optic nerve sheath diameter measurement for predicting raised intracranial pressure in adult patients with severe traumatic brain injury: a meta-analysis. J Crit Care. 2020;56:182–7.
71. Maas AI, Lingsma HF, Roozenbeek B. Predicting outcome after traumatic brain injury. Handb Clin Neurol. 2015;128:455–74.
72. Perel P, Wasserberg J, Ravi RR, Shakur H, Edwards P, Roberts I. Prognosis following head injury: a survey of doctors from developing and developed countries. J Eval Clin Pract. 2007;13(3):464–5.
73. Elahi C, Williamson T, Spears CA, Williams S, Nambi Najjuma J, Staton CA, et al. Estimating prognosis for traumatic brain injury patients in a low-resource setting: how do providers compare to the CRASH risk calculator? J Neurosurg. 2020;134(3):1285–93.
74. Hernandes Rocha TA, Elahi C, Cristina da Silva N, Sakita FM, Fuller A, Mmbaga BT, et al. A traumatic brain injury prognostic model to support in-hospital triage in a low-income country: a machine learning-based approach. J Neurosurg. 2019;132(6):1961–9.
75. Adil SM, Elahi C, Gramer R, Spears C, Fuller A, Haglund M, et al. Predicting the individual treatment effect of neurosurgery for TBI patients in the low resource setting: a machine learning approach in Uganda. J Neurotrauma. 2020;38(7):928–39.
76. Haig AJ, Im J, Adewole A, Nelson VS, Krabak B. Africa IRFCoPis. The practice of physical medicine and rehabilitation in sub-Saharan Africa and Antarctica: a white paper or a black mark? PM R. 2009;1(5):421–6.
77. WHO. The 2018 update, Global Health workforce statistics. Geneva: WHO; 2018.
78. WFOT. Global demographics of the occupational therapy profession. WFOT; 2020.
79. WHO. Mental health atlas 2017. Geneva: WHO; 2018.
80. WHO. Rehabilitation for persons with traumatic brain injury. Geneva: WHO; 2004.

81. Maas AIR, Menon DK, Adelson PD, Andelic N, Bell MJ, Belli A, et al. Traumatic brain injury: integrated approaches to improve prevention, clinical care, and research. Lancet Neurol. 2017;16(12):987–1048.
82. Steyerberg EW, Wiegers E, Sewalt C, Buki A, Citerio G, De Keyser V, et al. Case-mix, care pathways, and outcomes in patients with traumatic brain injury in CENTER-TBI: a European prospective, multicentre, longitudinal, cohort study. Lancet Neurol. 2019;18(10):923–34.
83. Yue JK, Vassar MJ, Lingsma HF, Cooper SR, Okonkwo DO, Valadka AB, et al. Transforming research and clinical knowledge in traumatic brain injury pilot: multicenter implementation of the common data elements for traumatic brain injury. J Neurotrauma. 2013;30(22):1831–44.
84. Clark D, Joannides A, Ibrahim Abdallah O, Olufemi Adeleye A, Hafid Bajamal A, Bashford T, et al. Management and outcomes following emergency surgery for traumatic brain injury – a multi-centre, international, prospective cohort study (the Global Neurotrauma Outcomes Study). Int J Surg Protoc. 2020;20:1–7.
85. Lingsma HF, Roozenbeek B, Li B, Lu J, Weir J, Butcher I, et al. Large between-center differences in outcome after moderate and severe traumatic brain injury in the international mission on prognosis and clinical trial design in traumatic brain injury (IMPACT) study. Neurosurgery. 2011;68(3):601–7. discussion 7-8
86. Huijben JA, Wiegers EJA, Lingsma HF, Citerio G, Maas AIR, Menon DK, et al. Changing care pathways and between-center practice variations in intensive care for traumatic brain injury across Europe: a CENTER-TBI analysis. Intensive Care Med. 2020;46(5):995–1004.
87. Bashford T, Clarkson PJ, Menon DK, Hutchinson PJA. Unpicking the Gordian knot: a systems approach to traumatic brain injury care in low-income and middle-income countries. BMJ Glob Health. 2018;3(2):e000768.

# Chapter 4
# The Role of Neurosurgery in Global Health Pediatrics

Nelci Zanon ⓘ, Eylem Ocal ⓘ, Martina Messing-Jünger, Souad Bakhti, Suchanda Bhattacharjee, and Wirginia Maixner

## Introduction

The word surgeon comes from the Greek *kheirourgos*, which means "done by the hand." Traditionally, a doctor at large may treat his/her patients by talking to them and prescribing medicine; hence, the Greeks considered surgeons to be specialized physicians. In 1929, a woman requested care for her child with a brain tumor from the father of neurosurgery, Dr. Harvey Cushing. He wrote her back and said: "The right thing is to have you take him to see Dr. [Franc] Ingraham at the Children's Hospital, and to abide unequivocally by what he says" [1].

N. Zanon (✉)
Pediatric Neurosurgeon, Department of Neurology and Neurosuregery, Federal University of São Paulo, São Paulo, Brazil
e-mail: nelcizanon@terra.com.br

E. Ocal
Pediatric Neurosurgeon, Little Rock, AR, USA
e-mail: eocal@uams.edu

M. Messing-Jünger
Pediatric Neurosurgeon, Head of neurosurgery, Chefärztin der Abteilung Neurochirurgie, Zentrum für Kinderchirurgie, -orthopädie und -neurochirurgie, Sankt Augustin, Germany
e-mail: m.messing@asklepios.com

S. Bakhti
Neurosurgery department, Neurosurgery Algiers Medical School University, Algiers, Algeria

S. Bhattacharjee
Nizams Institute of Medical Sciences (NIMS), Hyderabad, India

W. Maixner
Neurosurgeon at the Royal Children's Hospital Melbourne, Parkville, VIC, Australia
e-mail: wirginia.maixner@rch.org.au

I. M. Germano (ed.), *Neurosurgery and Global Health*,
https://doi.org/10.1007/978-3-030-86656-3_4

33

Worldwide, "pediatric neurosurgery…developed *pari passu* with the general acceptance that children's diseases are best understood and treated in an environment specially centered to their unique requirements" [2]. This is reflected in the establishment of children-specific hospitals, in the recognition of the unique care needs of children and their families, and in the establishment of pediatric neurosurgery as a subspecialty of neurosurgery.

Pediatric neurosurgery is still not recognized "officially" as a subspecialty in several countries. This is mainly due to undefined training requirements and inadequate expertise and/or other resources such as pediatric anesthesiologists, pediatric intensive care units with intensivists, pediatric nurses, and special equipment for pediatric surgery. Pediatric neurosurgery requires a multidisciplinary approach. Therefore, scaling up pediatric neurosurgical care especially in LMIC will also require increasing the workforce with a broader team approach.

## Defining the Pediatric Neurosurgery Specialty Through History

The first trepanation was performed around 6500 BCE. Early evidence of pediatric neurosurgery comes from the practice of trephination as well. A skull of an 11-year-old was excavated in Iran which dated back to 1100 BCE. Even though surgeries were performed on children with "large heads" since Hippocrates, Persian physician Muhammad ibn Zakariya al-Razi (854–925) was the founder of general pediatrics as a medical branch. It wasn't until the nineteenth century that "modern" children's hospitals emerged. These included the Hôpital Necker-Enfants Malades, Paris, in 1802; the Nikolai Hospital for Children, St. Petersburg, in 1834; the St. Anne's Children's Hospital, Vienna, in 1837; the Hospital for Sick Children, Great Ormond Street, London, in 1852; the Children's Hospital of Philadelphia in 1855; and the Children's Hospital of Boston in 1869 [3]. With these came an increasing recognition of the unique needs of children and the emergence of pediatrics as a specialty. Neurosurgery is one of the youngest specialties. It was the foundation of the freestanding large children's hospitals making the development of subspecialties necessary, including pediatric neurosurgery. These hospitals were looking for committed physicians including surgeons to expand their services to children with their own conditions and problems rather than treated as small adults.

Vesalius's description of a 2-year-old girl with a large head in the seventeenth century is evidence that these conditions were known and treated in children at the dawn of modern medicine. However, the foundation of pediatric neurosurgery had to wait until 1913 for Dr. Harvey Cushing's recruitment to the Peter Bent Brigham Hospital (PBHH) in Boston [4]. Dr. Cushing began operating on children with neurosurgical conditions who were brought for surgery from nearby Boston Children's Hospital (BCH). It did not take too long for Dr. Cushing to realize that the pediatric neurosurgery needed to be a dedicated subspecialty. He appointed one of his students – Dr. Franc D. Ingraham – to perform surgeries on pediatric patients [4–6].

Dr. Ingraham was recruited to PBHH in 1929 after finishing his medical studies at Harvard Medical School and surgical residency with Dr. Cushing. The neurosurgery department at BCH was established upon his return from Oxford, which thus became the first dedicated pediatric neurosurgery service in the world [7]. He was instrumental in training many talented neurosurgeons focused on pediatric neurosurgery including Dr. Donald Matson, Dr. Bruce Hendrick, and Dr. John Shillito who became the pioneers of pediatric neurosurgery in the USA, Canada, and internationally. The first textbook of pediatric neurosurgery *Neurosurgery of Infancy and Childhood* was published in 1954 by Dr. Ingraham and his student Dr. Donald D. Matson who became Ingraham's successor as chief of neurosurgery at BCH [7]. Dr. Ingraham operated on and published on a variety of pediatric neurosurgical conditions from spina bifida to tumors to hydrocephalus. With his momentum, the pediatric neurosurgery centers started to emerge in Europe, Latin America, the USA, and Canada.

By the 1960s, in North America, there were several freestanding dedicated children's hospitals like in Toronto, Chicago, Philadelphia, and Cincinnati. The protégés included prominent names in pediatric neurosurgery who ultimately established pediatric neurosurgical centers as chairpersons in the USA, Canada, and around the world. These centers in turn trained fellows nationally and internationally. One prominent figure is Dr. E. Bruce Hendrick who returned to Toronto in 1954 from his training in Boston. He was sent to Boston "for a lifetime opportunity" when he was serving as a postgraduate resident in neurological surgery at the University of Toronto. He became Canada's first dedicated pediatric neurosurgeon. The pediatric neurosurgery service was founded by Dr. Hendrick and his students Dr. Robin Humphreys and Dr. Harold Hofmann, hence the "3Hs."

Meanwhile, in Chicago Children's Memorial Hospital, which was founded in 1882, a neurosurgical service was established by Dr. Luis Amador in 1950. Dr. Amador trained international fellows like Dr. Kenneth Hill who then became a part of the founding team of pediatric neurosurgery service at the Hospital for Sick Children in London, UK. He was trained in Boston as well as Chicago and brought the influence from the USA to the UK. Sanat Bhagwati was another international fellow at Children's Memorial who became a pioneer in the development of pediatric neurosurgery in India [4–6, 8, 9]. The second dedicated pediatric neurosurgery service in the USA was in Children's Hospital of Philadelphia. Eugene Spitz was put in charge in 1957 to establish the clinic. He recruited Luis Schut as an associate in 1962 to work full time at the Children's Hospital [10].

## The Modern Era and the Birth of Organized Pediatric Neurosurgery

Pediatric neurosurgery arose as a subspecialty in the 1950s through the work of Ingraham and Matson in Boston, Amador and Raimondi in Chicago, Till in London, Dott and Shaw in Edinburgh, Rougerie in Paris, Keith and Hendrick in Toronto, and Spitz and Schut in Philadelphia. All of these worked in freestanding children's hospitals with dedicated neurosurgical subspecialization (subunits). Neurosurgeons evolved from general surgeons since the 1930s and 1950s into the era of pediatric specifically trained neurosurgeons in the 1970s and to the "second generation" of pediatric neurosurgeons in the 1980s and 1990s [4].

The modern era of pediatric neurosurgery started after 1970 when pediatric neurosurgery became organized separately within the neurosurgery. It was pioneered by Dr. Anthony Raimondi, born and raised in Chicago, trained with Amador in Chicago where he returned as the chief of the pediatric neurosurgical department at the Children's Memorial Hospital in 1968. Raimondi was essential for the foundation of organized pediatric neurosurgery and the International Society for Pediatric Neurosurgery (ISPN). He trained surgeons particularly from Europe, Japan, India, and Korea. Other countries such as China and Taiwan were also influenced by their counterparts in the USA especially from Chicago [7, 8]. Raimondi was knighted by the president of Italy in 1980 for his treatment of children with brain disorders.

The advancement of the field was accelerated by organized societies, which in turn brought a much more structured curriculum to pediatric neurosurgery training in addition to bringing pediatric neurosurgeons under one roof for further advancement of the field including surgical techniques, research, collaboration, and sharing knowledge and advancing medical technology (Table 4.1). The European Society of Pediatric Neurosurgery (ESPN) was the first pediatric neurosurgical society, founded in 1967 in Vienna, Austria. The AANS/CNS Joint Section of Pediatric Neurosurgery was established in 1972 after the foundation of ESPN [10] and was the first subspecialty section within the AANS. The same year, the ISPN was

**Table 4.1** Pediatric neurosurgery societies' history

| Year established | Society name | Acronym |
|---|---|---|
| 1967 | The European Society of Neurosurgery | ESPN |
| 1972 | AANS Section of Pediatric Neurosurgery[a] | |
| 1972 | International Society for Pediatric Neurosurgery | ISPN |
| 1972 | Japanese Society for Pediatric Neurosurgery | JPN |
| 1987 | Korean Society for Pediatric Neurosurgery | KSPN |
| 1990 | Indian Society for Pediatric Neurosurgery | IndSPN |
| 1998 | Brazilian Society of Pediatric Neurosurgery | SBNPed |
| 2013 | Asian-Australasian Society of Pediatric Neurosurgery | AASPN |
| 2017 | Latin American Society of Pediatric Neurosurgery | ESPN |

[a]Subsequently renamed: AANS/CNS Joint Section on Pediatrics

established in Chicago. Founding members were Raul Carrea (Argentina), Maurice Choux (France), Steen Flood (Norway), Bruce Hendricks (Canada), Wolfgang Koos (Austria), Satoshi Matsumoto (Japan), Jean Pecker (UK), Antony J. Raimondi (USA), Jacques Rougerie (France), John Shaw (UK), and K. Till (UK) [11].

Other national and international organizations followed as pediatric neurosurgery separated itself as a subspecialty in respective countries in the 1990s. The Indian Society for Pediatric Neurosurgery (IndSPN) was formed in 1990 after hosting the 17th Annual Conference of International Society for Pediatric Neurosurgery in 1989 in Bombay. The Society has steadily grown in strength and now has more than 500 members [12]. In Latin America, the Brazilian Society of Pediatric Neurosurgery (SBNPed) was established in 1998, as a progression from the pediatric section of Brazilian Society of Neurosurgery (SBN), currently with more than 150 members [13, 14]. More recently, the Latin American Society of Pediatric Neurosurgery was created in 2017, in continuity with the pediatric chapter of Latin American Federation of Neurosurgical Societies (FLANC) [15, 16]. Lastly, the Asian-Australasian Society of Pediatric Neurosurgery (AASPN) was founded in 2013 [17]. It includes many organizations under its roof: the Chinese Society for Pediatric Neurosurgery, Indian Society for Pediatric Neurosurgery, Japanese Society for Pediatric Neurosurgery, Korean Society for Pediatric Neurosurgery, and Taiwan Society for Pediatric Neurosurgery.

With the formation of multiple organizations specifically including pediatric neurosurgeons and as the number of fellowship-trained pediatric neurosurgeons began to grow, the demand for a specialty journal arose. The official journal of ISPN was founded in 1972 as *Child's Brain* and in 1985 became known as *Child's Nervous System*. Through the efforts of the editorial board led by Concezio Di Rocco, the journal became the official publication of many international pediatric organizations [19]. Ultimately, the *Journal of Pediatric Neurosurgery* was created in 2004 by the efforts of Dr. Jerry Oakes and Dr. John Jane Sr. These two are the main journals for pediatric neurosurgeons to publish their scholarly work in all aspects of pediatric neurosurgery.

The World Federation of Neurosurgical Societies (WFNS) was founded in 1955 [18]. With its foundation and due to the hard work of the pioneers, pediatric neurosurgery gained more recognition as a specialty. Many pediatric neurosurgeons now serve as officers of the WFNS. A separate pediatric neurosurgical committee was also established with a mission to promote education in pediatric neurosurgery, which now has become an essential part of the WFNS education program.

## Pediatric Neurosurgical Training

Between 1970 and 2000, many training programs for pediatric neurosurgery were established. However, as the pediatric neurosurgical practice broadened, it was evident that the education of pediatric neurosurgeons was inadequate to meet the needs. In some centers, there was not enough clinical volume even for resident training as well as faculty expertise. The surgical curriculum was not standard, both in North American centers and internationally. Training and supervising neurosurgeons taking care of children became an essential discussion in organized neurosurgery by the leaders. Especially in the USA and Canada, the idea of a certified fellowship training after completion of a neurosurgical residency training had been discussed but met resistance by prominent figures mainly for "political reasons" [4].

The attempts for identifying and certifying pediatric neurosurgeons waited until 1991 in North America. To establish and codify the optimum training and practice requirements for pediatric neurosurgeons, 40 senior pediatric neurosurgeons from the USA and Canada met in Chicago O'Hare Airport in 1991. By unanimous vote, they founded the American Board of Pediatric Neurological Surgery (ABPNS) to fulfill these functions. Subsequently, the Accreditation Council for Pediatric Neurosurgical Fellowships (ACPNF) was created in 1992 to oversee and regulate pediatric neurosurgical training/fellowship programs in the USA and Canada. The ABPNS is a nonprofit corporation that is now a well-established and well-accepted certifying body and has become the standard accreditation authority for pediatric neurological surgery in the USA and Canada [4].

In Europe, no official specialist degree for pediatric neurosurgeons exists. So far, there is no unified education system that defines a standard for European pediatric neurosurgery either. Approximately 90% of self-identifying pediatric neurosurgeons in Europe report in a survey that they received a formal pediatric neurosurgical training. This essentially consists of clinical training either as a fellow in a dedicated unit or in additional postgraduate training courses organized by the ESPN or national groups (e.g., German course run by the Pediatric Section of the German Neurosurgical Society). There are no course-related examinations. In general, pediatric neurosurgery is more or less integrated in mandatory specialist examinations run by the national medical associations or the EANS (European Association of Neurosurgical Societies) [20].

In Latin America, until the 1990s, the neurosurgeons were seeking pediatric neurosurgery fellowship training in Europe or in the USA. Nowadays, there are pediatric neurosurgery training centers in the large cities in several countries. There is no formal certification or an official necessity to be board certified. However, the recommendation is to complete a year of pediatric neurosurgery fellowship after completing residency and, additionally, to complete the Latin American Pediatric Neurosurgical Course [13].

In Australia, training in pediatric neurosurgery is supervised through the Neurosurgical Society of Australasia Training Board, regulated by the Royal Australasian College of Surgeons, and is part of the core neurosurgical training. Postgraduate training is typically undertaken at international pediatric neurosurgical centers; however, three centers – Westmead Children's, Queensland Children's, and the Royal Children's Hospitals – offer fellowships. The Neurosurgical Society of Australasia oversees and more recently Asian-Australasian Society of Pediatric Neurosurgery conduct all educational and administrative needs for pediatric neurosurgery in the region. Workshops in pediatric neurosurgery are conducted every 2 years [21].

The general lack of neurosurgeons in Africa led to a deficit in trained pediatric neurosurgeons [22]. There are very few countries where there is formal pediatric neurosurgery training. Best examples are Egypt and South Africa. In Egypt, before being qualified as pediatric neurosurgeons, the trainees have to be affiliated to the university children's hospital under supervision of one of the professors of pediatric neurosurgery. During this period, they have to perform at least 2 cases per week and more than 80 cases per year (Prof. Mohamed El Beltagy at Children's Cancer Hospital Egypt, personal communication, 2020). In Morocco, Algeria, and Tunisia, pediatric neurosurgery is not established as a subspecialty, but there are pediatric divisions where working general neurosurgeons are used to treating children.

In sub-Saharan countries, only a few have specialized children care facilities, such as the CURE Children's Hospital in Uganda. African neurosurgery leaders realized early on that training outside Africa was not an answer to the lack of neurosurgeons in the continent (most of the African trainees in Western countries did not return to their countries) and that it was necessary to have local programs of training and centers of training inside the continent. Currently, 15 countries of sub-Saharan Africa have a national program, while Nigeria has 7 [23]. The WFNS Rabat Training Center was created in 2001, and other countries (Algiers, Nairobi, Dakar, and Cairo) have been accredited by WFNS for training in the field under the program "100 for Africa," directed by Prof. Samii [24].

In India, the last decade has seen many neurosurgical centers offering pediatric neurosurgery fellowships for a period of 1–2 years. Some are certified by the provincial universities and some under the aegis of the IndSPN. Currently, there are almost seven centers offering pediatric neurosurgery fellowships. There is disbursement of knowledge by regular courses conducted by ISPN and IndSPN and AASPN. Additionally, courses on focused topics in pediatric neurosurgery and hands-on workshops like endoscopy and craniosynostosis are offered each year from time to time [11].

Overall in Asia, the mission of pediatric neurosurgery training is also being taken care by the AASPN. However, still in many countries, the formal training in pediatric neurosurgery is by apprenticeship in a pediatric neurosurgery center or doing fellowships from abroad.

## The Current Status of the Pediatric Neurosurgical Workforce Around the Globe

Pediatric neurosurgery is probably the most interdisciplinary specialty and represents 20–25% of the activity in most neurosurgical departments. In most countries, neurosurgeons practice both general neurosurgery and pediatric neurosurgery, and a few countries such as the USA, Canada, France, and Germany have exclusive pediatric neurosurgery units. The "cutoff" age for patients to be cared for in a pediatric unit is arbitrary, ranging from younger than 21 years to younger than 12 years.

Table 4.2 summarizes the estimated pediatric population around the globe. The United Nations the reference age are from zero to 14 years old. Table 4.2 shows the estimated pediatric population worldwide. As of mid-2020, about 26 percent of the world's population were under 15 years old.

## Africa

Africa is a continent of 30 million km² area and a population of 1,346,345,000 people representing 18.2% of the world population [25]. It is the youngest region in the world with a middle age of 19.7 years [25]. Twenty-two countries among 23 that have the highest rate of population under 15 years (31–45%) are African [26]. So we can consider that a big proportion of sick children in the world is in Africa. Hydrocephalus and spina bifida are very frequent diseases in the continent [27]. However, cancers are not uncommon and consequently brain tumors since they are the second cause of cancers in children [28]. The real incidence of brain tumors in Africa is probably underestimated because they are often underdiagnosed or not diagnosed [29]. Another cause of neurosurgical care in children is head/spine trauma secondary to traffic accidents. Africa has the highest number of deaths caused by motor vehicle accidents with 26.6 deaths/100,000 habitants, 44% of these are pedestrians and cyclists, and it is well known that a large proportion of these are children [30].

**Table 4.2** Estimated pediatrica population around the globe

| Geographical region | Pediatric population (0–14 years) | Year | Ref |
|---|---|---|---|
| Worldwide | 1.983.649.000 | 2019 | https://population.un.org/wpp/Publications/ *Suggested citation: United Nations, Department of Economic and Social Affairs, Population Division (2019). World Population Prospects 2019, Online Edition. Rev. 1.* |
| Africa | 540.830.000 | 2019 | https://population.un.org/wpp/Publications/ |
| Asia | 1.089.632.000 | 2019 | https://population.un.org/wpp/Publications/ |
| Australia/NZ | 5.906.580 | 2020 | https://www.nationmaster.com/country-info/ compare/Australia/New-Zealand/People |
| Europa | 298.000 | 2020 | https://ec.europa.eu/eurostat/cache/digpub/ demography/bloc-1c.html?lang=en |
| North America | 125.026.420 | 2020 | https://www.populationpyramid.net |
| Latin America | 189.771.239 | 2020 | https://www.populationpyramid.net |

Considering the dereferences "cutoff" age for patient population, Africa, the pediatric population represents almost half (47%) of the total population. It is currently estimated at 580 million children. This is four times the size of the European child population, 25% of children in the world; www.unicef.org (2017)

Over the past 20 years, the number of neurosurgeons has significantly increased in Africa with a reported neurosurgeon/population ratio of 1/1,066,666 in 1998 to 1/691,000 in 2016 [24]. Nonetheless, the lack of neurosurgeons in most of African countries persists with a degree of variability in availability of pediatric care. This is best available in North African countries, Morocco, Algeria, Tunisia, and Egypt, and the Republic of South Africa. There are very few countries where there are dedicated pediatric neurosurgeons. Egypt has officially 176 pediatric neurosurgeons that perform more than 80 cases per year (Prof. Mohamed El Beltagy at Children's Cancer Hospital Egypt, personal communication, 2020).

While trying to increase the neurosurgical workforce in Africa, it is also important to develop pediatric neurosurgery. This can be achieved by instituting training in pediatric neurosurgery as in Egypt; this kind of training can be done in many African countries (North, South, and some sub-Saharan countries). However, all these options of training need funds for scholarships, and this is also a difficult issue in Africa. National societies of neurosurgery have also a role to play by creating pediatric sections as in Egypt and South Africa which will lead to promote pediatric neurosurgery (Table 4.3).

## Asia

In the current scenario, pediatric neurosurgery is very well developed in Japan and South Korea; moderately developed in India, China, Indonesia, and Malaysia; and developing in the Philippines, Bangladesh, Pakistan, and some other countries [31–38]. However, pediatric neurosurgery is hardly developed in countries like Myanmar, Cambodia, Vietnam, Sri Lanka, and a host of other smaller Asian countries [23, 37, 39–46].

Asia accounts for 36% of the world's children (population below 18 years of age), and it is estimated that around 80% of all pediatric cancer patients are present in the LMIC and Asia shares a huge burden of LMICs. The major disparities in these countries are related to differences in healthcare resources, healthcare organization and system, economic level, and barriers together with other issues that may limit the quality of care offered to these valuable populations.

Asia is the largest continent with 48 countries. The pediatric neurosurgery (PNS) services are not uniformly available throughout the continent. The seeds of PNS have been laid down by the Western countries. Most of the Asian countries owe their beginning to the USA and Canada from where the founders finished their fellowships in PNS and came back to start in their own country [37, 46]. Japan has contributed tremendously to world pediatric neurosurgery like in any other subspecialties. A good number of neurosurgeons practice only pediatric neurosurgery, and all varieties of pediatric neurosurgery happen in Japan in most of the cities [37, 38]. South Korea is an Asian country where PNS developed fast. Started in 1940 and after the Korean War gained momentum and by 1961, it was fully developed. In Korea, pediatric neurosurgery has its own journal of pediatric neurosurgery and society from the last two decades.

**Table 4.3** Estimated pediatric[a] percentage of the pediatric population related to the area

| World | Year | % of population (0–14 years) |
|---|---|---|
| Arab world | 2019 | 33 |
| Caribbean small states | 2019 | 23 |
| Central Europe and the Baltics | 2019 | 15 |
| East Asia and the Pacific | 2019 | 20 |
| Euro area | 2019 | 15 |
| Europe and Central Asia | 2019 | 18 |
| Europe and Central Asia (excluding high income) | 2019 | 21 |
| European union | 2019 | 15 |
| Fragile and conflict-affected situations | 2019 | 41 |
| Heavily indebted poor countries | 2019 | 43 |
| Latin America and Caribbean | 2019 | 24 |
| Latin America and Caribbean (excluding high income) | 2019 | 24 |
| Least developed countries (UN classification) | 2019 | 39 |
| Middle East and North Africa | 2019 | 30 |
| Middle East and North Africa (excluding high income) | 2019 | 31 |
| North America | 2019 | 18 |
| OECD members | 2019 | 30 |
| Pacific Islands small states | 2019 | 35 |
| South Asia | 2019 | 28 |
| Sub-Saharan Africa | 2019 | 42 |
| Sub-Saharan Africa (excluding high income) | 2019 | 42 |
| Income wise | | |
| World | Year | % of population (0–14 years) |
| High income | 2019 | 16 |
| Low and middle income | 2019 | 27 |
| Low income | 2019 | 42 |
| Lower middle income | 2019 | 30 |
| Middle income | 2019 | 26 |
| Upper middle income | 2019 | 21 |

[a]Estimated percentage of the pediatric population related to the world region

In China, currently roughly over 40 children's hospitals are present all over the mainland having their own department of pediatric neurosurgery. Almost each province has at least one children's hospital. More than 400 pediatric neurosurgeons are doing surgeries solely in children's hospitals. Another 200 neurosurgeons perform operations in both adults and children. Usually all kinds of neurosurgical surgeries are practiced in each children's hospital, including tumor, hydrocephalus, MMC, spinal lipoma, trauma, craniosynostosis, and functional surgeries, and an average of 800–1200 cases per year are performed in each center. Though the absolute height number of numberis high, the population number is also leaving an unmet need in the workforce [32, 33].

India is the second most populous country in the world with a geographical area of 3,287,263 Km² [47]. The pediatric neurosurgery services of India follow a diverse pattern. There are very few dedicated pediatric neurosurgery centers in the country, mostly in the major cities of Mumbai, Delhi, Chennai, Bengaluru, and Hyderabad, but all of them are stationed either in pediatric divisions of neurosurgery or in pediatric hospitals. Most of the tier one and two cities offer pediatric neurosurgery services as components of general neurosurgery services (Suchanda Bhattacharjee, personal communication, 2020).

In Russia, the PNS services are well developed in Moscow and still developing in other regions. In 2016, an association of senior specialists on pediatric neurosurgery was arranged, and there are designated pediatric neurosurgeons in all the regions overseeing the work in pediatric neurosurgery called pediatric neurosurgeons-in-chief of Russia [48]. Hence, we can infer that Russia has developing and systemized pediatric neurosurgery services.

Besides the five countries reviewed above, the other Asian countries have not so much prominent representation as far as pediatric neurosurgery work is concerned. Countries like Indonesia and Malaysia offer a significantly good pediatric neurosurgery coverage. The subspecialty is always along with the general neurosurgical specialty, and the majority does pediatric neurosurgery along with other subspecialties. There are very few neurosurgeons exclusively doing pediatric cases in these countries.

## Australia

Today, almost five million children less than 15 years of age are living in Australia [49] and almost one million in New Zealand [50]. Their neurosurgical needs are served through eight dedicated pediatric neurosurgical centers. However, there are only two full-time pediatric neurosurgeons in Australia, Wirginia Maixner and Alison Wray in the Royal Children's Hospital in Melbourne. The remainder of pediatric neurosurgeons have a substantive role in pediatric neurosurgery combined with adult neurosurgical care.

## Europe

In order to explain the role of pediatric neurosurgery in Europe, two major problems exist: first of all, the definition of Europe in terms of territorial versus cultural background (Eurasian continent). Data from Turkey and Russia are not included in most of the available statistics. The second problem reflects the fact that pediatric neurosurgery is not recognized as different from general neurosurgery in some European regions. Compared to other continents, the European population is getting older with a decreasing proportion of citizens younger than 18 years of age currently at

32% (in 2020, 143 million citizens out of 448 million). On the other hand, the number of doctors and hospitals per population is steadily growing in most European countries and the highest worldwide [51].

In 2017, on average, 3.7 physicians per 1000 inhabitants were available in the European Union (in 1990, it was 2.93) [52]. In 2016, in Europe, consisting of 51 countries, a total of 10,730 neurosurgeons were registered with a population of 912,065,031 people and a neurosurgeon/population ratio of 1/85,000. Yet, the population had decreased from 2014 with a negative population development (−4.16%). The neurosurgeon density per million is 11.76 only exceeded by the Western Pacific Region [53].

Pediatric neurosurgery in most European countries is often elective surgery. The spectrum differs significantly from the one described for LMIC. The true number of pediatric neurosurgeons can only be estimated. In most centers in Europe, a pediatric neurosurgery service is offered by specialized units inside a children's hospital or subdivisions and working groups of a department for general neurosurgery. Still a significant proportion of patients is treated in a general neurosurgical environment without specific pediatric expertise [23].

## Latin America

Latin America is a vast region, with 21,069,501 km$^2$, made up of 20 countries, which have different cultures, languages, traditions, and social structures. According to ECLAC (Economic Commission for Latin America and the Caribbean), part of the United Nations, in 2020, the Latin American population from 0 to 19 years old is 206,371 inhabitants [54]. Not all children and adolescents have access to equitable healthcare and treatment of neurosurgical diseases. In Brazil, in recent years, with the indiscriminate opening of new medical schools, we now have many more medical schools than more populous countries such as China, India, and the USA. Brazil is starting to train 35,000 doctors per year, for a population growth of 1.7 million new inhabitants (0.77% per year), that is, 1 new doctor for every 500 new inhabitants. WHO recommends 1 doctor for every 1000 inhabitants. In January 2018, despite having 452,801 doctors (ratio of 2.18 doctors per thousand inhabitants), Brazil has great inequality in the distribution of the medical population between regions, and the majority is concentrated in large urban centers (variation between 0.30 and 4.33/1000 inhabitants). Specialists are 61% of the physicians, and 3298 are neurosurgeons (1.59/100.000 inhabitants) [55].

Pediatric neurosurgery as a subspecialty is not certified in Brazil. It is not mandatory to have a certification to practice. However, in recent years, the specialty has been gaining prominence, and more neurosurgeons have been showing interest in improvement, specialization, and development within the specialty. The Brazilian Society of Pediatric Neurosurgery has stood out for its engagement, development of activities, and interest of members in improving and growing the specialty in Latin America. Within the ISPN, Brazil is the nation with the second largest number of members (45/493), after the USA (Shlomi Constantini, Membership Committee chair of ISPN, personal communication, 2020).

## North America (USA and Canada)

According to the population database in 2019, 22% of the population in the USA – which is 73 million of population – are children. The pediatric neurosurgical workforce was a topic of concern in the last two decades, and efforts of organizations especially the ACPNF contributed to the increasing fellowship-trained subspecialists. The number of accredited fellowships has increased to 31 in 2020, and the number of pediatric neurosurgeons trained from 1993 to 2020 with certification reached 434. The number of graduates per year has grown steadily over time. Of particular importance, the percentage of women who completed a pediatric fellowship and certified by ABPNS in 2019 was just over 40% in the USA with overall percentage (20.4%) of practicing pediatric neurosurgeons being female [56].

A recent study showed that the majority of these fellowship-trained pediatric neurosurgeons (67.8%) trained since 1993 are in an academic setting practicing all of pediatric neurosurgical conditions. Seventy percent of fellowship-trained pediatric neurosurgeons practice only pediatric neurosurgery which is different from most of their European and Asian counterparts [56].

## Middle Eastern Asia

The Middle East is the term used for more than ten countries with populations characterized by different ethnic roots and religions and with diverse political and economic dynamics. At the moment, the countries that have borders within the region are Turkey, Syria, Iraq, Iran, Lebanon, Jordan, Israel, Kuwait, Palestine, the United Arab Emirates, and Saudi Arabia.

It is probably the most unstable part of the whole world, having spent centuries with political struggles. Reflecting this political turmoil, the health problems and priorities in these countries are very different than those in Western countries. Medical associations, including neurosurgical associations, in most of these countries have very little communication with international societies compared with such associations in other parts of the world. Pediatric neurosurgery has been regarded as a subspecialty in some part of the Middle East countries for the last three decades. Although it is not well organized except in Turkey and Israel, most of the countries in this region now have neurosurgeons who give special attention to pediatric neurosurgery within their general neurosurgical practice. No country in the region has a special pediatric neurosurgery training program, and no single neurosurgeon is dedicated exclusively to pediatric neurosurgery except for Israel.

Israel has exclusive pediatric neurosurgery centers associated with the pediatric hospitals. Israel not only offers quality pediatric neurosurgery but also excels in research as seen by the number of articles which come out in the pediatric neurosurgery journals. The young account for a far higher percentage of the population than in the Western world, which means that more sick children are encountered than adults. Congenital and genetically inherited disorders, spinal dysraphism, and parasitic diseases are still public health problems because of the high birth rate and insufficient healthcare. For these reasons, the universal norms of pediatric neurosurgery need to be adapted to this area (Suchanda Bhattacharjee, personal communication, 2020).

The development of pediatric neurosurgical care is a priority in the Middle Eastern Asia for several reasons including the presence of unrests and the young mean age of the population. Children are inadvertently injured in combats or bombings or are deliberately used as human shields. In Afghanistan, the mean age of population is 18 years, and 43% of the population are <15 years [57]. As a result of the lessons learned from the management of >3500 infants and children in military hospitals in Afghanistan and Iraq, the US forces have initiated a program designed to train medical personnel in pediatric critical care before deployment. In addition, a chapter on pediatric critical care is inducted in the emergency surgery manual of the US military force. The data from the Syrian civil war reports that children are afflicted in 18% of cases. Traumatic brain injury in children accounted for 44% as reported by the military personnel's experience in French NATO hospital in Kabul, Afghanistan. The Association of Neurological Surgeons in Iraq, established in 2013, has launched several initiatives including the advancement of pediatric care by establishing subspecialty care and encouraging a prioritization toward the neurosurgical needs of children's conflict-torn zones, which may be through a global initiative (Suchanda Bhattacharjee, personal communication, 2020). The organization has also a woman in neurosurgery and a medical student chapter to empower diversity and specialty growth.

## Future Opportunities/Unmet Needs

The true number of pediatric neurosurgeons who take care of children and adolescents, either full or part time, can only be estimated. In 2017, Dewan et al. performed a worldwide survey on pediatric neurosurgical workforce, access to care, equipment, and training needs. They estimated that more than 1000 pediatric neurosurgeons are working in Europe and North America, which means that 1 neurosurgeon is responsible for 250,000 children, whereas 30 million children in Africa are treated by only 1 pediatric neurosurgeon [44].

In high-income countries (HIC), pediatric neurosurgeons are more often involved in surgeries for hydrocephalus, occult spinal dysraphism (OSD), craniofacial deformity, Chiari malformation, and brain tumor and in selected units also in functional neurosurgery (epilepsy surgery, spasticity treatment, and very rarely deep brain stimulation) compared to relatively few myelomeningocele and trauma cases which constitute most of the caseloads in LMIC. Additionally, there is a significant gap in the use of most recent surgical technology and availability of advanced medical treatments when servicing children with neurosurgical diseases. Providing advanced technology, training the next generation of neurosurgeons with most up-to-date knowledge, and research to elevate the care of children to equal high standards are of paramount importance.

The challenge of pediatric neurosurgery starts on a basic level. Around 51 million births remain unregistered every year in LMIC according to the UNICEF. Congenital malformations like spina bifida – one of the most complex neurological malformations – can be prevented with strategies created by the collaborative work of the pediatric neurosurgeons, medical societies, international organizations, and local governments. In several countries, the folic acid fortification has already resulted in a significant decrease of prevalence of spina bifida with cost-benefit already proven. Another way to prevent congenital defects is to provide basic prenatal care such as use of folic acid supplement before and during pregnancy. The World Health Organization (WHO) recommends that all women of childbearing age consume 400 µg of folic acid daily and that women with pregnancies previously affected by NTDs consume 5000 µg of FA daily [58]. These initiatives mainly depend on the political, cultural, and socioeconomic status of the countries like education, availability of the supplements, and individual and community awareness.

Trauma prevention also is another essential matter of education and collaboration between medical societies and public and private institutions. Per 2020 Child Mortality Report developed by the UN Inter-agency Group for Child Mortality Estimation in 2019 alone, 7.4 (7.2, 7.9) million children, adolescents, and youth died mostly of preventable or treatable causes. Most pediatric trauma deaths can be prevented. This is true for children who are victims of abuse, namely, non-accidental head traumas. Pediatric neurosurgeons should share the lead responsibility in preventing, detection, and appropriate referral of child victims of abuse in addition to treating related brain and spine injuries.

One of the most important advancements in treating patients with neurosurgical pathologies has been the invention of shunts for CSF diversion. The most prevalent pathology in pediatric neurosurgical units is hydrocephalus. However, disparities remain in accessing these endoscopic treatments and shunt procedures which are the standard treatment modalities. Although the complications are less frequent, more work needs to be done to decrease the shunt infection rates below 1% [59].

Theoretically and ideally, a single (or few) center in each LMIC should be fully equipped and staffed to act as a referral center for advanced pediatric neurosurgery. This has the theoretic advantage of improving the level of care and the outcomes. Emergency pediatric neurosurgery and majority of pediatric oncology surgeries should be performed in any neurosurgical center but by a pediatric neurosurgeon ideally. Aggregating and concentrating on the experience, equipment, and staff without repetition and standardizing the high level of service are the successful ways to overcome most of the difficulties and face the challenges in LMIC in the field of pediatric neurosurgery.

**Acknowledgment**

1. For the hard work of our medical students Eliana Kim, Gleice Salibe de Oliveira, and Milagros Niquen Jimenez who will be the future of neurosurgery
2. For the precious information: Dr. Nabil Taghlit (Algeria), Dr. Nobuhito Morota (Japan), Dr. K.C. Wang (South Korea), Dr. Suryaningtas Wihatso (Indonesia), Dr. Khalid-el-Kharazi (Kuwait), Dr. Pullivendhan Sellamuthu (Malaysia), Dr. Manas Panigrahi (India), and Dr. Sudipto Mukherjee (Bangladesh), Dr Ricardo Oliveira (Brazil)

# References

1. Scott RM. The history of pediatric neurosurgery. Neupsy Key. 2016; [cited 2020 Nov 9]. Available from: https://neupsykey.com/the-history-of-pediatric-neurosurgery/.
2. Humphreys RP. The history of paediatric neurosurgery. In: Albright AL, Pollack IF, Adelson PD, editors. Principles and practice of pediatric neurosurgery. Thieme; 2011.
3. Radbill SX. A history of children's hospitals. AMA Am J Dis Child. 1955;90(4):411–6. Available from: https://jamanetwork.com/journals/jamapediatrics/fullarticle/498210.
4. Scott RM. The history of pediatric neurosurgery. In: Principles and practice of pediatric neurosurgery. 3rd ed. Thieme; 2011.
5. Page LK. History of pediatric neurosurgery in the United States and Canada. Childs Nerv Syst. 1991;7(1):53–5.
6. Lohani S, Cohen AR, Franc D. Ingraham and the genesis of pediatric neurosurgery. J Neurosurg Pediatr. 2013;11(6):727–33.
7. Cohen AR. Boston children's hospital and the origin of pediatric neurosurgery. Childs Nerv Syst. 2014;30(10):1621–4. Available from: https://jhu.pure.elsevier.com/en/publications/boston-childrens-hospital-and-the-origin-of-pediatric-neurosurger.
8. Albright AL. The past, present, and future of pediatric neurosurgery. Matson lecture. J Neurosurg. 2004;101(2 Suppl):125–9.
9. Bhagwati SN. Paediatric neurosurgery in India. Childs Nerv Syst. 1999;15(11–12):802–6.
10. Humphreys RP. The modernization of pediatric neurosurgery. The Donald D. Matson Lecture 2003. Childs Nerv Syst. 2004;20(1):18–22.
11. Home [Internet]. International Society for Pediatric Neurosurgery (ISPN). 2020 [cited 2020 Nov 9]. Available from: https://www.ispneurosurgery.org/.
12. History [Internet]. The Indian Society for Pediatric Neurosurgery (INDSPN). 2020 [cited 2020 Nov 11]. Available from: https://www.indspn.org/history.
13. SBNPed: Home [Internet]. Sociedade Brasileira de Neurocirurgia Pediátrica. 2020 [cited 2020 Nov 1]. Available from: https://www.sbnped.com.br/pt/.
14. da Silva MC, Salomão JFM, Zanon N. História da neurocirurgia pediátrica no Brasil. Rev Bras Neurol E Psiquiatr. 2014;18(2). Available from: https://www.revneuropsiq.com.br/rbnp/article/view/73.
15. Da Cunha AHGB. Historical aspects of the foundation of the Latin American Society of Pediatric Neurosurgery. Childs Nerv Syst. 2018;34(11):2127–31. https://doi.org/10.1007/s00381-018-3932-5.
16. History of Pediatric Neurosurgery – Flanc Pediatría [Internet]. Capitulo Pediatrico. 2020 [cited 2020 Nov 11]. Available from: http://www.flancpediatria.org/Historia_de_la_Neurocirugia_Pediatrica.
17. About AASPN. [Internet]. Asian-Australasian Society for Pediatric Neurosurgery (AASPN). 2020 [cited 2020 Nov 9]. Available from: http://www.aaspn.org/.
18. WFNS History – About WFNS. [Internet]. World Federation of Neurosurgical Societies (WFNS). 2020 [cited 2020 Nov 9]. Available from: https://www.wfns.org/menu/5/wfns-history.

19. Society Journal [Internet]. International Society for Pediatric Neurosurgery (ISPN). 2020 [cited 2020 Nov 11]. Available from: https://www.ispneurosurgery.org/society-journal/.
20. EANS Courses [Internet]. The European Association of Neurosurgical Societies (EANS). 2020 [cited 2020 Nov 11]. Available from: https://www.eans.org/page/EANS-courses.
21. Hamilton DG. 100 years of paediatric surgery in Sydney. Med J Aust. 1980;2(13):721–6.
22. El Khamlichi A. Aperçu sur l'histoire de la neurochirurgie africaine. In: Emergence de la neurochirurgie Africaine; 2019. p. 58.
23. Dewan MC, Baticulon RE, Rattani A, Johnston JM, Warf BC, Harkness W. Pediatric neurosurgical workforce, access to care, equipment and training needs worldwide. Neurosurg Focus. 2018;45(4):E13.
24. El Khamlichi A. Le centre de référence de la WFNS à Rabat pour la formation des neurochirurgiens Africains. In: Emergence de la Neurochirurgie Africaine; 2019.
25. Population of Africa (2020) – Worldometer [Internet]. Worldometer. 2020 [cited 2020 Nov 1]. Available from: https://www.worldometers.info/world-population/africa-population/.
26. Sardon J-P. La population des continents et des États en 2016. Popul Avenir. 2016;730(5):18–23. Available from: https://www.cairn.info/revue-population-et-avenir-2016-5-page-18.htm.
27. Dewan MC, Rattani A, Mekary R, Glancz LJ, Yunusa I, Baticulon RE, et al. Global hydrocephalus epidemiology and incidence: systematic review and meta-analysis. J Neurosurg. 2018;1:1–15.
28. Stefan C, Bray F, Ferlay J, Liu B, Maxwell Parkin D. Cancer of childhood in sub-Saharan Africa. Ecancermedicalscience. 2017;11. Available from: https://www.ncbi.nlm.nih.gov/pmc/articles/PMC5574662/.
29. Magrath I, Steliarova-Foucher E, Epelman S, Ribeiro RC, Harif M, Li C-K, et al. Paediatric cancer in low-income and middle-income countries. Lancet Oncol. 2013;14(3):e104–16. Available from: https://www.thelancet.com/journals/lanonc/article/PIIS1470-2045(13)70008-1/abstract.
30. Bilan de la sécurité routière : exposé 2019 des statistiques par pays [Internet]. Atlas Magazine. 2020 [cited 2020 Nov 11]. Available from: https://www.atlas-mag.net/article/securite-routiere-en-2017.
31. Chidambaram B. Chandrashekhar Deopujari. Childs Nerv Syst. 2016;32(10):1757–9. https://doi.org/10.1007/s00381-016-3147-6.
32. Liu W, Tang J, Van Halm-Lutterodt N, Luo S, Li C. History and current state of pediatric neurosurgery at Beijing Tiantan Hospital Neurosurgery Center. Childs Nerv Syst. 2018;34(5):797–803.
33. Zhao J-Z, Zhou L-F, Zhou D-B, Tang J, Zhang D. The status quo of neurosurgery in China. Neurosurgery. 2008;62(2):516–20. discussion 520-521.
34. He X, Ma W, Zhao Y, Ma C, Ma J. Chinese Society for Pediatric Neurosurgery (CSPN): a new society promoting pediatric neurosurgery in China. Childs Nerv Syst. 2013;29(12):2327–9.
35. Choi J-U. The promotion of pediatric neurosurgery throughout the world. Childs Nerv Syst. 2007;23(9):929–36.
36. Khan AH, Hossain AM, Shalike N, Barua KK. Evolution of neurosurgery in Bangladesh. Bangladesh J Neurosurg. 2019;8(2):57–62. Available from: https://banglajol.info/index.php/BJNS/article/view/42345.
37. Sato O. Pediatric neurosurgery around the world–Asia and Australasia. Childs Nerv Syst. 1988;4(6):317–20.
38. Maki Y. My memories of Japanese pediatric neurosurgery. Childs Nerv Syst. 1997;13(8):448–53. https://doi.org/10.1007/s003810050118.
39. Wong T-T. My living history to pediatric neurosurgery. Childs Nerv Syst 2010;26(10):1253 9.
40. Abbassioun A. Perspectives in international NeurosurgeryNeurosurgery in Iran. Neurosurgery. 1981;9(2):205–7. Available from: https://academic.oup.com/neurosurgery/article/9/2/205/2746928.
41. El Chehab H, Agard E, Dot C. Cephalic region war injuries in children: experience in French NATO hospital in Kabul Afghanistan. Injury. 2018;49(9):1703–5.

42. Mauer UM, Freude G, Schulz C, Kunz U, Mathieu R. Pediatric neurosurgical care in a German Field Hospital in Afghanistan. J Neurol Surg Part Cent Eur Neurosurg. 2017;78(1):20–4.
43. Jean WC, Huynh T, Pham TA, Ngo HM, Syed HR, Felbaum DR. A system divided: the state of neurosurgical training in modern-day Vietnam. Neurosurg Focus. 2020;48(3):E2.
44. Dewan MC, Baticulon RE, Ravindran K, Bonfield CM, Poenaru D, Harkness W. Pediatric neurosurgical bellwether procedures for infrastructure capacity building in hospitals and healthcare systems worldwide. Childs Nerv Syst. 2018;34(10):1837–46.
45. Di Rocco C. Joon-Uhn Choi: the 2005–2006 ISPN president. Childs Nerv Syst. 2007;23(9):925–8. https://doi.org/10.1007/s00381-007-0402-x.
46. Erbengi A. Pediatric neurosurgery in the Middle East: present and future. Childs Nerv Syst. 1999;15(11):814–6. https://doi.org/10.1007/s003810050477.
47. India Population [Internet]. Worldometer. 2020 [cited 2020 Nov 11]. Available from: https://www.worldometers.info/world-population/india-population/.
48. Gorelyshev S. First all-Russian conference on pediatric neurosurgery. Childs Nerv Syst. 2004;20(4):253–4.
49. 3101.0 – Australian Demographic Statistics, Jun 2019 [Internet]. Australian Bureau of Statistics. c=AU; o=Commonwealth of Australia; ou=Australian Bureau of Statistics; 2019 [cited 2020 Nov 1]. Available from: https://www.abs.gov.au/ausstats/abs@.nsf/0/1CD2B1952 AFC5E7ACA257298000F2E76?OpenDocument.
50. Stats on Kids [Internet]. Office of the Children's Commissioner of New Zealand. 2020 [cited 2020 Nov 11]. Available from: https://www.occ.org.nz/our-work/statsonkids/.
51. Bevölkerung Europa – Statistisches Bundesamt [Internet]. Statistisches Bundesamt. 2020 [cited 2020 Nov 11]. Available from: https://www.destatis.de/Europa/DE/Thema/Bevoelkerung-Arbeit-Soziales/Bevoelkerung/_inhalt.html.
52. Physicians (per 1,000 people) – European Union | Data [Internet]. World Bank. 2020 [cited 2020 Nov 11]. Available from: https://data.worldbank.org/indicator/SH.MED.PHYS. ZS?locations=EU.
53. Mukhopadhyay S, Punchak M, Rattani A, Hung Y-C, Dahm J, Faruque S, et al. The global neurosurgical workforce: a mixed-methods assessment of density and growth. J Neurosurg. 2019;4:1–7.
54. CEPALSTAT Home: Databases and Statistical Publications [Internet]. Economic Commission for Latin America and the Caribbean (ECLAC). 2020 [cited 2020 Nov 11]. Available from: https://estadisticas.cepal.org/cepalstat/portada.html?idioma=english.
55. Scheffer M. Demografia Médica no Brasil 2018 [Internet]. Sao Paulo, SP: FMUSP, CFM, Cremesp; [cited 2020 Nov 11]. Available from: http://www.flip3d.com.br/web/pub/cfm/ind ex10/?numero=15&edicao=4278.
56. Nadel JL, Scott RM, Durham SR, Maher CO. Recent trends in North American pediatric neurosurgical fellowship training. J Neurosurg Pediatr. 2019;04:1–6.
57. Afghanistan auf einen Blick [Internet]. Lexas Länderinformationen. 2020 [cited 2020 Nov 11]. Available from: https://www.lexas.de/asien/afghanistan/index.aspx.
58. Peña-Rosas JP, De-Regil LM, Dowswell T, Viteri FE. Daily oral iron supplementation during pregnancy. Cochrane Database Syst Rev. 2012;12:CD004736.
59. Choux M, Genitori L, Lang D, Lena G. Shunt implantation: reducing the incidence of shunt infection. J Neurosurg. 1992;77(6):875–80.

# Chapter 5
# The Role of Neurosurgery in Global Health Cerebrovascular Surgery

**Mehmet Osman Akçakaya, Aneela Darbar, Marco Cenzato, Mahmood Qureshi, Guiseppe Lanzino, and Talat Kırış**

## Introduction

Although neurosurgical development has been rapid and impressive in high-income settings, low- and middle-income countries (LMICs) have lagged behind. According to the Lancet Commission and World Bank report in 2015, there is a shortage of essential surgical care for five to six billion people worldwide [1]. Of the overall necessary-surgery burden-related annual mortality of 147 million, 47 million can be prevented through adequate and timely surgical intervention [2]. Of the reported number of annual surgical procedures worldwide (approximately 250 million), only 3.5% are performed in the poorest 33% world population [3].

The number of practicing neurosurgeons worldwide was 49,940 in 2018 [4], of which 18,000 are practicing in the Western Pacific area mainly in China and Japan. Overall, 44% of these neurosurgeons are working in high-income countries (HICs) [4]. On the other hand, in a survey conducted in 2016, the number of neurosurgeons

M. O. Akçakaya
Neurosurgical Department, Florence Nightingale Hospital, Demiroglu Bilim University, Istanbul, Turkey

A. Darbar
Aga Khan University Hospital, Karachi, Pakistan

M. Cenzato
Neurosurgical Department, Grande Ospedale Metropolitano Niguarda, Milano, Italy

M. Qureshi
Yaya Centre, Nairobi, Kenya

G. Lanzino
Department of Neurological Surgery, Mayo Clinic, Rochester, MN, USA

T. Kırış (✉)
Neurosurgery Department, American Hospital and Koc University, Istanbul, Turkey

in Africa was 1727 for a population of 1.12 billion, yielding a ratio of 1:654,000. Of these, South Africa had 171 neurosurgeons (ratio 1:420,000), North Africa had 1187 neurosurgeons (ratio 1:131,000), and sub-Saharan Africa (SSA) had 369 neurosurgeons (ratio 1:2,395,000) [5]. Despite the disparities in distribution, there has been some progress in the distribution of neurosurgeons [6]. Recent data show a ratio is 1/80,000 in HIC [7]. So, we might say that there is a significant lack of neurosurgeons in LMIC.

Also the condition of infrastructure for healthcare services is poor in LMIC. A recent evaluation by the United Nations documented that steady electricity was found in only 35% of surveyed district hospitals in 12 SSA countries and oxygen sources were only available for 40% of surveyed surgical hospitals in East Africa [8]. The availability of consistent running water, which is an essential component, was found in only 20% of surveyed hospitals in Sierra Leone [8]. Before advancing with the evaluation, we want to underline the truth: "Healthcare infrastructure in LMIC is insufficient to even meet basic needs."

Cerebrovascular diseases (CD) are a global health problem. CD are the second cause of death in developed countries, the first cause of disability in adults, and the second cause of dementia [9]. Stroke constitutes a major health problem with 15 million people afflicted each year, resulting in 5 million deaths annually (10% of all deaths worldwide) leaving an additional 5 million people with a permanent disability [10]. The burden of cerebrovascular diseases for the economy of developing countries is heavy. Over the past decades, HICs have seen a significant decrease both in incidence (29%) and mortality (25%) for stroke [10]. It is expected that with the aging of the general population, developing countries will suffer more and more from the economic burden of these disease processes and must therefore organize their resources to manage patients both in the acute emergency setting and chronic patient care [10]. Another problem in the management of CD is the challenging nature of cerebrovascular surgery. Surgeries for aneurysm or arteriovenous malformations need careful preoperative evaluations in order to understand the hemodynamics of the vascular lesions as well as normal and pathologic anatomy. The surgical technique needs to be refined requiring long periods of surgical training. Yet this specialized surgery is often required in an emerging setting.

## Brief History of Cerebrovascular Neurosurgery

Cerebrovascular pathologies and their impact on society have been known throughout the centuries. The Egyptian physician Imhotep performed anatomic observations and described for the first time an arterial aneurysm in *Ebers Papyrus* [11]. Anatolian physicians like Flaenius Rufus of Ephesus described a posttraumatic aneurysm for the first time, and Galen of Pergamum also made important contributions to the history of cerebrovascular diseases [11]. However, modern understanding of cerebral vasculature and first attempts of surgical treatment based on scientific background date back only to the eighteenth century, when John Hunter proposed treatment of an aneurysm through ligation of the proximal feeding artery in 1748, referred to this day as Hunterian ligation [12]. Cooper, Cogswell, and Horsley modified this technique [11, 12]; however, mortality and morbidity rates continued to be very high. Harvey Cushing further advanced the treatment of intracranial aneurysms and described "wrapping" and "packing" techniques. He formulated the idea of silver surgical clips in 1911 [12], although his "rival" Walter Dandy is credited to be the first one to utilize a surgical clip in 1945 to treat an internal carotid artery aneurysm [13].

Hunter was also known for the first description of an extracranial arteriovenous malformation (AVM) [14]. However, Rudolf Virchow, a German pathologist, was the first to describe and differentiate AVMs in 1863 [14]. In 1888, D'Arcy Power, during an autopsy, was the first surgeon to recognize a Sylvian fissure AVM with associated hemorrhage which had resulted in the patient death [14]. Davide Giordano, an Italian surgeon, in 1889, was the first one to attempt surgical treatment of an AVM by ligating proximal feeding arteries [14]. Dandy, Cushing, and Percival Bailey from the USA reported surgically treated cases in the 1920s which were associated with very high mortality and morbidity rates [14]. Herbert Olivecrona from Sweden was the first neurosurgeon to successfully and totally remove a cerebellar AVM in 1932 and was able to operate on several others with a much lower mortality than his predecessors [14].

A major impetus for the further refinement of diagnosis and treatment of cerebrovascular diseases came with the invention of cerebral angiography by Egas Moniz in 1927 [11]. The impact of cerebral angiography was enormous for better understanding of the pathology and the anatomy underlying these conditions which enabled surgeons to better plan their surgery. In 1944, Dandy reported a mortality rate of 25% in 36 surgically treated aneurysm patients [13]. However, despite these technological advances, surgical morbidity and mortality rates remained considerably high in the 1950s and 1960s. The surgical approaches for aneurysms mainly consisted of a large bicoronal scalp flap, a unilateral frontal or bifrontal craniotomy, and a subfrontal or frontolateral approach [12]. The introduction of the surgical microscope with the goal of improving both illumination and visualization of the surgical field was a revolutionary step which paved the way to the development of microneurosurgery as we know it today. Kurze, Pool, and Colton, Rand and Janetta, and Lougheed and Marshall were among the pioneers who published their early experiences with microscopic technique [12]. It was not until the monumental work of M. Gazi Yaşargil that the advantages of the microscope were fully recognized and the microscope became routinely adopted and utilized around the world [15–17]. Yaşargil was also the first neurosurgeon in 1969 to publish his results on AVMs treated with pure microsurgical technique with excellent outcomes [14]. Several other surgeons, including Pia, Wilson, Malis, Stein, Parkinson, Sundt, and Nornes, followed establishing the modern microsurgical treatment of AVMs [14]. Albert Rhoton Jr. with his studies on the microsurgical anatomy of the brain and its vasculature played a critically important role in our understanding and further refinement of cerebrovascular anatomy as it applies to microneurosurgery [18–21]. Simultaneously, Charles G. Drake pioneered and refined bold approaches to challenging posterior circulation aneurysms [12]. Thanks to these efforts, a new generation of neurosurgeons, including among others Dolenc, Tew, Samson, and Spetzler, became very proficient and further contributed to the development of the specialty [11, 12]. Very impactful and highly cited were the contributions of Robert Spetzler to our understanding of AVM angioarchitecture and their classification to plan surgical strategies and better predict surgical risk and outcomes [14].

Developments of imaging technologies, primarily the introduction of CT scanners in the 1970s and later MRI, were instrumental in increasing the indications for and improving the safety of surgery. Moreover, further refinements of digital subtraction angiography and development of microcatheters able to be navigated safely through the tortuosities of the intracranial vasculature led to the development of a brand new field, surgical neuroradiology or interventional neuroradiology. Milestones in this process were the seminal work by Serbinenko in the 1970s who reported successful treatment of intracranial aneurysms and caroticocavernous fistulas with detachable balloons and by Guglielmi who developed detachable coil embolization system in 1990 [11]. Nowadays, endovascular techniques allow us to treat effectively many intracranial aneurysms; dural, spinal, and intracranial fistulas; extra- and intracranial stenosis; and acute ischemic stroke and are a valid adjunct in the treatment of intracranial AVMs [11]. More technological advances in the field of functional MRI (fMRI) and diffusion tensor imaging (DTI) have improved surgical management and planning especially as it applies to AVMs and cavernous angiomas.

## Current Status of Vascular Neurosurgery

Over the last two decades, there has been further evolution of the instruments and technical armamentarium available to neurosurgeons which brought important changes to vascular neurosurgery. Perhaps the top three major improvements include the "non-stick" bipolar forceps [22], the intraoperative angiography (with indocyanine green or the more recent sodium fluorescein) [23, 24], and the improved safety of surgery through the utilization of intraoperative neuromonitoring [25]. Other improvements worth mentioning include newer aneurysm clips which have increased enormously the angle of approach to intracranial aneurysms, intraoperative imaging techniques such as the ultrasound with micro-bubble contrast, and intraoperative Angio suite as part of "hybrid" rooms. Where intraoperative angiography is not sufficient to put at rest the surgeon's mind, intraoperative micro-Doppler flow meter can ensure that the flow is sufficient and there is no risk for an ischemic event [26, 27].

Contemporary surgery has routinely become minimally invasive, especially for aneurysms with reduced use of retractors and consequential less brain damage with improvements especially of cognitive outcomes thanks to these techniques. In the next few paragraphs, we will specifically address some of the newer developments as they apply to AVM surgery, aneurysm surgery, cavernous angioma surgery, and carotid surgery.

## AVM Surgery

After an initial decline following the shock generated by the ARUBA study [28] and the animated discussion which followed this controversial study, attention toward invasive treatment of AVMs has increased and progressively oriented toward concentration of cases in centers with high caseload. The concentration of the disease in centers with greater expertise has always been a key for better clinical results but difficult to achieve. The consequences of the critical re-evaluation of AVM treatment following the ARUBA study have shifted definitive treatment primarily toward surgical and radiosurgical treatment, with an overall reduction of endovascular techniques as a curative option, although these trends are highly variable depending on local logistics.

New instrumentation ("non-stick" bipolar – laser) and intraoperative visualization devices (NA$^+$ fluorescein – ICG – Ecography) have had an important impact on surgical outcomes allowing safer surgical resection. AVM treatment is a true example in medicine of multidisciplinary treatment in which the different potential of each available treatment (surgical, endovascular, and radiosurgical) is integrated into a therapeutic path that must be defined from the beginning. The European consensus conference [29] has highlighted the risk of initiating treatment without a well-defined a priori strategy.

Furthermore, the combined treatment of selective embolization procedures and radiosurgery scheduled over the course of months or years allows some AVMs judged inoperable until a few years ago to be reduced in size so that they can be surgically resected with good clinical results. In recent years, transvenous endovascular and even surgical approaches focused on the "venous" component of the AVM have been proposed and represent an interesting and evolving field.

## Aneurysm Surgery

Aneurysm surgery has massively declined in numbers in HICs. There has been a clear shift toward endovascular procedures for several reasons. Since the International Subarachnoid Aneurysm Trial (ISAT) study [30], technological evolution of intravascular devices (extra- and intrasaccular flow diverters, low-profile stents, etc.) has further expanded endovascular indications and treatment options. Endovascular procedures require less time than open surgery. The treatment of a ruptured aneurysm can be safely completed in half an hour, compared to an average of 3–4 hours for surgical clipping. Surgical clipping of aneurysms still constitutes the very end of training for neurosurgeons and requires hours and hours of dedication and a caseload to maintain adequate skills that nowadays is very difficult to achieve for younger generations [31]. The opposite is happening in endovascular procedures that continue to improve and be highly dependent on technology and have a shorter learning curve. Busy neurosurgeons are also more inclined to refer challenging aneurysm cases to endovascular specialists. This is happening despite the fact that aneurysm microsurgery has undergone positive changes over the past few years which have reduced surgical invasiveness with greatly reduced postoperative hospital stays. The increasingly widespread use of intraoperative monitoring and intraoperative ICG fluorescein angiography and minimal use of mechanical retractors make aneurysm surgery very safe minimizing the risks of inadvertent compromise of the parent artery, closure of a perforating vessel, or brain damage.

On the other end, endovascular therapies are effective in preventing rebleeding as long-term follow-up of ruptured and unruptured intracranial aneurysms shows that the risks of rebleeding are not as high as originally feared despite some degree of compaction after coiling or small recurrences after intrasaccular flow disrupters. There are no important differences in outcome between the two methods, particularly for anterior circulation as confirmed by the Collaborative Unruptured Endovascular versus Surgery Trial 2017 (CURES) [32]. In recent years, there has been also a progressive decrease in the number of treatment of small, unruptured aneurysms given their exceedingly low risk of rupture, while imaging studies of the aneurysm wall are being developed, even though at present their role remains purely speculative. After aneurysmal subarachnoid hemorrhage (SAH), the use of pharmacological agents either intravenously or intraarterially through direct catheter injection and cerebrospinal fluid removal has greatly reduced the incidence of malignant vasospasm.

The need of bypasses for giant aneurysms has decreased with the development of effective flow diverter stents. Nevertheless, it remains a valid option in selected cases which further reinforces the need for concentrating this pathology in a few tertiary and quaternary referral centers where surgeons can maintain the required dedicated skills.

## Cavernous Angioma Surgery

The literature shows that cavernous angiomas have a relatively low morbidity after bleeding when compared to other intracranial vascular pathologies. This consideration stresses the importance of paying very close attention to indications for invasive surgical treatment especially in asymptomatic patients or in those with symptomatic deep lesions or in high eloquent locations. Surgery of cavernous angiomas of the brainstem continues to be characterized by an important rate of complications given the high eloquent area despite marked improvements in surgical techniques and anatomical knowledge and widespread use of neurophysiological monitoring. Therefore, surgical indications even for a cavernous angioma which has bled only once and does not come to a brain or ependymal surface should be carefully considered [33, 34].

Initial enthusiasm for the pharmacological interventions with drugs such as propranolol which seemed to reduce the risk of bleeding in anecdotical cases or small series was probably unfounded, and clinical trials are required to show effectiveness of other drugs such as aspirin, which paradoxically seems to be a promising agent in reducing the incidence of bleeding from symptomatic and asymptomatic cavernous angiomas. The role of radiosurgery in the control of cavernoma bleeding is still controversial, although an increasing number of centers are reporting encouraging results suggesting possible reduction in bleeding episodes over the years following treatment. Radiosurgery may be considered a possible alternative to surgery in truly inoperable lesions. Further developments in the understanding of cavernous angiomas and their treatment will emerge as the role of the associated deep venous anomaly (DVA) in the genesis and recurrence of cavernous angiomas is better defined and the role of genetic factors better understood.

## Carotid Surgery

Treatment of carotid artery stenosis has received a lot of attention in the past few decades due to the completion of multiple multicenter randomized clinical trials which have defined indications for invasive treatment and the respective role of medical, surgical, and endovascular treatment. Treatment of carotid stenosis consists of best medical treatment (BMT) and carotid revascularization by either carotid endarterectomy (CEA) or carotid artery stenting (CAS). Revascularization techniques carry procedural risks, which reinforces the importance of proper patient selection. National and International Societies guidelines have been developed to guide treatment decisions and continue to be updated as new information emerges. Overall, CEA is indicated in symptomatic patients with recent symptoms and greater than 50% carotid stenosis. Carotid angioplasty and stenting is a valid alternative to CEA in patients considered to be high-risk surgical candidates such as those with prior radiation to the neck, restenosis after prior CEA, "hostile neck," and high-riding bifurcation and those with important medical comorbidities. Treatment of asymptomatic carotid stenosis is controversial irrespective of the degree of stenosis because of the very low risk of ipsilateral ischemic event with best medical therapy [35]. Invasive treatment of asymptomatic patients should be considered with caution and only in very selected cases, while participation of these patients in some of the ongoing trials comparing best medical therapy to revascularization should be considered and encouraged.

## Acute Ischemic Stroke

The treatment of acute ischemic stroke has undergone a revolution in the past few decades. Immediate evaluation of patients with acute ischemic stroke for possible administration of intravenous thrombolysis and consideration of mechanical thrombectomy in those with large vessel occlusion have become mainstay of treatment in developed countries, and this approach has been supported by large-scale randomized clinical trials. The ability of providing organized and prompt care under urgent circumstances in these patients has represented and still represents an ongoing challenge for healthcare organizations throughout the globe and has led to the development of primary stroke centers. Moreover, the risk of intraparenchymal hemorrhage after pharmacological and endovascular treatment of acute ischemic stroke requires the immediate availability of neurosurgeons able to deal with such complications. Decompressive craniectomy in selected patients with malignant middle cerebral artery infarct has also been affirmed in well-conducted studies and has become an integral part of the therapeutic management of acute ischemic stroke.

## Current Status of Cerebrovascular Surgery Across the Globe

Despite the advances above summarized, the distribution and availability of cerebrovascular surgery varies greatly across the world. In an attempt to have a snapshot of the current status of cerebrovascular surgery in 20 different nations and areas of the 5 continents, we have conducted an informal survey in preparation of this chapter.

The World Federation of Neurosurgical Societies (WFNS) cerebrovascular committee, under the chairmanship of Prof. Talat Kiris, was requested to provide an overview of neurovascular services available globally, with special emphasis on resources in LMIC. In order to address this rather ambitious task, colleagues from each continental region were selected. This chapter reflects the efforts undertaken by this group. It is hoped that this will provide an opportunity to understand the current status and, hopefully, lead to a broader discussion among global neurosurgical leaders. The ultimate aim of any such endeavor is, of course, to address the challenges faced in many regions of the world, in an attempt to provide an acceptable level of care to its respective population. This modest study does not in any way wish to provide a readily available solution. In seeking to highlight the current status, it is hoped that attempts will follow to determine how best the neurosurgical community may work together to find solutions to improve the care of patients with neurovascular pathologies across the world.

The group commenced its agenda, by formulating a survey that was sent out through its committee members to all continental societies, with a plea to have the survey conducted in as many centers as possible, within their respective jurisdiction. Table 5.1 shows the characteristics of the survey responders. A large body of

**Table 5.1** Survey responders' characteristics

| | Yes | No |
|---|---|---|
| National neurosurgical societies (NNS) in LMIC | 94.30% | 5.70% |
| NNS member of the continental society | 83.10% | 9.70% |
| NNS member of the World Federation of Neurosurgeon (WFNS) | 84.60% | 14.60% |

respondents belong to a neurosurgical society and were represented within their national and/or continental association, which in turn was represented in the World Federation (WFNS) in over 84.6% of respondents. This is encouraging, as it indicates the possibility for such services to be enhanced, especially in LMICs, through initiatives channeled through the WFNS and its committees.

Figure 5.1 shows the distribution of neurosurgeons and neurosurgical centers within each teaching facility that participated to the survey. Approximately 1/3 of patients with SAH (Fig. 5.2) and with ischemic stroke must travel more than 100 km to reach a facility with cerebrovascular or endovascular center, respectively. A similar trend was noted for patients sustaining an embolic stroke, whereby over 67% would be required to travel more than 400 km to access a facility that had the capacity to offer mechanical thrombectomy. The percentage of hospital with facilities able to perform endovascular thrombectomy is shown in Fig. 5.3. The ratio of clipping versus coiling is summarized in Fig. 5.4. Table 5.2 summarizes the distribution of facilities that can perform open or closed treatment of cerebrovascular aneurysms. Table 5.3 shows that 17% of responders did not have facilities with endovascular capabilities, while only 1% did not have capability to perform open surgery to

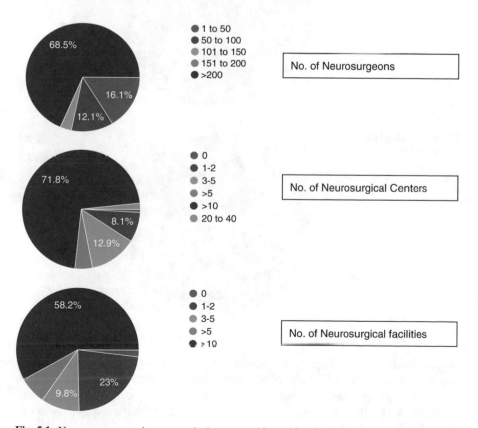

**Fig. 5.1** Neurosurgeons and neurosurgical centers with teaching facilities

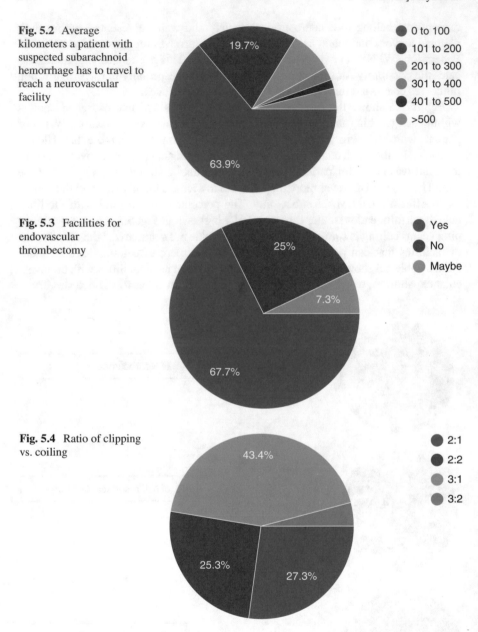

**Fig. 5.2** Average kilometers a patient with suspected subarachnoid hemorrhage has to travel to reach a neurovascular facility

- 0 to 100
- 101 to 200
- 201 to 300
- 301 to 400
- 401 to 500
- >500

**Fig. 5.3** Facilities for endovascular thrombectomy

- Yes
- No
- Maybe

**Fig. 5.4** Ratio of clipping vs. coiling

- 2:1
- 2:2
- 3:1
- 3:2

clip an aneurysm. In the operating rooms, 89% of neurosurgeons responding to this survey had an advanced or highly advanced microscope to clip aneurysms, with only 7% having manual microscopes without coaxial eyepiece or camera. Postoperatively, 10% of respondents noted that they do not have access to rehabilitation facilities for their patients.

**Table 5.2** Neuro-interventional procedures

|  | 0 | 1–5 | 6–10 | >10 |
|---|---|---|---|---|
| Neurovascular facilities that can embolize an aneurysm | 16.50% | 28.10% | 6.60% | 48.80% |
| Neurovascular facilities that can clip an aneurysm | 0.80% | 30% | 9.20% | 605 |

**Table 5.3** (A) Availability of endovascular neuroradiology equipment and physicians. (B) Endovascular neuroradiology physicians

(A)

|  | 0 | 1–2 | 3–5 | >5 | >10 | 20 to 40 |
|---|---|---|---|---|---|---|
| Neurosurgical centers that have facilities for CT *angiography*? | 1.60% | 6.50% | 11.30% | 4% | 75% | 1.60% |
| Neurosurgical centers that have facilities for MR *angiography*? | 1.60% | 10.50% | 5.60% | 5.60% | 75% | 1.60% |
| Neurosurgical centers that have facilities for digital subtraction angiography | 7.30% | 10.50% | 4.80% | 16.90% | 58.90% | 1.60% |
| Neurosurgical centers in your country that have facilities for monoplane cath labs | 7.30% | 8.60% | 12.90% | 21.60% | 46.60% | 1.70% |
| Number of interventional neurosurgeons in LMIC | 7.30% | 9.70% | 8.10% | 17.70% | 2.40% | 52.45 |
| Bi-plane cath labs in LMIC | 11% | 25.40% | 5.90% | 15.30% | 40.7 | 1.70% |
| (B) | | | | | | |
|  | 0 | 1–2 | 3–5 | >5 | >10 | 20 to 40 |
| Interventional physicians (neurosurgeons) | 7.30% | 11.40% | 17.90% | 10.60% | 51.20% | 1.60% |
| Interventional physicians (neuroradiologists) | 9.70% | 9.70% | 8.10% | 17.70% | 2.40% | 52.40% |
| Interventional physicians (neurologists) | 38.80% | 12.40% | 10.70% | 6.60% | 29.80% | 38.80% |

While the cost of neurovascular treatment in private care facilities is understandably high, due to absence of government support to the private care institutions (Fig. 5.5), the cost remains prohibitive even in public sector institutions, where the government pays for the care (Fig. 5.6). This implies that for such care, even if facilities are available in public sector hospitals in LMIC, the service may actually not be available consistently due to low budget allocation in LMICs.

The availability of neurosurgical equipment remains a challenge in LMIC regions, as does the facilities for effective neurorehabilitation (Figs. 5.7 and 5.8, respectively).

In summary, and not surprisingly, the survey points to a three-tier categorization of cerebrovascular services globally:

- Tier 1 – Absence of neurovascular facilities, mainly in LMIC regions. This appears to be a smaller percentage than one would have expected and may be

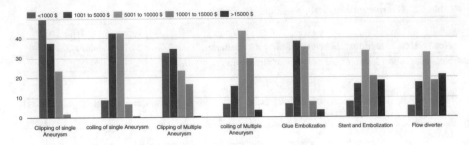

**Fig. 5.5** Approximate cost in private sector

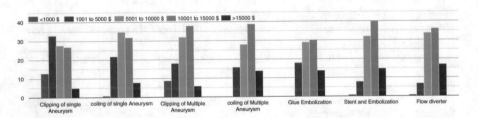

**Fig. 5.6** Approximate cost in public sector

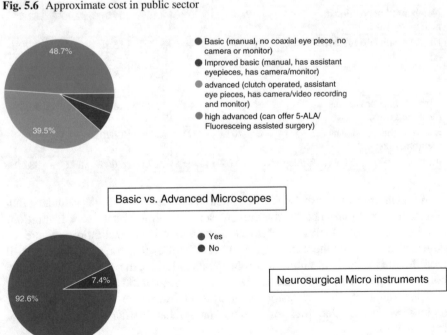

**Fig. 5.7** Neurosurgical instruments

**Fig. 5.8** Neurorehabilitation facilities

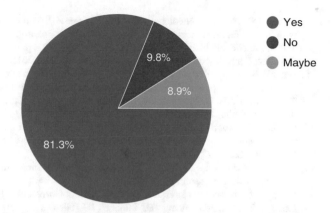

reflected by the nature of our survey. In reality, this Tier 1 group is likely to be much larger. A broader survey may be required to identify this group.

- Tier 2 – This appears to be the majority, whereby medium-level care is available to patients, but is not readily available within a reasonable distance.
- Tier 3 – These countries are largely in Western regions. A smaller global population has access to the highest level of care within acceptable distances and utilizing expensive and state-of-art facilities.

The challenge faced by cerebrovascular surgeons is to develop ways as a global community to ensure that the larger majority of patients residing in LMIC regions have improved access to acceptable levels of care. A collaborative effort with our national and continental societies to achieve this goal is desirable to meet this goal. Coordination of care focusing resources in centralized centers with adequate expertise and technological support is key to make this objective possible.

# References

1. Park KB, Johnson WD, Dempsey RJ. Global neurosurgery: the unmet need. World Neurosurg. 2016;88:32–5.
2. Meara JG, Hagander L, Leather AIM. Surgery and global health: a Lancet Commission. Lancet. 2014;383:12–3.
3. Ravindra VM, Kraus KL, Riva-Cambrin IK, Kestle JR. The need for cost-effective neurosurgical innovation – a global surgery initiative. World Neurosurg. 2015;84:1458–61.
4. Dewan MC, Rattani A, Fieggen G, Arraez MA, Servadei F, Boop FA, Johnson WD, Warf BC, Park KB. Global neurosurgery: the current capacity and deficit in the provision of essential neurosurgical care. Executive summary of the Global Neurosurgery Initiative at the Program in Global Surgery and Social Change. J Neurosurg. 2018; https://doi.org/10.3171/2017.11. JNS171500.
5. El Khamlichi A. Emerging Neurosurgery in Africa, Jun 2019. p. 173.
6. Dempsey RJ. Neurosurgery in developing world: specialty service and global health. World Neurosurg. 2018;112:325–7.

7. Servadei F, Rossini Z, Nicolosi F, Morselli C, Park KB. The role of neurosurgery in countries with limited facilities: facts and challenges. World Neurosurg. 2018;112:315–21.
8. Millennium development goal & taking stock of the global partnership for development. MDG Gap Task Force Report 2015. New York: United Nations; 2015.
9. Bejot Y, Benatru I, Rouauda O, Fromont A, Besancenot JP, Moreau T. Epidemiology of stroke in Europe: geographic and environmental differences. J Neurol Sci. 2007;262:86–8.
10. Zuaznabar MAB, Concepcion OF, Marre GC, Vidal RMT. Epidemiology of cerebrovascular diseases in Cuba, 1970 to 2006. MEDICC Rev. 2008;10(2):33.
11. Peschillo S, Caporlingua A, Caporlingua F, Gugliemi G, Delfini R. Historical landmarks in the management of aneurysms and arteriovenous malformations of the central nervous system. World Neurosurg. 2016;88:661–71.
12. Lai LT, O'Neill AH. History, evolution and continuing innovations of intracranial aneurysm surgery. World Neurosurg. 2017;102:673–81.
13. Dandy WE. Intracranial arterial aneurysms. Ithaca: Cornstock; 1944.
14. Colby GP, Coon AL, Huang JD, Tamargo RJ. Historical perspective of treatments of cranial arteriovenous malformations and dural arteriovenous fistulas. Neurosurg Clin N Am. 2012;23:15–25.
15. Yasargil MG. Microsurgery applied to neurosurgery. Stuttgart: Georg Thieme; 1969.
16. Yasargil MG, Fox JL. The microsurgical approach to intracranial aneurysms. Surg Neurol. 1975;3:7–14.
17. Yasargil MG. A legacy of microneurosurgery: memoirs, lessons and axioms. Neurosurgery. 1999;45:1025–92.
18. Rhoton AL. Rhoton cranial anatomy and surgical approaches. Philadelphia: Lippincott Williams & Wilkins; 2003.
19. Gibo H, Carver CC, Rhoton AL Jr, Lenkey C, Mitchell RJ. Microsurgical anatomy of the middle cerebral artery. J Neurosurg. 1981;54:151–69.
20. Perlmutter D, Rhoton AL Jr. Microsurgical anatomy of the anterior cerebral-anterior communicating recurrent artery complex. J Neurosurg. 1976;45:259–72.
21. Saeki N, Rhoton AL Jr. Microsurgical anatomy of the upper basilar artery and the posterior circle of Willis. J Neurosurg. 1977;46:563–78.
22. Elliott-Lewis EW, Mason AM, Barrow DL. Evaluation of new bipolar coagulation forceps in a thermal damage assessment. Neurosurgery. 2009;65(6):1182–7.
23. Raabe A, Beck J, Gerlach R, Zimmermann M, Seifert V. Near-infrared indocyanine green video angiography: a new method for intraoperative assessment of vascular flow. Neurosurgery. 2003;52(1):132–9. discussion 139
24. Rey-Dios R, Cohen-Gadol AA. Technical principles and neurosurgical applications of fluorescein fluorescence using a microscope-integrated fluorescence module. Acta Neurochir. 2013;155:701–6.
25. Chemtob G, Kearse LA Jr. The use of electroencephalography in carotid endarterectomy. Int Anesthesiol Clin. 1990;28(3):143–6.
26. Firsching R, Synowitz HJ, Hanebeck J. Practicability of intraoperative microvascular Doppler sonography in aneurysm surgery. Minim Invasive Neurosurg. 2000;43:144–8.
27. Scienza R, Pavesi G, Pasqualin A, et al. Flowmetry-assisted aneurysm clipping. A cooperative study. In: The proceedings of the 12 European congress of neurosurgery; 2003. p. 309–314.
28. Mohr JP, et al. Medical management with or without interventional therapy for unruptured brain arteriovenous malformations (ARUBA): a multicentre, non-blinded, randomised trial. Lancet. 2014;383(9917):614–21.
29. Cenzato M, Boccardi E, Beghi E, Vajkoczy P, Szikora I, Motti E, Regli L, Raabe A, Eliava S, Gruber A, Meling TR, Niemela M, Pasqualin A, Golanov A, Karlsson B, Kemeny A, Liscak R, Lippitz B, Radatz M, La Camera A, Chapot R, Islak C, Spelle L, Debernardi A, Agostoni E, Revay M, Morgan MK. European consensus conference on unruptured brain AVMs treatment (Supported by EANS, ESMINT, EGKS, and SINCH). Acta Neurochir. 2017;159(6):1059–64.

30. Molyneux AJ, Kerr RSC, Yu L-M, et al. International subarachnoid aneurysm trial(ISAT) of neurosurgical clipping versus endovascular coiling in 2143 patients with ruptured intracranial aneurysms: a randomized comparison of effects on survival, dependency, seizures, rebleeding, subgroups, and aneurysm occlusion. Lancet. 2005;366:809–17.
31. Lai L, Morgan MK. The impact of changing intracranial aneurysm practice on the education of cerebrovascular neurosurgeons. J Clin Neurosci. 2012;19:81–4. https://doi.org/10.1016/j.jocn.2011.07.008.
32. Darsaut TE, Findlay JM, Magro E, et al. Surgical clipping or endovascular coiling for unruptured intracranial aneurysms: a pragmatic randomised trial. J Neurol Neurosurg Psychiatr. 2017;88:663–8.
33. Awad IA, Polster SP. Cavernous angiomas: deconstructing a neurosurgical disease. J Neurosurg. 2019;131(1):1–13.
34. Akers A, Al-Shahi Salman R, Awad I, Dahlem K, Flemming K, Hart B, Kim H, Jusue-Torres I, Kondziolka D, Lee C, Morrison L, Rigamonti D, Rebeiz T, Tournier-Lasserve E, Waggoner D, Whitehead K. Synopsis of guidelines for the clinical management of cerebral cavernous malformations: consensus recommendations based on systematic literature review by the Angioma Alliance Scientific Advisory Board clinical experts panel. Neurosurgery. 2017;80(5):665–80.
35. Salzler GG, Farber A, Rybin DV, Doros G, Siracuse JJ, Eslami MH. The association of Carotid Revascularization Endarterectomy versus Stent Trial (CREST) and Centers for Medicare and Medicaid Services Carotid Guideline Publication on utilization and outcomes of carotid stenting among "high-risk" patients. J Vasc Surg. 2017;66(1):104–111.e1.

# Chapter 6
# The Role of Neurosurgery in Global Health Oncology

Claire Karekezi, Fumio Yamaguchi, Di Meco Francesco, Marcos Maldaun, and Edjah K. Nduom

## Introduction

Primary brain tumors and other central nervous system (CNS) malignancies are quite rare; the overall incidence rate is estimated as 11/100,000 persons per year, with estimates of incidence rates ranging from 00.1/100,000 (pineal tumors) to 26/100,000 (all primary brain tumors) [1]. Their worldwide incidence is, on the other hand, not well documented. Available data may not reflect the real picture due to incomplete information among various regions, countries, and continents (Fig. 6.1) [2]. CNS tumors are very heterogeneous and vary by histological types [1, 3]. They are categorized into 29 histologic groups according to the World Health Organization (WHO) classification of tumors of the CNS. Histological types also vary significantly not only in their incidence but also in their presentation, treatment regimens, and prognosis [4, 5]. Gliomas account for the largest proportion of malignant brain tumors. CNS tumors affect both children and adults. They can be located in all CNS anatomical regions, with the vast majority (>90%) occurring in the brain, the rest occurring in the meninges, spinal cord, and cranial nerves [3].

C. Karekezi
Rwanda Military Hospital, Kigali, Rwanda

F. Yamaguchi
Nippon Medical School, Department of Neurosurgery for Community Health, Tokyo, Japan

D. M. Francesco
Department of Neurosurgery, Fondazione IRCCS Istituto Neurologico Carlo Besta, Milan, Italy

M. Maldaun
Society of Neuro-Oncology Latin America (SNOLA), Sao Paulo, Brazil

E. K. Nduom (✉)
Department of Neurosurgery, Emory University School of Medicine, Atlanta, GA, USA
e-mail: enduom@emory.edu

© The Author(s), under exclusive license to Springer Nature Switzerland AG 2022
I. M. Germano (ed.), *Neurosurgery and Global Health*,
https://doi.org/10.1007/978-3-030-86656-3_6

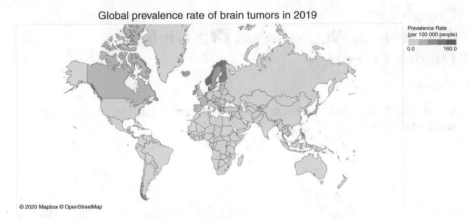

**Fig. 6.1** 2019 estimated global prevalence rate of brain tumors. (Data from the Global Burden of Disease [2])

In addition to primary brain tumors, the CNS is also affected by metastatic brain tumors. Brain metastases are the most commonly diagnosed CNS tumor in North America, with an estimated occurrence 10 times as frequent as malignant primary brain tumor. Their incidence has been increasing over the years. Factors responsible for this increase include the increased population longevity, the increased overall survival of patients with primary cancers due to improved treatments, and the greater sensitivity/availability of diagnostic modalities.

Although rare compared to other tumors, brain and other CNS tumors cause morbidity and mortality that are disproportionate to their incidence. They are very destructive, interfering with the normal function of the nervous system [4–6]. The field of neuro-oncology and neurosurgical oncology, which study primary and metastatic brain tumors and their treatment, has seen tremendous evolution over the past 30 years. The growth and success of this field has been made possible due to the research focused on better understanding these tumors, but additional work is needed. The continued development of emerging therapeutic strategies will require the constant scientific work of dedicated physicians and scientists [6].

In the early 1970s, few physicians and researchers were studying brain tumors; the first Conference on Brain Tumor Research and Therapy held at Asilomar, CA (USA), in 1975, attracted only 35 scientists [6]. The breakthroughs achieved since then in the deep understanding of brain anatomy, advances in neuroimaging and neuronavigation, continued evolution of microsurgical techniques, data on the importance of extent of resection, improved brain mapping, and introduction of new therapeutics, technologies, and innovations led to the implementation of modern subspecialized neurosurgical oncology, with significant positive impact on the field of neuro-oncology. There are now neuro-oncological organizations in Africa, Asia, Europe, and North/South America with combined membership estimates numbering in the thousands worldwide.

Beyond neurosurgical techniques, imaging, and diagnostic improvements, one of the most significant advances in neuro-oncology in recent years has been the understanding of the biology and molecular patterns of different CNS tumor types and subtypes. This led to the most recent revision of the WHO classification of CNS tumors that includes, for the first time, results from molecular diagnostic testing as part of the final integrated diagnosis [5]. These developments had an impact not only on how we treat patients with brain tumors after surgery, but it has also changed the surgical approach in selected patients [7, 8].

## Neuro-oncology Across the Globe

### Africa

#### The Neuro-oncology Disease Burden in Africa

The global burden of cancer has been increasing progressively, according to the World Health Organization [9]. The GLOBOCAN 2018 estimated globally 18.1 million new cases of cancer and 9.6 million deaths from cancer at the end of 2018 [10]. The current situation regarding any cancer remains quite challenging in Africa; according to predictions from the International Agency for Research on Cancer (IARC), there is an ever-increasing cancer burden over the next decades, particularly in low- and middle-income countries (LMIC), with over 20 million new cancer cases expected globally, annually as early as 2025 [10].

CNS tumors have been thought to be uncommon in Africa. However, with the current increase in life expectancy across the continent, we have seen the incidence of brain tumors increasing. Accordingly, the perception about rarity of brain tumors in the African population has changed. Unfortunately, the lack of organized national and continent-wide databases of CNS tumors makes their incidence unclear [11]. Challenges also exist at different levels from underdiagnoses/improper assessment, lack of appropriate medical imaging, poor histopathological diagnosis, and insufficient neurosurgical treatment to radiotherapy and oncology service deficiencies. Currently, these cases are often managed by generalists, and the lack of specialized team management of these tumors remains a huge barrier to successful neuro-oncological management that would lead to equivalent clinical results to those achieved in HICs [12–14]. Little information exists on the incidence of CNS cancer and brain tumors in Africa especially the sub-Saharan African region. The available data in the literature are not homogeneous, and they largely arise from various reports of single institutions. The paucity of reliable and adequate brain tumor registries makes the true incidence of CNS tumors on the African continent unknown.

Morocco and Egypt dominate the **North African** literature on CNS tumors, but series remain mixed and heterogeneous. An Egyptian team [15] which reviewed the incidence of CNS tumors over 5 years, all ages included, in one tertiary hospital in Cairo reported 996 cases, combined. They found a high proportion of gliomas

(35%), followed by meningiomas (33.3%) and pituitary adenoma (15.6%); most tumors were found in the adult population. A previously published manuscript on the epidemiology of pediatric intracranial neoplasms in Egypt [16] found 451 cases over a period of 3 years aged between 0 and 14 years, and most tumors were reported to be infratentorial, and the majority were astrocytomas (35%), medulloblastomas (18.8%), and craniopharyngiomas (11%). A similar study done in Morocco [17] reviewed pediatric patients aged from 0 to 19 years in the two big cities of Rabat and Casablanca and found 542 cases; medulloblastoma was the most common brain tumor (34.5%), followed by pilocytic astrocytoma (17.3%) and diffuse astrocytoma grade II (12.5%).

In the **West African** literature, Nigeria, the country with the largest population in Africa and approximately 1 neurosurgeon for every 2.4 million people, has more papers published from different neurosurgical centers with existing neuro-oncology care. The first study on CNS tumors in Nigeria was published in early 2000 [18] from Ibadan (southwestern Nigeria); this study reviewed brain tumor cases over a period of 10 years (1980–1990); there were 210 histologically confirmed CNS cases among them. 172 of these lesions were primary and 48 secondary neoplasms. The majority of patients were adults (135 adults vs 75 children, ratio 1.8:1). Gliomas accounted for the largest group of tumors followed by metastases to the brain; craniopharyngioma was the most common tumor in children.

In **East and Central Africa**, little data exist. The CURE Children's Hospital neurosurgical team in the northern part of Uganda reported 172 pediatric tumor cases over a period of 8 years (2002–2012). Glial tumors were the most common [60] (34.8%). Other tumors included ependymal tumors [28] (16.3%), embryonal tumors [26] (15.2%), craniopharyngiomas [17] (9.9%), and choroid plexus tumors [16] (9.3%). They estimated average annual incidence of less than 0.1 per 100,000 of pediatric brain tumors in their region [19].

One of the largest studies [20] on pediatric brain tumors conducted at the University of Cape Town in **South Africa** reviewing pediatric tumor cases over 20 years from 1996 to 2017 revealed about 554 cases, primary brain tumors were more common among males (55.4%), and most tumors were located supratentorially (52%). Commonest tumors revealed to be astrocytomas (20.3%) followed by medulloblastomas (19.1%) and craniopharyngiomas (9.8%).

## Limitations in the Accurate Assessment of the Neuro-oncology Disease Burden

There is no complete data describing the status of brain tumors on the African continent, as the above series are not representative of whole continent. The observed variations in the incidence of CNS tumors by countries seem to be related to different levels of resources and could partly be explained by contrasts in health system infrastructure, access to care, and availability of diagnostic services [12–14]. Regions and cities within countries also differ in numbers; this is due to the disparity that exists between the well-established field of neurosurgery in the northern/

southern part of Africa and the rest of SSA [12, 15, 18]. For most SSA countries, access to neuro-oncology care remains insufficient; diagnosis and treatment options are extremely limited by constraints of economy, infrastructure, and security [13, 14]. In addition, the ratio of neurosurgeons or other dedicated physicians to population is still low; most neurosurgical pathologies will go misdiagnosed with the majority of brain tumors diagnosed at very late stages. These late diagnoses lead to high morbidity and mortality rates. Additionally, the high rate of patients lost to follow-up also makes the little available data incomplete.

**Neuro-oncology Education and the Way Forward**

The number of neurosurgeons is gradually increasing in Africa. Recent reports count more than 1300 neurosurgeons (WFNS Map) for 1.349 billion people on the continent [21]. However, their distribution remains non-homogeneous on the continent. There is a severe deficit of neurosurgeons in SSA countries who have only around 512 neurosurgeons. These neurosurgeons are mostly occupied with responding to the high trauma burden on the continent due to poor transportation infrastructure. Experts with exclusive dedication to the neuro-oncology field are still very few. Medical centers with established neuro-oncology facilities and oncologic centers are even more scarce, and only a few medical professionals have had further subspecialty training in neuro-oncology. The creation of societies like SNOSSA (Society for Neuro-Oncology Sub-Saharan Africa), formally established at its first meeting in July of 2018, will boost the education on brain/spinal cord tumors by allowing collaboration and exchange with other established worldwide societies. We hope that this interaction will provide a blueprint to foster better care for patients with CNS tumors in the region in the future.

## Asia

**The Neuro-oncology Disease Burden in Asia**

Asia is a large and diverse continent, with several countries having a range of health infrastructure and neurosurgical workforce. In Asia, there are many countries which have different development status. The equivalent age to global average 65-year-olds varies from 76.1 years of Japan and 66.0 of China to 59.6 of India [22]. The incident cases of CNS cancer in 2016 are high in East Asia (10,800) followed by Western Europe (49,000) and South Asia (31,000) [23]. Age-standardized incident rate of CNS cancer is especially high in China (106,207). Age-standardized disability-adjusted life years (DALYs) of CNS cancer in Asia are as follows, 44.76 (Japan), 53.65 (Vietnam), 65.83 (India), 69.65 (South Korea), 88.47 (Philippines), 70.14 (South Asia), 84.60 (Southeast Asia), 131.54 (East Asia), 132.67 (China), 148.34 (Central Asia), and 164.52 (Turkey), compared to 118.94 (USA). These values are largely different depending on areas and countries which have different medical standards. Here, we focus on Japan, due to the author's familiarity with the country and the high standard of neurosurgical quality in the country, comparable to the United States and European countries.

## Brief History of Neuro-oncology in Japan

Japanese modern neurosurgery started in the Meiji era (1868 to 1912). Prior, most medical knowledge was imported from China, Portugal, and the Netherlands. The Meiji Restoration changed the structure of medical administration of Japan, and then German and British medicines were introduced to the country. Unlike other medical fields, most neurosurgical training techniques were introduced from the United States by the pioneers of Japanese neurosurgery. According to the literature, the history of modern neuro-oncological surgery in Japan started with a brain tumor resection in 1905 [24]. This was followed by resections of spinal tumors (1911) [25], transsphenoidal surgery (TSS) for pituitary tumor (1914), transcranial pituitary surgery (1925), and glioma resections using "Bovie" electrocautery in 1931.

The Second World War slowed down medical research activity in Japan. However, after the end of war, neurosurgical research activity resumed. The first academic meeting of Japanese neurosurgery was held in 1948, hosted by Dr. Makoto Saito. Then, Dr. Mizuho Nakata [26], one of the pioneers of Japanese neurosurgery, reported the total resection of pineal tumors in 1952. In radiotherapy, the first boron neutron capture therapy in Japan was performed in 1968 [27]. In 1975, the first CT scan was introduced at Tokyo Women's Medical University [25]. Following this, diagnostic capabilities significantly progressed. The number of neurosurgical patients in Japan has increased due to this increase in capabilities. Japanese surgeons reported the resection of acoustic tumors via an extended middle cranial fossa approach in 1976 [28].

Basic research by Japanese neurosurgeons also gradually progressed in this time period; Japanese neurosurgeons reported on the method of diagnosis and treatment for brain tumors by monoclonal antibody in 1983 [29] and reported CSF PLAP as a tumor marker in intracranial germinoma in 1988 [30, 31]. Further, another group provided proof of hypoxia in malignant brain tumors in 1991 [32]. Technological development is a hallmark of Japanese neurosurgeons [25]. The world's first neuronavigation machine was developed in 1987, followed by reports of radiosurgery by LINAC (1992) [33], awake surgery using propofol (1995) [34], and gene therapy for malignant brain tumors (2000) [35].

## The Japanese Brain Tumor Registry

The Japanese registry of brain tumors started in 1973, and it has been updated every 3 years [36].

Recently, the 14th edition was published in 2017 [37]. Based on this database, the number of primary brain tumor and metastatic brain tumor is 16,277 and 3200 individually in 2005–2008. Primary brain tumors consist mainly of glioma (23.9%), meningioma (23.9%), neurinoma (8.6%), and pituitary adenoma (16.8%). The number of glioblastoma patients is 2006, and its median overall survival (mOS) and median progression-free survival (mPFS) are 18.0 and 11.0 months individually. The detailed information of every tumor is in the database which can be downloaded from the journal. Furthermore, the Japan Neurosurgical Society has started to request to register all hospital-admitted patients in Japan Neurosurgical Database (JND). Those activities accelerate comprehension of the current situation of neurosurgical patients in Japan.

## Neuro-oncology Care in Japan

The present form of the Japanese universal healthcare system was started in 1961. All citizens of Japan have access to advanced medical care through this health insurance system. However, free medical care for elderly patients over 65 years old has ended, due to Japanese financial stringency. Currently, 10–30% of the cost of care is self-covered, on an income-based scale. The government does fully support the medical care of the poor people of Japan.

There are 2472 hospital-based neurosurgical services in Japan, covering 32.0% of all hospitals in Japan. In Japan, there are 95 university hospitals and 32 cancer centers, and these have neurosurgical departments providing neuro-oncological services. In total, asia neurosurgical clinics number is 1562, representing 1.6% of all clinics in Japan. The number of Japanese board-certified neurosurgeons is approximately 6000, with a population of 127 million in 2018, and Japan has a neurosurgeon/inhabitant ratio of 1/21,000. Not all neurosurgeons perform surgery, since Japanese neurosurgeons also treat diseases such as headache, dizziness, epilepsy, and cerebral infarction, which are dealt by neurologists in the United States and many Western countries. Since there are no neuro-oncologists in Japan, neurosurgeons cover not only surgery but also postoperative chemotherapy for CNS tumor patients. Boosted by rapid economic growth, Japanese medical devices have greatly increased, recently. In 2017, the ratio of CT scanner to population was 111.49/1 million, and the ratio for MRIs was 51.7/1 million, exceeding the ratio in the United States.

Although the number of CT and MRI machines is quite high, that of radiotherapeutic device is relatively low with a ratio of 6.83/1 million compared 11.73/1 million in the United States. Due to the diversification of radiation therapy for CNS tumors in recent years, the technologies, such as LINAC, IMRT, Gamma Knife, and CyberKnife, are all available and used according to the disease and location.

## Neuro-oncology Education

The board examination for certified neurosurgeons is one of the most difficult examinations in Japan. It contains highly detailed questions also on neuro-oncology. The education of neuro-oncology is usually included in the neurosurgical residency program, and there are no independent neuro-oncological training courses or fellowships. It is offered annually, and the pass rate is approximately 60 to 70%. The education for residents and certified neurosurgeons is conducted by the Japan Neurosurgical Society (JNS) and the Japanese Congress of Neurological Surgeons (JCNS). To maintain the qualification as a certified neurosurgeon, attendance to academic meetings and training courses authorized by JNS and JCNS and periodical reports of one's clinical practice are required. According to the coming unprecedented aging society in Japan, the number of aged CNS tumor patients is expected to increase. This will increase the demand for neurosurgical oncology services.

## *Europe*

### The Neuro-oncology Disease Burden in Europe

In Europe, the standardized (world) incidence of primary CNS malignant brain tumors ranges from 4,5 to 11.2 cases per 100,000 men and from 1.6 to 8.5 per 100,000 women. The two most common CNS cancers, high-grade glioma and brain metastasis, occur more frequently during adulthood and especially among the elderly. In Europe, the peak of incidence is 18.5/100,000 in people aged 65 years; the relative frequency of CNS tumors is, however, highest during childhood, when they account for 23% of all tumors diagnosed [38]. In Europe, the 5-year survival rate in adults for the primary CNS tumor is 17% for men and 19% for women (1995–2002) [39], with differences across European regions [Table 6.1] [40]. Survivorship is higher among young European patients (63%) as compared to the elderly ones [41].

In Europe, as for most Western countries, meningiomas are among the most common intracranial tumors, with an estimated incidence of 8 cases per 100,000 persons per year. Up-to-date and detailed population-based data on the burden of meningiomas from European regions are sparse. A recent paper from Holleczek et al. [42, 45] reported incidence, mortality, and outcome of meningiomas from a German population study. Data from 992 patients who were diagnosed between 2000 and 2015 were included. In this study, the age-standardized incidence rate was found to be 2.5 and 5.8 cases per 100,000 men and women per year, respectively. Between 2000 and 2015, the incidence remained constant in both female and male populations with a ratio of 2.53. Mean age at diagnosis was 63 years. WHO grading (2007 WHO classification) was available for 80% of the patients, of whom 70% had a benign meningioma (WHO grade I), 28% had an atypical meningioma (grade II), and 2% had an anaplastic meningioma (grade III). Higher proportions of atypical and anaplastic meningiomas occurred in men (39%) than in women (27%), respectively.

**Table 6.1** Incidence (AAAIR, average annual age-adjusted incidence rate) per histology and region [3]

| Histology and region | All ages | Children (0–14) | AYA (15–39) | Older adults (40+) |
|---|---|---|---|---|
| *Astrocytic tumors* | | | | |
| Northern Europe | 2.98 | 0.58 | 1.38 | 6.63 |
| Western Europe | 3.59 | 0.50 | 1.38 | 8.45 |
| Southern Europe | 3.01 | 0.63 | 1.22 | 6.86 |
| *Oligodendroglial tumors and mixed gliomas* | | | | |
| Northern Europe | 0.45 | 0.07 | 0.42 | 0.79 |
| Western Europe | 0.61 | 0.10 | 0.57 | 1.04 |
| Southern Europe | 0.37 | – | 0.36 | 0.62 |
| *Ependymal tumors* | | | | |
| Northern Europe | 0.22 | 0.25 | 0.16 | 0.27 |
| Western Europe | 0.23 | 0.26 | 0.18 | 0.28 |
| Southern Europe | 0.20 | 0.23 | 0.16 | 0.23 |
| *Medulloblastoma* | | | | |
| Northern Europe | 0.16 | 0.45 | 0.09 | 0.02 |
| Western Europe | 0.18 | 0.48 | 0.13 | 0.02 |
| Southern Europe | 0.22 | 0.58 | 0.16 | 0.02 |

## Average Estimated Brain Tumor Economic Burden

According to Pugliatti et al. [43], the total economic burden for brain tumors is about 567 million in purchasing power parity (€PPP). In particular, the costs are subdivided into *direct costs*, *direct non-medical costs*, and *indirect costs*. *Direct costs* include healthcare costs, such as inpatient care, outpatient care, drug costs, and tests, and amount to 150 €PPP millions, approximately 25% of total cost.

Direct non-medical costs include costs associated with assistance from community or social services; purchases like bed lift, rails, walking aids, wheelchairs, and house adaptation; and informal care amounting to 36 €PPP millions, approximately 6% of total costs. *Indirect costs* including lost production from absenteeism from work as well as early retirement amount to 373 €PPP millions, approximately 69% of total cost. Interestingly, as reported by Wittchen et al., an increase in total expenditure for brain tumors in recent years has been noted [44]. Interestingly, as reported by Gustavsson et al., an increase in total expenditure for brain tumors has been noted in recent years, raising from 4586 €PPP millions in 2004 to 5174 €PPP millions in 2010 [44].

## Neuro-oncology Training in Europe

Because of the composite cultural background among different nations, European neurosurgical training programs are quite heterogeneous [45]. This poses difficulties in comparing the different training regimens. Furthermore, the reduction of working hours for professionals (European community directive 2003/88/EC10) has led to a contraction of trainees' operating room attendance and surgical load exposure [46, 47]. Reulen and Marz, in a thoughtful article on training conditions at a major German neurosurgical department, estimated that an annual caseload of 250–300 procedures per resident would be required for adequate training, but it is unclear whether European trainees meet those expectations [48].

Currently, in an effort to achieve uniformity among training programs, the EANS (European Association of Neurosurgical Societies) and the UEMS (Union Européenne des Médecins Spécialistes) meet regularly to evaluate and improve the training of neurosurgical trainees in Europe [49]. Since 1994, UEMS has adopted its own charter of postgraduate training, a document containing a series of recommendations valid throughout Europe to ensure good medical training. This is composed of six chapters: five are common to all specialties; the latter is specific to each discipline. This document emphasizes the importance of a training portfolio that collects the surgical curriculum of trainees. UEMS has also published a list of key procedures that the future neurosurgeon must acquire, with the minimum and optimal number of specific procedures including oncological ones. For the time being, however, across Europe, there are no structured subspecialty programs in neuro-oncology.

## North America

### The Neuro-oncology Disease Burden in North America

Treatment for brain and spine tumors in North America, generally, and the United States, specifically, harken back to the days of Harvey Cushing, after he returned from his education in Europe [50]. While he practiced broadly in medicine and neurosurgery, his 2000 brain tumor surgeries argue quite strongly for his nomination as the first true subspecialized neurosurgical oncologist [51]. Here, we will explore the epidemiology of brain and spine tumors in North America, with a focus on the United States, and the case for further subspecialization of care for our brain tumor patients.

CNS tumors present a significant burden on the United States [52]. There is an incidence of 6.4 new cases of brain and other nervous system cancers per 100,000 men and women per year in the United States, with a death rate of 4.4 deaths per 100,000 people per year. There were an estimated 168,494 people living with CNS cancer in the United States in 2017. While these CNS cancers are the 16th in terms of incidence in the United States, CNS tumor deaths are disproportionately high, being the 7th highest source of cancer death. In children aged 0–14 years, brain and other spinal tumors are the most common cancer site, at 5.74 per 100,000 people per year. They are also the most common cause of cancer death in children. Within brain tumors, meningiomas account for almost 40% of tumors, while nerve sheath tumors account for approximately 8.6 percent of those seen. Sellar lesions represent approximately 18% of these lesions, whereas tumors of neuroepithelial tissue are about 28% of the total presented. About 10% of the lesions represented in the CBTRUS survey were located in the spinal cord/cauda equina [53]. The cost of caring for patients with CNS tumors has been estimated as high as $4.5 billion [54].

Interestingly, the reported incidence rates of brain and spine tumors are higher in Canada, with a reported incidence of 8.71 malignant brain and other CNS tumors diagnosed in the Canadian population from 2009 to 2013, which may be related, in part, to comprehensive data collection in the Canadian national health program. We were unable to review cancer deaths in Mexico, as, in our extensive English literature search, there were single-center studies which discussed the incidence of brain tumors, but no population-based studies. This search was limited, as we did not perform an extensive search of the Spanish literature, beyond PubMed.

## Training in Neuro-oncology in North America

With regard to training in neurosurgical oncology, all neurosurgery training programs in the United States will expose trainees to some measure of neurosurgical oncology. Current American Board of Neurological Surgery (ABNS) standards mandate a minimum of 60 adult craniotomies for tumor during basic neurosurgical residency training, along with 20 sellar tumors. For pediatrics, five brain tumor cases are expected for completion of residency. As a result of this exposure, general neurosurgeons in private practice in the United States will often operate on these lesions on their own, without referral to a tertiary center. Current estimates suggest that the majority of brain tumors are not operated on by self-identified brain tumor specialists.

The American Board of Neurological Surgery and the American Board of Medical Specialties currently recognize three areas of focused practice in neurosurgery – Neurocritical Care, Neuroendovascular Surgery, and Pediatric Neurosurgery. There is no existing certification for a neurosurgical oncologist. However, practicing neurosurgeons can now opt to select tumor as a subspecialization in the American Board of Neurological Surgeons Oral Examination. If this is selected, the candidate will have one session on general cases in neurosurgery but then an additional session which rigorously examines the breadth of neurosurgical oncology, specifically. Finally, their exam includes an hour review of their own cases, which would include established neurosurgical oncologists for those selecting the tumor specialty. At this time, there is no data to suggest how this subset of certification has affected the practice of young neurosurgical oncologists in the United States.

With regard to additional subspecialization in neurosurgical oncology, there are several neurosurgical oncology training programs in the United States. Most of these take residents primarily after the completion of their residency training, and the duration of training is 1 year. Separately, there are several skull base fellowships in the United States and Canada, most of which also are 1 year (Table 6.1). Within the skull base fellowships, there are several differences, with some focusing on anterior skull base/endoscopic training, others focusing on open skull base cases, and some focusing mainly/solely on tumors, while yet others include vascular lesions or are focused solely on the operative management of vascular lesions.

Studies have long suggested that subspecialization is beneficial for brain and spine tumor patients, with increased volume leading to improved outcomes [55, 56]. Benefits for patients treated by a subspecialists may include access to clinical trials and access to new and improved surgical techniques. While it is not yet practical for all brain and spine tumor patients to be treated at tertiary referral centers, this is a goal of patient advocacy groups, like the National Brain Tumor Society. To continue to improve outcomes for patients with brain tumors, just as Dr. Cushing did all those years ago, we believe that we should champion subspecialization in neurosurgery and the establishment of regional centers of excellence.

## Latin America

### The Neuro-oncology Disease Burden in Latin America

Similar to other regions of the world, in Latin America, brain and CNS cancers represent a significant burden [3] but as observed for Africa; little data exist on the real incidence of these pathologies in this part of the world. All data found is from individual researchers or institutional databases with the expected bias that this creates. The situation of neuro-oncology in Latin America is changing. For the last decades, this subspecialty never existed. Efforts from many fronts are trying to change this scenario and to improve assistance to our CNS tumor patients. This includes providing continuing education on the topic, establishing multidisciplinary teams, and conducting research in the field. At the present time, there are still huge differences among countries, and within each country, there are variations among regions, big versus small cities, private versus public hospitals, cancer-dedicated hospitals versus general hospitals, and isolated specialists versus a multidisciplinary team/practices.

Checking with all official organizations in Brazil and with some colleagues in Latina America, we could not find comprehensive information regarding brain or spine tumor data. All data found is from individual studies or institutional databases with lots of bias. In Latin America, CNS tumors don't require compulsory notification, like one seen in regions covered by the Central Brain Tumor Registry of the United States (CBTRUS). Additionally, diagnosis codes are not routinely and accurately applied to cases. There is no governmental interest in developing brain tumor teams separate from general oncologists due to lower numbers of cases and the higher treatment cost.

### Neuro-oncology Care in Latin America

There are differences in degree of care when comparing patients who are treated in dedicated tumor centers compared to general hospitals, private versus public assistance. There are also differences among different countries. If we consider a "standard of care treatment" for a GBM as maximal safe resection, proper pre- and postoperative imaging following RANO criteria [57], pathology with molecular and genetic markers like IDH and MGMT status [58, 59], and chemoradiation starting up to 30 days after surgery and 6 cycles of temozolomide like Stupp protocol [60], only few centers could afford it. Even with notable surgeons and oncologists and increasing tools and technology like intraoperative MRI (iMRI), intraoperative ultrasound (IOUS), 5-aminolevulinic acid (5-Ala), MRI, and new radiation devices and techniques, most Latin American countries struggle to reach the standard pattern of assistance with some island of excellence in big centers.

When considering second-line treatments for patients with GBM, the disparities in treatment availability are worse. Despite the creation of the Society for Neuro-oncology Latin America (SNOLA), established in 2015, and some surgical or onco-logical societies' efforts to improve governmental rules and policies to CNS tumors, there are still significant work and improvements to accomplish. In the last Brazilian national estimation for patients with GBM (around 6000 cases/year), only 80% of patients could get any basic assistance, and in a recent SNOLA research, only 15% can receive the complete standard multidisciplinary treatment. There has, however, been a progressive improvement in all spheres of treatment in the last years.

## Neuro-oncology Education

At the present time, there are many skilled general neurosurgeons performing excel-lent surgeries but few tumor dedicated ones. The existing 5-year neurosurgical resi-dency training can only provide basic tumor instruction, just enough for a young neurosurgeon to start her/his practice after residency. Fortunately, neurosurgical societies are announcing courses, observerships, and fellowships in neurosurgical oncology. To the best of our knowledge, there are dedicated neurosurgical CNS tumor training programs in Argentina, Mexico, and Brazil. On the other hand, the high demand level mainly in cancer centers and big cities is increasing the need for subspecialization.

SNOLA is also working hard to spread the important concept of a multidisci-plinary approach to CNS tumors, stimulating tumor boards; promoting satellite meetings all over Latin America, beyond the big biannual congress; and referring many colleagues to international experience expecting to create leaders in neuro-oncology. SNOLA currently counts 315 active members. Its mission is to become a truly international multidisciplinary society embracing specialists from neurology, neurosurgery, radiology, pathology, radiation oncology, and oncology and research-ers promoting neuro-oncological education, policies, and research. Another exam-ple to highlight is the Latin American Brain Tumor Board (LATB) teleconference, initiated in August 2013, which now connects 6 global pediatric neuro-oncologists from children's hospitals and cancer centers in the United States, Canada, and Spain with pediatric subspecialists from 20 Latin American countries. This is a great step in improving pediatric neuro-oncology [61, 62]. Accordingly, the LATB aims to both provide support and education and promote a multidisciplinary approach and second pathology and radiology reviews.

During the pandemic period, webinars were initiated and coordinated with other societies worldwide to keep education in neuro-oncology active. These included collaborations between SNOLA and the European Association for Neuro-Oncology (EANO), the Asian Society for Neuro-oncology (ASNO), and the Society for Neuro-Oncology (SNO) for all support and friendship. Besides continued medical education programs, two other aspects are pivotal to continue improving the growth of neuro-oncology in Latin America. These are research and clinical trials. At the present time, there are only a few centers in Latin America where research can be performed using organized clinical databases along with brain tumor bench and translational work. The SNOLA consortium and Latin American Cooperative Oncology Group (LACOG) Neuro Cancer Group are also open to start multicenter clinical trials, crucial to increase industry and government interest in neuro-oncology. We hope that in the near future, Latin America will be able to provide promising and useful translational research while providing excellence care for brain tumor patients.

## Australia

On average, approximately 1750 brain cancers are diagnosed each year in Australia; that is roughly one person diagnosed with brain cancer every 5 hours [63]. Brain cancer kills more children in Australia than any other disease [64]. It also kills more people under 40 in Australia than any other cancer. Approximately 1250 people die each year from brain cancer, which is about 1 every 7 hours. Death related to brain cancer has shown a modest steady increase over the past two decades from 21% (1995–1999) to 23% (2000–2004) to 25% (2005–2009) [64]. Brain cancer costs more per person than any other cancer because it is highly debilitating, affects people in their prime, and often means family members cannot work if they become carriers (Fig. 6.2) [65]. For those aged 35–44 years, brain cancer accounted for the highest proportion of cancer expenditure, totaling $32 million [66].

### Neuro-oncology Education

Post-fellowship neurosurgical education and training in Australasia is governed by the Neurosurgical Society of Australasia (NSA). Such fellowships must be a minimum of 12 months of length. Neuro-oncology fellowships are one type of fellowship offered by the NSA. There are several reports that are collected from fellows during their fellowship program to ensure that their neurosurgical oncology training is, ultimately, adequate for specialization. The only accredited Post-Fellowship Education and Training fellowship program in Australasia, according to the NSA, is currently at the Royal Melbourne Hospital and Melbourne Private Hospital. Given

## Index of lifetime cost per patient

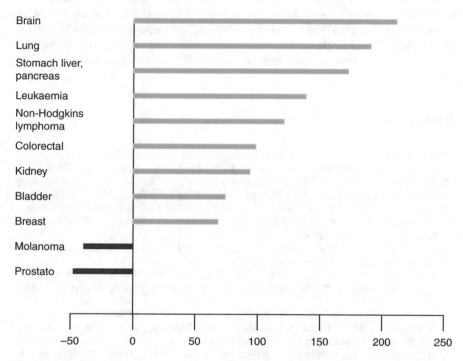

**Fig. 6.2** The cost of brain cancer in New South Wales (NSW), Australia [65]

the population of this region, it would be preferable, in the future, for additional accredited programs to be established to enhance subspecialization in neurosurgical oncology.

## Conclusion

The progressive increase in the number of neurosurgeons worldwide, the recent technological advancements, and the multidisciplinary approach to management have significantly improved the safety of patients suffering from CNS tumors worldwide. Successful neuro-oncology practice requires a multidisciplinary team, made up of neurosurgeons, neurologists, nursing providers, medical oncologists, radiation oncologists, neuroradiologists, neuropathologists, and palliative care specialists. The paucity of these specialists in the general pool still makes sole dedication to the neuro-oncology field difficult. We all believe that subspecialization is the way forward for neuro-oncology, and increased international cooperation will continue to make this a reality.

The World Federation of Neurosurgical Societies (WFNS), the Foundation for International Education in Neurological Surgery (FIENS), and other national and continental neurosurgery societies are making efforts to improve neurosurgical oncology training worldwide through the ongoing development of training courses. During the COVID-19 pandemic, ongoing virtual educational offerings have tried to help raising the level of neurosurgical care of CNS tumors worldwide.

# References

1. de Robles P, Fiest KM, Frolkis AD, et al. The worldwide incidence and prevalence of primary brain tumors: a systematic review and meta-analysis. Neuro-Oncology. 2015;17(6):776–83.
2. GBD Results Tool | GHDx. Accessed 11 Dec 2020. http://ghdx.healthdata.org/gbd-results-tool?params=gbd-api-2019-permalink/b57ec9435d00dd319b77698bc08eed2a.
3. Leece R, Xu J, Ostrom QT, Chen Y, Kruchko C, Barnholtz-Sloan JS. Global incidence of malignant brain and other central nervous system tumors by histology, 2003–2007. Neuro-Oncology. 2017;19(11):1553–64.
4. Louis DN, Ohgaki H, Wiestler OD, et al. The 2007 WHO classification of tumours of the central nervous system. Acta Neuropathol (Berl). 2007;114(2):97–109.
5. Louis DN, Perry A, Reifenberger G, et al. The 2016 World Health Organization classification of tumors of the central nervous system: a summary. Acta Neuropathol (Berl). 2016;131(6):803–20.
6. Levin VA. Neuro-oncology: an overview. Arch Neurol. 1999;56(4):401–4.
7. Molinaro AM, Hervey-Jumper S, Morshed RA, et al. Association of maximal extent of resection of contrast-enhanced and non–contrast-enhanced tumor with survival within molecular subgroups of patients with newly diagnosed glioblastoma. JAMA Oncol. 2020;6(4):495–503.
8. Beiko J, Suki D, Hess KR, et al. IDH1 mutant malignant astrocytomas are more amenable to surgical resection and have a survival benefit associated with maximal surgical resection. Neuro-Oncol. 2014;16(1):81–91.
9. Mathers C, Fat DM, Boerma JT, World Health Organization, editors. The global burden of disease: 2004 update. World Health Organization; 2008.
10. Bray F, Ferlay J, Soerjomataram I, Siegel RL, Torre LA, Jemal A. Global cancer statistics 2018: GLOBOCAN estimates of incidence and mortality worldwide for 36 cancers in 185 countries. CA Cancer J Clin. 2018;68(6):394–424.
11. Murray CJ, Barber RM, Foreman KJ, et al. Global, regional, and national disability-adjusted life years (DALYs) for 306 diseases and injuries and healthy life expectancy (HALE) for 188 countries, 1990–2013: quantifying the epidemiological transition. Lancet. 2015;386(10009):2145–91.
12. Park KB, Johnson WD, Dempsey RJ. Global neurosurgery: the unmet need. World Neurosurg. 2016;88:32–5.
13. Dewan MC, Rattani A, Fieggen G, et al. Global neurosurgery: the current capacity and deficit in the provision of essential neurosurgical care. Executive summary of the Global Neurosurgery Initiative at the Program in Global Surgery and Social Change. J Neurosurg. 2018;130(4):1055–64.
14. Mukhopadhyay S, Punchak M, Rattani A, et al. The global neurosurgical workforce: a mixed-methods assessment of density and growth. J Neurosurg. 2019;130(4):1142–8.
15. Hewedi I, Ibrahim R, Elserry T, et al. Frequency of primary central nervous system tumors in a tertiary hospital, Cairo, Egypt.
16. El-Gaidi MA. Descriptive epidemiology of pediatric intracranial neoplasms in Egypt. Pediatr Neurosurg. 2011;47(6):385–95.

17. Karkouri M, Zafad S, Khattab M, et al. Epidemiologic profile of pediatric brain tumors in Morocco. Childs Nerv Syst. 2010;26(8):1021–7.
18. Olasode BJ, Shokunbi MT, Aghadiuno PU. Intracranial neoplasm in Ibadan, Nigeria. East Afr Med J. 2000;77(1):4.
19. Stagno V, Mugamba J, Ssenyonga P, Kaaya BN, Warf BC. Presentation, pathology, and treatment outcome of brain tumors in 172 consecutive children at CURE Children's Hospital of Uganda. The predominance of the visible diagnosis and the uncertainties of epidemiology in sub-Saharan Africa. Childs Nerv Syst. 2014;30(1):137–46.
20. Arnold-Day C. Paediatric brain tumours: The University of Cape Town experience from 1996–2017. Published online 2019.
21. Emerging trends in the neurosurgical workforce of low- and middle-income countries: a cross-sectional study - ScienceDirect. Accessed 17 Oct 2020. https://www.sciencedirect.com/science/article/pii/S1878875020315886.
22. Chang AY, Skirbekk VF, Tyrovolas S, Kassebaum NJ, Dieleman JL. Measuring population ageing: an analysis of the Global Burden of Disease Study 2017. Lancet Public Health. 2019;4(3):e159–67. https://doi.org/10.1016/S2468-2667(19)30019-2.
23. Patel AP, Fisher JL, Nichols E, et al. Global, regional, and national burden of brain and other CNS cancer, 1990–2016: a systematic analysis for the Global Burden of Disease Study 2016. Lancet Neurol. 2019;18(4):376–93. https://doi.org/10.1016/S1474-4422(18)30468-X.
24. Katsura S, Suzuki J, Wada T. A statistical study of brain tumors in the neurosurgical clinics in Japan. J Neurosurg. 1959;16(5):570–80.
25. Kobayashi S, Morita A. The history of neuroscience and neurosurgery in Japan. Int Neurosci J. 2015;1(1):31–40.
26. Y U. Memories of the late Dr. Mizuho Nakata. Rinsho Shinkeigaku. 1975;15(11):783.
27. Kanda K. Experience of boron neutron capture therapy in Japan. In: International conference neutrons in research and industry, vol. 2867. International Society for Optics and Photonics; 1997. p. 27–30.
28. Shiobara R, Ohira T, Kanzaki J, Toya S. A modified extended middle cranial fossa approach for acoustic nerve tumors: results of 125 operations. J Neurosurg. 1988;68(3):358–65.
29. Yoshida J, Wakabayashi T, Mizuno M, et al. Tumor-specific binding of radiolabeled G-22 monoclonal antibody in glioma patients. Neurol Med Chir (Tokyo). 1992;32(3):125–9.
30. Edwards MS, Hudgins RJ, Wilson CB, Levin VA, Wara WM. Pineal region tumors in children. J Neurosurg. 1988;68(5):689 97.
31. Shinoda J, Yamada H, Sakai N, Ando T, Hirata T, Miwa Y. Placental alkaline phosphatase as a tumor marker for primary intracranial germinoma. J Neurosurg. 1988;68(5):710–20.
32. Kayama T, Yoshimoto T, Fujimoto S, Sakurai Y. Intratumoral oxygen pressure in malignant brain tumor. J Neurosurg. 1991;74(1):55–9.
33. Terao H, Nishikawa H, Ooishi H, Endo T, Kaneko I, Kogure T. A new principle and device for radiosurgery using a linear accelerator; its principle, devices and clinical trials. No Shinkei Geka. 1992;20(5):583–92.
34. Fukaya C, Katayama Y, Yoshino A, Kobayashi K, Kasai M, Yamamoto T. Intraoperative wake-up procedure with propofol and laryngeal mask for optimal excision of brain tumour in eloquent areas. J Clin Neurosci. 2001;8(3):253–5. https://doi.org/10.1054/jocn.2000.0866.
35. Yoshida J, Mizuno M, Fujii M, et al. Human gene therapy for malignant gliomas (glioblastoma multiforme and anaplastic astrocytoma) by in vivo transduction with human interferon β gene using cationic liposomes. Hum Gene Ther. 2004;15(1):77–86.
36. Shibui S. Report of brain tumor registry of Japan (2001–2004). Neurol Med Chir (Tokyo). 2014;54(suppl. 1):1.
37. Japan C. of BTR of. Report of brain tumor registry of Japan (2005–2008). Neurol Med Chir Tokyo. 2017,57(Suppl 1):9–102.
38. Kaatsch P. Epidemiology of childhood cancer. Cancer Treat Rev. 2010;36(4):277–85. https://doi.org/10.1016/j.ctrv.2010.02.003.

39. Sant M, Allemani C, Santaquilani M, et al. EUROCARE-4. Survival of cancer patients diagnosed in 1995-1999. Results and commentary. Eur J Cancer. Published online 2009. https://doi.org/10.1016/j.ejca.2008.11.018.
40. Sant M, Minicozzi P, Lagorio S, et al. Survival of European patients with central nervous system tumors. Int J Cancer. Published online 2012. https://doi.org/10.1002/ijc.26335.
41. Crocetti E, Trama A, Stiller C, et al. Epidemiology of glial and non-glial brain tumours in Europe. Eur J Cancer. Published online 2012. https://doi.org/10.1016/j.ejca.2011.12.013.
42. Holleczek B, Zampella D, Urbschat S, et al. Incidence, mortality and outcome of meningiomas: a population-based study from Germany. Cancer Epidemiol. Published online 2019. https://doi.org/10.1016/j.canep.2019.07.001.
43. Pugliatti M, Sobocki P, Beghi E, et al. Cost of disorders of the brain in Italy. Neurol Sci. 2008;29(2):99–107. https://doi.org/10.1007/s10072-008-0868-7.
44. Gustavsson A, Svensson M, Jacobi F, et al. Cost of disorders of the brain in Europe 2010. Eur Neuropsychopharmacol. Published online 2011. https://doi.org/10.1016/j.euroneuro.2011.08.008.
45. Omerhodzic I, Tonge M, Matos B, et al. Neurosurgical training programme in selected European countries: from the young neurosurgeons' point of view. Turk Neurosurg. Published online 2012. https://doi.org/10.5137/1019-5149.JTN.5133-11.0.
46. Maxwell AJ, Crocker M, Jones TL, Bhagawati D, Papadopoulos MC, Bell BA. Implementation of the European working time directive in neurosurgery reduces continuity of care and training opportunities. Acta Neurochir. Published online 2010. https://doi.org/10.1007/s00701-010-0648-z.
47. Stienen MN, Bartek J, Czabanka MA, et al. Neurosurgical procedures performed during residency in Europe—preliminary numbers and time trends. Acta Neurochir. Published online 2019. https://doi.org/10.1007/s00701-019-03888-3.
48. Reulen HJ, März U. 5 years' experience with a structured operative training programme for neurosurgical residents. Acta Neurochir. Published online 1998. https://doi.org/10.1007/s007010050237.
49. Lindsay K. Accreditation of neurosurgical training programmes in Europe: report of JRAAC. Acta Neurochir. Published online 2012. https://doi.org/10.1007/s00701-012-1337-x.
50. Canale DJ. William Osler and "the special field of neurological surgery". J Neurosurg. 1989;70(5):759–66.
51. Black PM. Harvey cushing at the Peter Bent Brigham hospital. Neurosurgery. 1999;45(5):990–1001.
52. Institute, N.C., https://seer.cancer.gov/statfacts/html/brain.html. 2017. - Yahoo Search Results. Accessed 18 Oct 2020.
53. Ostrom QT, Cioffi G, Gittleman H, et al. CBTRUS statistical report: primary brain and other central nervous system tumors diagnosed in the United States in 2012–2016. Neuro-Oncology. 2019;21(Supplement_5):v1–v100. https://doi.org/10.1093/neuonc/noz150.
54. Mariotto AB, Robin Yabroff K, Shao Y, Feuer EJ, Brown ML. Projections of the cost of cancer care in the United States: 2010–2020. J Natl Cancer Inst. 2011;103(2):117–28.
55. Barker FG 2nd, Curry WT Jr, Carter BS. Surgery for primary supratentorial brain tumors in the United States, 1988 to 2000: the effect of provider caseload and centralization of care. Neuro-Oncology. 2005;7(1):49–63. - Yahoo Search Results. Accessed 18 Oct 2020.
56. Luther EM, McCarthy D, Berry KM, et al. Hospital teaching status associated with reduced inpatient mortality and perioperative complications in surgical neuro-oncology. J Neuro-Oncol. 2020;146(2):389–96.
57. RANO criteria for glioblastoma | Radiology Reference Article | Radiopaedia.org. Accessed 23 Oct 2020. https://radiopaedia.org/articles/rano-criteria-for-glioblastoma.
58. Combs SE, Rieken S, Wick W, et al. Prognostic significance of IDH-1 and MGMT in patients with glioblastoma: one step forward, and one step back? Radiat Oncol. 2011;6(1):115.
59. Juratli TA, Kirsch M, Geiger K, et al. The prognostic value of IDH mutations and MGMT promoter status in secondary high-grade gliomas. J Neuro-Oncol. 2012;110(3):325–33.

60. Stupp R, Mason WP, van den Bent MJ, et al. Radiotherapy plus concomitant and adjuvant Temozolomide for Glioblastoma. N Engl J Med. 2005;352(10):987–96. https://doi.org/10.1056/NEJMoa043330.
61. Abu Arja MH, Coven S, Stanek JR, et al. DEV-07. The Latin-American Brain Tumor Board (LATB) teleconference: results of a web-based survey to evaluate participant experience and the program. Neuro-Oncology. 2018;20(suppl_2):i46.
62. Osorio DS, Lassaletta A, la Madrid AEM, et al. DEV-14. Impact of a Latin America-wide Teleconferenced Brain Tumor Board. Neuro-Oncology. 2018;20(Suppl 2):i47.
63. Cancer in Australia 2017, Table of contents. Australian Institute of Health and Welfare. Accessed 11 Dec 2020. https://www.aihw.gov.au/reports/cancer/cancer-in-australia-2017/contents/table-of-contents.
64. Causes of Death, Australia, 2019 | Australian Bureau of Statistics. Published October 23, 2020. Accessed 11 Dec 2020. https://www.abs.gov.au/statistics/health/causes-death/causes-death-australia/latest-release.
65. costofcancer_summary.pdf. Accessed 11 Dec 2020. https://www.cancercouncil.com.au/wp-content/uploads/2010/11/costofcancer_summary.pdf.
66. Health system expenditure on cancer and other neoplasms in Australia 2008–09, Table of contents. Australian Institute of Health and Welfare. Accessed 11 Dec 2020. https://www.aihw.gov.au/reports/health-welfare-expenditure/health-system-expenditure-cancer-2008-09/contents/table-of-contents.

# Chapter 7
# The Role of Neurosurgery in Global Spine Health

**Mehmet Zileli, Salman Sharif, Marcos Masini, Oscar L. Alves, and Scott Robertson**

## Abbreviations

| | |
|---|---|
| CAANS | Continental Association of African Neurosurgical Societies |
| CME | Continuous medical education |
| DOPS | Direct observation of procedural skills |
| FIENS | Foundation for International Education in Neurological Surgery |
| LMIC | Lower-middle-income country |
| MESS | Middle East Spine Society |
| MiniCeX | Mini-clinical examination |

M. Zileli (✉)
Ege University, Izmir, Turkey

WFNS Spine Committee, Izmir, Turkey

S. Sharif
WFNS Spine Committee, Izmir, Turkey

Liaquat National Hospital & Medical College, Karachi, Pakistan

M. Masini
School of Medicine Faciplac, Brasília, Brazil

Hospital Lago Sul, Brasilia, Brazil

O. L. Alves
Neurosurgery Department, Centro Hospitalar de Gaia/Espinho, Vila Nova de Gaia, Portugal

Neurosurgery Department, Hospital Lusiadas Porto, Porto, Portugal

S. Robertson
Neurosurgery Department, Laredo Medical Center, University of the Incarnate Word School of Osteopathic Medicine, Laredo, TX, USA

© The Author(s), under exclusive license to Springer Nature Switzerland AG 2022
I. M. Germano (ed.), *Neurosurgery and Global Health*,
https://doi.org/10.1007/978-3-030-86656-3_7

NASS        North American Spine Society
VR          Virtual reality
WFNS        World Federation of Neurosurgical Societies
WSCS        World Spinal Column Society

# Introduction

Spinal disorders are a primary source of global disability and are a considerable burden on society. People in low- and middle-income countries (LMICs) are significantly affected. Disability caused by back pain has escalated by 54% between 1990 and 2015 [25, 30]. A significant rise in back pain has happened in LMIC since there is an increase in population and aging. Back pain should be considered a significant financial burden toward the expenses associated with health care, lack of productivity, and loss of work due to illness. Similar problems exist for other spinal disorders [25]. However, there is a shortage of health resources and professionals required to address the increasing burden of chronic diseases in underdeveloped countries [28]. Despite these facts, spine health care has not to date received the attention required to change and recognize spine problems as a global burden and priority.

# Brief Historical Background

Until the beginning of the twentieth century, spine surgery pioneers cannot be distinguished as orthopedic or neurosurgery, since specialization did not occur during history. Neurosurgery, as a medical discipline, has started at the beginning of the twentieth century. However, after Cushing's early papers in the 1920s, brain surgery has taken the primary interest, and the spine has been a neglected topic by neurosurgeons. Despite this fact, there have been many contributions of neurosurgeons to the evolution and advancement of spine surgery.

The evolution of spine surgery can be divided into four steps: (1) decompression (mainly laminectomy) of the spinal cord and nerve roots, (2) stabilization of unstable spine, (3) deformity correction, and (4) minimally invasive techniques.

## *Decompression Techniques*

Although laminectomy was applied in the nineteenth century, the surgeries were very complicated, and outcomes were worse. Anesthetics, antibiotics, and pain killers should be developed to improve the results. Victor Horsley is one of the earliest neurosurgeons who did the first successful operation to remove an extramedullary tumor of the spinal cord in 1888 [21]. The invention of X-rays by German physicist Wilhelm Roentgen in 1885 led to better diagnosis of spinal disorders. In 1905, Cushing [13] operated a patient with an intramedullary tumor, but he decided to perform a myelotomy in the dorsal column without removal. In 1907, von Eiselsberg successfully resected an intramedullary tumor.

Taylor (Taylor) has developed the hemilaminectomy technique in 1910, after early aggressive laminectomies in trauma and tumor surgeries. Contributions of Harvey Cushing to the history of neurosurgery have been tremendous. Cushing has developed hemostatic clips, other hemostatic agents, coagulants, and suction mechanisms [42]. Charles A. Elsberg has published his first series of laminectomies in 1913 [18]. Elsberg was one of the first to remove a cervical disk by a posterior approach in 1925 [19]. Walter E. Dandy [14] published a description of two cases of herniated lumbar disks causing a cauda equina syndrome in 1929. But, the first disk herniation surgery was reported by Mixter and Barr [40].

## Stabilization Techniques

Orthopedic spine surgeons have mainly developed thoracolumbar stabilization techniques. However, in the development of the cervical spine fixations, neurosurgeons have played significant roles. In 1910, silk sutures were used to fixate atlantoaxial instability [39]. Gallie first developed C1–C2 wiring in the 1950s, then Brooks [6] in the 1970s, and then Sonntag and Dickman in the 1980s [17].

Goel has first described a plate fixation of the lateral masses of C1 and C2 in 1994 [20]. This technique allowed the reduction of C1 subluxation on C2 and is safer than Magerl's transarticular screw fixation by preventing vertebral artery injury. Goel has then improved his approach, did classification of basilar invagination, and achieved a posterior reduction by placing a spacer between the atlantoaxial joint. It was a paradigm shift by making a transoral odontoid resection surgery unnecessary.

Neurosurgeons historically achieved many improvements in cervical spine surgery. In 1958, Cloward pioneered the ventral approach to the cervical spine [10]. With his technique, it was easy to remove the disk and fuse the level by placing a bone dowel in between the vertebral bodies. Caspar [8] has popularized the anterior cervical plating system. Howard H. Hepburn, a British neurosurgeon, has designed skull tongs for cervical spine traction in the middle of the 1920s for treating wounded soldiers in World War I [47], long before Crutchfield's publication in 1933 [12].

In the 1990s, neurosurgeons were mainly performing cervical spine fixations, but orthopedic spine surgeons developed pedicle screw fixation for the thoracic and lumbar spine. Usage of pedicle screws by neurosurgeons took the time [58].

*Deformity Correction*

Orthopedic spine surgeons also pioneered deformity correction, especially scoliosis surgery.

*Minimally Invasive Spinal Surgery*

Yasargil [60] and Caspar [9] have pioneered discectomies under a microscope. The microendoscopic tubular system was introduced in 1997 and became famous for performing discectomies and laminectomies [48]. After the first description of Scoville's posterior cervical discectomies in 1976 [51], a similar technique was adapted to tube-guided surgery by Adamson in 2001 [2]. Foley's group has adjusted the transforaminal interbody graft and cage placement by tubes in 2005 [50].

## Current Status of Spinal Neurosurgery

*Spinal Neurosurgery Clinical Practice*

Spine surgery is a major part of the neurosurgical practice. In the USA, it is estimated that, of all neurosurgical operations, 77% are performed for spinal cases, and this percentage is growing as of 2013 [11]. Traditionally, they were good in the decompression of spine neural elements, whereas orthopedic surgeons surpassed in the spine stabilization domain. Neurosurgeons practice more on degenerative disorders, cervical spine trauma, and intradural pathologies, while orthopedic surgeons practice more on trauma and deformity. However, recently, more and more neurological spine surgeons are performing all types of surgeries, including deformity.

*Spinal Neurosurgery Research*

Since the seminal biomechanical works of Edward Benzel et al. [4], which influenced the modern training of younger generations, neurosurgeons can nowadays excel in treating spine disorders. As a result of this rather holistic vision and understanding, neurosurgeons are very well placed to steer spine research. Publication metrics show that neurosurgeons, or research groups led by them, produce a significant percentage of papers published in spine journals. Especially the fields like nanotechnology, molecular engineering, and stem cell research for spinal diseases and pathology are in neurosurgeons' scope. Some areas, such as regenerative therapies on spinal cord injury, have been the primary interest of neurosurgery departments.

An excellent example of that is the laboratory of Charles Tator in Toronto [54]. Advances in basic science offer hope for further reconstruction of the spinal cord in the future, the development of genetic repair treatments, the introduction of chitosan channels for rebuilding the spinal cord structure, and stem cell transplantations and neurotrophic factors to stimulate spinal cord repair. Besides, developments in nano-technology and bionics offer new opportunities for restoration of function in para-lyzed sections.

Biomechanical concepts and studies on the cadaveric spine are mainly developed in biomechanical engineering laboratories [46]. Optical markers and reference points were used to investigate load distributions of cadaveric specimens and new implant designs, and the effect of some surgical approaches were investigated [46]. Basic science laboratories and biomechanical laboratories have also been estab-lished and pioneered in neurosurgical departments [26, 56]. The spine biomechan-ics books of Edward C. Benzel have been fundamental to understand many concepts on managing spinal disorders [4]. The first edition of the book *Biomechanics of Spine Stabilization* is first published in 1995, and the 3rd edition is dated 2015.

An expert spine surgeon should better devote more than 85% of his/her practice exclusively to spine cases to gather a meaningful volume of patients and be up to date with the specific scientific literature. As in any specific medical arena, it is impossible to become a proficient scientist without sound knowledge. Additionally, a spinal neurosurgeon-scientist can be defined as a neurosurgeon spending some of his/her time performing research in the spine arena.

When dealing with the most valuable currency – time – the logical question is if a dual neurosurgeon-scientist career is feasible. The degree of commitment depends more on the funding and the infrastructures allocated locally to research than any other factor. There is a need for the development of research networks at local, regional, or international levels. A substantial number of the top-cited articles in spine surgery journals are the product of these collaborative networks.

A neurosurgeon-scientist is a bridge affectionate, redirecting knowledge from preclinical bench science to the patient's bedside and back again. From biomateri-als, implants, and cell regeneration to biomechanics, numerous examples arise from areas where the neurosurgeon-scientist can identify the need for a better under-standing of the clinical dilemmas.

Researching, in addition to clinical duties, will undoubtedly improve patients' outcomes. In general, establishing an academic program of spine surgery compared with historical records showed a significant improvement in health-care quality indexes, such as decreased morbidity, mortality, hospital stay, re-admission, and re-OP rates. This may not result from better operating skills, but applying the scien-tific method to clinical practice.

Other essential constraints to become a neuro-spine surgeon-scientist, besides the financial considerations – double of workload not proportional to the income – are the difficulties in nurturing research involvement during the neurosurgical resi-dency. Among those, lack of training with research tools, lack of influential mentors, failure to establish a network of researchers, difficulty in getting research grants at an individual level, and perceived lack of reward play a role. Additionally, the shortage in neurosurgeon's labor force and emergency coverage deficits present a barrier to neurosurgeons becoming involved in spine research.

Ideally, spine surgeons should receive formal research training in preclinical and clinical research. A research fellowship of at least 3 months should be part of the formal training program, also integrating basics on public health and health economics due to the impact of spine surgery on medicine's overall costs. Formal research training correlates with future research productivity, funding, and a higher probability of getting a chair position in a neurosurgical department.

In summary, there is a profound clinical need for neurosurgeons who conduct original translational research in the spine arena, as there is still a lack of good treatment strategies for spine disorders. It is essential for the progress of spine surgery and the preservation of the academic spine neurosurgeon paradigm. Performing research brings personal gratification, benefits patients, and advances the field. The WFNS Spine Committee should propel the research competencies and needs within the neuro-spine community.

## Spinal Neurosurgery Publications

The first publications on spine have appeared in the *Transactions of the American Orthopaedic Association* in 1887 and *Journal of Neurosurgery* in 1944 [41]. "Spine" journal began publication in 1976. It was the first dedicated spine journal. Among the most cited 100 articles, neurosurgical journals such as *Journal of Neurosurgery*, *Journal of Neurosurgery-Spine*, *Neurosurgical Review*, and *Neurosurgery* have had many of them [41]. Cloward's paper describing a new technique "The Anterior Approach for Removal of Ruptured Cervical Disks" was one of the most cited surgical technique papers [10].

There are currently neurosurgical journals dedicated to the spine such as *Journal of Neurosurgery: Spine* and *Neurospine*. The *Journal of Neurosurgery: Spine* started publication four times a year in 1999. *Neurosurgery* has been the source of many consensus guidelines on spine surgery [58].

## *Guidelines and Recommendations*

Neurosurgical societies have established and published numerous spine-related guidelines for managing various spinal disorders and injury. The North American Spine Society (NASS) has developed eight guidelines in different topics [43]. The Congress of Neurological Surgeons (CNS) and AANS/CNS Spine Section have developed four spine-related guidelines [1]. The WFNS Spine Committee has prepared recommendations on four topics after consensus meetings: cervical spondylotic myelopathy, lumbar spinal stenosis, cervical spine trauma, and spinal cord injury [59].

## Spinal Neurosurgery Education

Neurosurgery is a swift evolving discipline, so then the education of neurosurgeons evolves. Educating the next generation of humanitarian neuro- and spine surgeons, armed with the lessons of those who have come before, will strengthen the field's efforts.

## *The Evolution of Spine Neurosurgery Education*

Education in medicine has done revolutionary changes in the last 150 years. From the Scottish model going through Humboldt's German concept, most universities in the world follow similar models. The idea of making the university a research center was the first major revolution in biomedical education.

Another great revolution in medical education took place when students were selected only on merit and were subjected to regular tests throughout the period in which they were enrolled. The current residency program or "specialization" was added to the educational scheme by William Halsted. He has created the concept of subspecialty in medicine [35]. Problem-based learning (PBL) is an innovative pedagogical method implemented in education and medical education over the last 20 years. Realistic simulation models for training teams attending emergencies can also be applied to spine problems [27]. Spine surgery has always been an integral part of neurosurgery training. The advantages of neurosurgeons are their familiarity with a neurological examination and nerve root and spinal cord manipulations during surgery.

Beginning in the 1980s, spinal surgery was becoming a staple of neurosurgical residency training. Since it is a significant product line for the practicing general neurosurgeon, spinal surgery became the focal point of innovation and energy in neurosurgical practice. Neurosurgical training programs would flourish as functional, pediatric, cerebrovascular, oncological, traumatic, and spinal and peripheral nerve surgery as subspecialties. Spinal surgery became a part of the neurosurgical residency curriculum from the beginning of formal neurosurgical training. It has kept pace with and participated in the advances that have occurred. Kelly has pointed out that "All neurosurgery residents are spinal surgeons by definition, even if they ultimately migrate to another subspecialty. Neurosurgeons are the only spinal surgeons that can be trained in their residency." [32].

The competency-based objectives for spinal surgery in residency training include the entire spine, from the craniovertebral junction to the sacrum, as a required curriculum, as published in the Resident Curriculum Guidelines for Neurosurgery in the USA [55].

The role of societies in the education of spine surgery has been significant. Among those, WFNS Spine Committee, NASS, Spine Society of Europe (SSE),

EANS, Latin American Federation of Neurosurgical Societies (FLANC), Middle East Spine Society (MESS), ACNS, and CSRS can be counted.

## Spinal Neurosurgery Education in Latin American: A Pioneer Example

The structure of medical education in Latin America received influences from European and American schools. The Brazilian Society of Neurosurgery (SBN) has a pioneering role in structuring resident training systems in Latin America [38]. The structure of each educational program includes three features: (1) competency-based training, which guarantees a real preparation to solve the patient's problems, (2) several nonpesific and implied subjects, such as ethics, compliance, cultural knowledge, etc., are also necessary to form an adequate professional profile and must be included in the resident training process, and (3) information integration process within the programs, which could improve both trainees and teachers [35]. The expansion of scientific medical knowledge extends physicians' training who work with new information and complex technologies. However, the emerging of defensive medicine due to excess of legal claims for medical malpractice causes a restructuring of the existing training structure.

For these reasons, the Federation of Latin American Neurological Surgery (FLANC) Education Committee has adopted a more suitable system for specialization in spinal neurosurgery [37]. For example, we regularly update the existing/active training reference centers in Latin America on specific spinal neurosurgery topics, such as pain, degenerative, tumor, and congenital deformities. Besides, these centers are required to focus on laboratory research and epidemiological studies. The association of online theoretical courses with periods organized in face-to-face format reduces financial investment, thus obtaining similar or even better results [53].

Keeping the intersection with similar projects in orthopedics spine training centers is accomplished with the Ibero-American Column Society of Ibero-Latin American Column (SILACO), which brings together neurosurgeons and orthopedic surgeons. SILACO is composed of all Latin American spine societies and the Iberian Peninsula (Spain and Portugal), using two official languages, Spanish and Portuguese [34].

There is also the Latin American Center for Research and Training in Minimally Invasive Surgery (CLEMI), www.clemi.edu.co, in Bogotá. This educational center, founded in 2006, dedicated not only to the spine but also other clinical subspecialties interested in advancing minimally invasive surgery. To date, CLEMI has hosted more than 100 hands-on endoscopic spine surgery workshops, training close to 1200 specialists among neurosurgeons and orthopedists from all over Latin America. The participants have also implemented their ESS programs in their respective countries. Equally noteworthy are the well-known microsurgery laboratories of Prof. Evandro Oliveira, in São Paulo, Brazil, and Prof. Alvaro Campero, in Buenos Aires, Argentina.

The FLANC Education Committee currently develops training and certification of young neurosurgeons and residents to strategically and financially support their participation in reference centers accredited by FLANC. Those centers are recertified every 2 years. Forty-eight active centers are participating in the program from the following countries, Argentina, Belgium, Bolivia, Brazil, Chile, Colombia, Cuba, Mexico, Peru, Spain, Uruguay, and the USA, being 27 of them prepared for training in spine surgery [36].

Annually FLANC Foundation allocates over $50,000 on scholarship and professional visits to ten fellows previously selected and mandatorily appointed by member societies. Applicants must meet the prerequisites set out in the Candidate Manual drawn up by the Education Committee (www.e-FLANC.org). This system allowed the training of 91 young neurosurgeons in the last 5 years.

## Global Spinal Neurosurgery Education

Many eminent spinal surgeons have worked tirelessly over the last decades to establish a training program in countries with limited resources. The World Federation of Neurosurgical Societies (WFNS) established training programs in Rabat (Morocco) and Nairobi (Kenya) to train young African neurosurgery residents in collaboration with various countries. Additional organizations, like the Foundation for International Education in Neurological Surgery (FIENS), established 50 years ago, have grown over time to also offer in developing regional neurosurgical training programs, including the spine. Multiple committees of WFNS, including the WFNS Spine Committee, FIENS, Continental Association of African Neurosurgical Societies (CAANS), World Spinal Column Society, Eurospine, NASS, and Middle East Spine Society (MESS), have put immense effort in LMICs. World Spine Care is a nonprofit organization established in 2008 to improve the lives of the underprivileged population. It aimed to work for the provision of sustainable solutions toward spine care. World Spine Care initiated spinal programs in Botswana, the Dominican Republic, India, and Ghana [24].

"Global Spine Education" is defined by interventions that highlight skills transfer, teaching medical students/residents/neurosurgeons by giving lectures, Internet-based teaching, assessments before and after, and providing educational materials such as books, pamphlets, and videos. These education programs seek to improve the quality of care provided in the country. It is distinct from training, which comprises a scheduled method of a specific duration, meant to increase the number of spine surgeons or spine surgery-capable professionals. Most surgeons in the low- and middle income countries have been functioning below their capacity due to limited resources. Hence, they might as well require some level of education when modern equipment is brought in. Secondly, there are significant challenges encountered in the education of young aspiring professionals in the spine. This program facilitates training in visiting residencies and fellowships through online certification courses with experts in the area to counter this aspect. This is to increase the number of trained professionals affiliated with spine care and enhance their skill set [23].

The suggested education program for LMICs is shown in Table 7.1. For the next generation of students' education, a program with multiple specialties should be in place. As stated in the conclusion of a WFNS special symposium for neuro- and spine surgery, in 2018, "The equality in the access to the neurosurgical treatments by all individuals should be the ultimate aim in structuring education, human resources, and facilities in all countries across the globe" [31].

## Benefits of Global Spinal Neurosurgery Education

A real spine training program is truly a partnership with society and the government [15]. Starting a spine program with a small number of trainees can greatly affect any region not having the spine service. Such a program could improve the trauma, congenital disability, and spine tumor care of their population. The effective spine care system must provide appropriate care of the spine and return healthy patients as contributing members of society.

Pain, spinal deformity, and cancer care are impossible to treat completely using modern techniques without spine surgeons. The benefits of involving specialized surgical care were presented in the Lancet Commission's landmark presentations on global surgery and the World Bank reports in 2015 [52]. The Lancet Commission reasoned that access to essential surgical care could be life-saving and return productive citizens to society, lacked billions of people worldwide. Evidence places access to crucial surgery on a par with access to clean water, antibiotics, and freedom from war or famine in its importance to world health.

The globalization of spine surgery has brought astonishing benefits to the developed world. The transference of information between Europe, Asia, and the Americas has resulted in the unrivaled quality of care. Modern telecommunication has resulted in the rapid propagation of new techniques, scientific developments, and a worldwide impetus for excellence. Global neurosurgery and specifically spine surgery will benefit the developing world. The humanitarian neurosurgery has been an essential component of global spine surgery in addressing the worldwide disparities in health care and bringing the collective benefits of a developing country in establishing a steady health-care system [15, 16].

## Spinal Neurosurgery and Community Education

People-centered, culturally competent health care can be integrated throughout the system, such as educational interventions, clinical encounters, health promotion programs and services, and processes at the systems level [30]. People-centered

**Table 7.1** Spine education tiers

| | Concerns | Providers | Interventions | Prevention |
|---|---|---|---|---|
| Community and public education | Lack of safety road awareness, safety harness, protective railings for toddlers and elderly | School teachers, media (print, social, and others), and community health workers | Community awareness program, school/factory/corporate visits for awareness program | Health education programs |
| Primary spine education | Nonspecific back and neck pain, myalgias, depression, anxiety, posture care | General physician and first responders | Seminar, webinars, CMEs, workshops | Reduce risk factor and patient handling, awareness regarding posture |
| Secondary spine education | Chronic pain/neurologic deficit affecting daily life activities | Residents and trainees, rheumatologist, physiotherapist | Specialty care, workshops and certificate courses, CME | Reduce severity and address risk factors |
| Tertiary spine education | Spine trauma, deformity, and infection | Spinal surgeons/societies/governments/institutions | Societies helping governments and having sister institutions/spine fellowship programs, spine symposiums, webinars | Prevent morbidity and mortality |

care contains a wide variety of community participants, including the individual, caregivers, families, and communities, as participants in the health-care process. It includes not only the clinical encounter but also health policy and services. This approach is participatory; therefore, there is greater accountability to local stake-holders and disadvantaged populations. Success metrics include community health outcomes, such as population health outcome measures and value of care indicators.

## Spinal Neurosurgery and Residents' Training

Surgical education of spine surgery residents in the operating room forms an integral part of their surgical training. However, patient safety need not be sacrificed in the place of education [57]. By viewing recordings of the previous surgeries repeatedly, one can master all the necessary steps involved in the procedure. Sound knowledge of anatomical landmarks may serve as a replacement for neuronavigation. A standard uniform curriculum of global neurosurgery should be designed to arrest the decline in the neurosurgical training across the globe. Accurate tracking of resident performance parameters by semester and complementing the educators' feedback is an essential part of resident training. Standardized tools to educate and evaluate trainees should also be considered [7, 29].

The ideal residents' training should not be limited to acquiring textbook knowledge and laboratory work but also skillful in the surgical and non-surgical management of patients with spinal diseases. Spine surgery training should be divided into five levels. The first and second years of training should focus on strengthening the core concepts of neurophysiology and neuroanatomy. Midlevel residents are required to apply the knowledge into practice. The surgical skills and ability to make an accurate diagnosis are essential at this level. As a senior resident in the third phase, one is required to perform surgical procedures under supervision ("Shows How" phase). The fourth phase is for unsupervised practice ("Does" phase). The final level of training is becoming an innovator ("Does Better" phase).

Models of training initiated by high-income countries (HIC) for the LMIC are not self-sustainable financially. Those programs are funded by various donors, foundations, grants, and partnerships, whereas a self-reliance program must be designed for LMIC in collaboration between the WHO and the governments [5, 16]. The initiatives carried out by HIC to train neurosurgeons from LMIC for the past 10 years have successfully accelerated neurosurgery education and training. More important is the long-term mentorship that has been established between mentors from HIC with a mentee from the LMIC. Besides having been trained as a competent neurosurgeon, one should also be trained as a good neurosurgery teacher. In his paper, Edward Benzel stated that we retain 90% of what we do or teach while only keeping 50% of what we hear and see [16, 44]. It is the senior neurosurgeons' responsibility to train the next generation of neurosurgeons, especially from the developing countries, to decrease the disparity in world neurosurgical services level, which includes the effort to provide better equipment and resources to the developing countries [16].

## Interactive Spinal Neurosurgery Learning, e-Learning, and Digital Technology

Interactive learning methods that encourage the active participation of learners have shown to boost the level of education. Problem-based learning is one such modality, which utilizes clinical scenarios to teach problem-solving skills. Compared with lecture-based training, problem-based learning has shown superior performance in improving the medical educational environment. Despite this, lecturing is the most widely used method of teaching in CME. This has changed in recent times. The series of webinars being conducted by various organizations, with leading experts worldwide, have contributed immensely toward imparting the pearls and tips and tricks of the neurosurgery trait. To attract the participants and have a weightage of these CME activities, they started with pre- and post-evaluation and interactive discussion between participants and the experts [32].

The ongoing pandemic affected the medical community worldwide. It also paused all in-person educational activities. During this time, many international societies, including WFNS and Pakistan Society of Neurosurgeons, initiated interactive and thought-out webinars with renowned spinal surgeons worldwide. According to unpublished data from these webinars, it was evident that e-learning significantly influences the spine surgery training and practice. Most participants felt that online education is an adequate substitution of traditional teaching methods and wanted to continue this practice post-pandemic. Digital education is an emerging tool in spine surgery education with free and low-cost mobile content with a high educational impact [16, 33]. Examples are summarized in Table 7.2.

**Table 7.2** Examples of digital opportunities available to enhance the training of spinal neurosurgeons

| Digital content channels | Links |
| --- | --- |
| WFNS Young Neurosurgeons Forum | https://www.youtube.com/channel/UCyINk2dpT5N00ZWcdCRIKOQ |
| Brainbook | https://www.youtube.com/channel/UCnbPqck6c4yydPKVK0Faf6w |
| NeuroMind | https://surgicalneurologyint.com/apps/neuromind/ |
| UpSurgeOn | http://www.upsurgeon.com/ |
| The Neurosurgical Atlas | https://www.neurosurgicalatlas.com/ |
| Touch Surgery | https://www.touchsurgery.com/ |
| The 100 UCLA Subjects in Neurosurgery | https://podcasts.apple.com/us/podcast/ucla-100-subjects-in-neurosurgery/id434135906 |
| Neurosurgical Survival Guide | https://neurosurgerysurvivalguide.com/ |
| Neurosurgical TV | https://www.youtube.com/user/DigitalHealthHome |
| Neurosurgery LNH | https://www.youtube.com/neurosurgerylnh |
| WFNS Spine Committee Webpage | www.wfns-spine.org |

## Education via Spine Neurosurgery Simulation and Virtual Reality

Technological innovations and their widespread dissemination have met educational sciences' needs, providing powerful tools to enhance and shorten the learning curve in several fields, including medicine. The first attempts at an immersive, multimodal simulation of the reality date back to 1968 with Morton Heilig's milestone Sensorama, a machine that included a vibrating seat, fans, stereo sound, and stereoscopic video systems. This complex machine simulated a motorbike ride involving the user in a multisensory experience. Educational training in medicine is pressed in between two urgent needs: (1) to ensure the uppermost level of safety for the patient ("primum non nocere") and (2) to provide the highest level of competence for health-care professionals through an efficient, reproducible, and measurable transfer of expertise.

Virtual reality (VR) has been used in medicine, initially as a positive reinforcement for more traditional educational pathways (classroom lectures, cadaver labs, live tissue courses) and, more recently, as their potential substitute. Le et al. compared three different teaching method ancillaries to the standard anatomy theory classroom course for medical students: "manikin" (pictures, plastic models, specimens), "cadaver" (dead human bodies), and virtual reality (3D virtual reality simulation). They found that VR technology in teaching was more efficient in terms of knowledge transfer than the use of cadavers and plastic manikins and less expensive since the latter two modalities required frequent replacements to ensure satisfactory quality of the didactic materials [32].

Over the last decade, virtual reality (VR) has been tested, first as an addition to traditional education and, more recently, as their potential substitute. VR has been frequently sampled in medicine, initially as a positive reinforcement for more conventional educational tracks (classroom lectures, cadaver labs, live tissue courses) and, more recently, as their potential substitute. Some evidence supports the efficacy of VR training in skills acquisition and competence transfer: specifically, this innovative learning pathway showed its applicability in spinal surgery [3, 32]. Further improvements, already under testing, include the opportunity to simulate the procedure on different anatomic grounds to increase the number of possible variables of the procedure (unusual neurovascular anatomy, degenerative changes of the spine such as degenerative scoliosis or disk height reduction, reciprocal relationship between the lumbar spine and iliac crest). VR-based training in spine surgery holds promise to be of value for residents and inexperienced surgeons.

## Future Plans and Recommendations

### Global Spine Health

In a recent collaborative work called "Global Spine Care Initiative," discrepancies between high-income and low- and middle-income countries have been stressed and some recommendations created. The global spine care initiative model emphasizes people-centered health-care systems, which refocuses the health-care system on the people's needs in the community and society. This model engages community representatives as stakeholders [24, 30]. The key points were taken from the Global Spine Care Initiative paper [24]:

(a) Spinal disorders, including spinal pain, are the primary cause of disability in the world. Disability disproportionately impacts woman, older populations, rural populations, poorer quintile of populations, and low-income countries.
(b) An interdisciplinary, international team, consisting of 68 members from 24 countries, collaborated to develop an evidence-informed, practical, and sustainable spine health-care model for communities around the world, which could be implemented with various levels of resources.
(c) The team developed reviews of the literature on assessment, noninvasive management, invasive management, public health, psychological and social issues, and osteoporosis management.
(d) From these reviews, a classification system, care pathway, list of resources, and care model were developed through a consensus process.

What are the risk factors for common spinal disorders in high-income countries and moderate- to lesser-income countries? Green et al. [22] have developed recommendations for prevention interventions for spinal disorders that could be delivered globally, especially in underserved areas and low- and middle-income countries.

Biological, psychosocial, non-modifiable, and exposure variables existed in the risk factor and association categories with interactions between these categories mentioned frequently in the literature [22]. Nordin et al. [45] have tried to develop recommendations for assessing spine-related complaints in medically underserved areas with limited resources. Their advice to clinicians in low- and middle-income countries are (1) take a clinical history to determine signs or symptoms suggesting severe pathology (red flags) and psychological factors (yellow flags); (2) perform a physical examination (musculoskeletal and neurological); (3) do not routinely obtain diagnostic imaging; (4) obtain diagnostic imaging and/or laboratory tests when serious pathologies are suspected, and/or presence of progressive neurologic deficits, and/or disabling persistent pain; (5) do not perform electromyography or nerve conduction studies for diagnosis of intervertebral disk disease with radiculopathy; and (6) do not perform discography for the assessment of spinal disorders. They can also be applied to all areas of the world. Besides, we must stress the cost-effectiveness ratio of any treatment technique, especially surgical procedures.

## Neurosurgery Spine Education

LMICs are suffering from a lack of access to spine care. These large gaps cannot be filled with episodic service missions from developed countries. Self-sustaining spine programs must be locally developed in the countries of need. International support should be built on "Service through Education." The success of sustainable, locally championed neurosurgery educational programs will be dependent on the simultaneous, parallel development of all associated services. They will require the thoughtful collaboration of all major spine societies with a compassionate emphasis while championing the local surgeons, who must assume leadership.

Some suggested recommendations aiming the future of spine education are below summarized:

- Promote the reorganization and unification of training courses in every country [49].
- Stress the importance of neurosurgical societies in the control of final exam and in the recertification.
- Try to improve the number and quality of reference training centers all around the world.
- Encourage bilateral association between societies, associations, and university centers from other continents aiming at the exchange of experiences of residents and young neurosurgeons in medical practices in different cultures.
- Find suitable and legal ways we can grant fellowships financed by the medical industry avoiding conflict of interest.
- Promote more intensively the dissemination of basic disease prevention projects aiming at the prevention of spinal cord, brain, and other traumatic injuries through education, research, and advocacy guided by the success of experiences of ThinkFirst, USA, and Think Well, Brazil. Top spine prevention areas include nervous system deformities in children, neurotrauma in young adults, and stroke prevention for gait preservation in elderly patients.
- Systematize the residency and specialization training services, including spine diseases, respecting the rules of the country of each affiliated society, but providing the structural bases for the training.
- Sponsor a support system for professional visits and scholarships at reference centers of different geographical areas so that the exchange of experiences can be focused on local needs.
- Recognize and evaluate the growing importance of distance learning methods, virtual medical care, and special procedures.

## Conclusions

### *Clinical Spine Neurosurgery*

The field of spine surgery has undergone one of the most significant transformations in medicine over the last century. Over the past three decades, the most significant advancement has come with the evolution of spinal instrumentation and fusion. In this chapter, we tried to capture only specific components of many monumental milestones, each of which likely required the dedication of many unnamed surgeons, scientists, engineers, and entrepreneurs. Both neurosurgical and orthopedic contributions have been tremendous, with continued daily innovation, particularly in navigation, robotics, materials science, and spinal biomechanics. These contributions have allowed for safer, more productive, and more efficient methods of treatment, improving outcomes and quality of life for patients. Looking at the history of spine surgery and its incredible recent journey provides excitement for continued progress in the future.

## Spinal Neurosurgery Education

Global spine surgery is a flourishing arena in which its key players endeavor to make a difference through surgical camps, educational programs, training programs, health system strengthening projects, health policy changes/development, and advocacy. In recent times, massive strides have been taken to develop a coherent voice for this work. This large-scale collaboration via multilateral, multinational engagement is the only correct solution. The leading players have begun to come together toward this powerful solution. With this, the future of sustainability and improvement of the spine education program is bright. A mixture of such efforts and advancement in educational tools will continue to globally sustain and improve spine education.

## References

1. AANS/CNS Spine Section Guidelines www.spinesection.org/guidelines
2. Adamson TE. Microendoscopic posterior cervical laminoforaminotomy for unilateral radiculopathy: results of a new technique in 100 cases. J Neurosurg. 2001;95(1 Suppl):51–7.
3. Arnold P, Bohm P. Simulation and resident education in spinal neurosurgery. Surg Neurol Int. 2015;6(1):33.
4. Benzel EC. Biomechanics of spine stabilization. 3rd ed. New York/Stuttgart/Delhi/Rio: Thieme Verlag; 2015. p. 568. ISBN: 978-1-60406-924-2
5. Berjano P, Villafañe J, Vanacker G, Cecchinato R, Ismael M, Gunzburg R, et al. The effect of case-based discussion of topics with experts on learners' opinions: implications for spinal education and training. Eur Spine J. 2017;27(S1):2–7.
6. Brooks AL, Jenkins EB. Atlanto-axial arthrodesis by the wedge compression method. J Bone Joint Surg Am. 1978;60:279–84.
7. Carr S. The Foundation Programme assessment tools: an opportunity to enhance feedback to trainees? Postgraduate Med J. 2006;82(971):576–9. https://doi.org/10.1136/pgmj.2005.042366
8. Caspar W, Barbier DD, Klara PM. Anterior cervical fusion and Caspar plate stabilization for cervical trauma. Neurosurgery. 1989;25:491–502.
9. Caspar W. A new surgical procedure for lumbar disc herniation causing less tissue damage through a microsurgical approach. In: Wüllenweber M, Brock J, Hamer M, et al., editors. Lumbar Disc Adult Hydrocephalus. Berlin: Springer; 1977. p. 74–80.
10. Cloward RB. The anterior approach for removal of ruptured cervical disks. J Neurosurg. 1958;15:602–17.
11. Cote DJ, Karhade AV, Larsen AM, et al. United States neurosurgery annual case type and complication trends between 2006 and 2013: an American College of Surgeons National Surgical Quality Improvement Program analysis. J Clin Neurosci. 2016;31:106–11.

12. Crutchfield WG. Skeletal traction for dislocation of the cervical spine. South Surg. 1933;2:156–9.
13. Cushing H. The special field of neurological surgery. Bull Johns Hopkins Hosp. 1905;16:77–87.
14. Dandy WE. Loose cartilage from the intervertebral disc simulating tumour of the spinal cord. Arch Surg. 1929;19:660–72.
15. Dempsey R, Buckley N. Education-based solutions to the global burden of neurosurgical disease. World Neurosurg. 2020;140:e1–6.
16. Dewan MC, Onen J, Bow H, Ssenyonga P, Howard C, Warf BC. Subspecialty pediatric neurosurgery training: a skill-based training model for neurosurgeons in low-resourced health systems. Neurosurg Focus. 2018;45(4):E2. https://doi.org/10.3171/2018.7.FOCUS18249
17. Dickman CA, Hadley MN, Browner C, Sonntag VK. Neurosurgical management of acute atlas-axis combination fractures. A review of 25 cases. J Neurosurg. 1989;70:45–9.
18. Elsberg CA. Experiences in spinal surgery. Surg Gynecol Obstet. 1913;16:117–32.
19. Elsberg CA. The extradural ventral chondromas (enchondroses), their favorite sites, the spinal cord and root symptoms they produce, and their surgical treatment. Bull Neurol Inst N Y. 1931;1:350–88.
20. Goel A, Laheri V. Plate and screw fixation for atlanto-axial subluxation. Acta Neurochir. 1994;129:47–53.
21. Gowers WR, Horsley VA. A case of tumour of the spinal cord: removal; recovery. Med Chir Trans. 1888;53:379–428.
22. Green BN, Johnson CD, Haldeman S, et al. The Global Spine Care Initiative: public health and prevention interventions for common spine disorders in low- and middle-income communities. Eur Spine J. 2018;27(Suppl 6):838–850. https://doi.org/10.1007/s00586-018-5635-8. Epub 2018 Aug 11.PMID: 30099669
23. Haglund M, Fuller A. Global neurosurgery: innovators, strategies, and the way forward. J Neurosurg. 2019;131(4):993–9.
24. Haldeman S, Nordin M, Chou R, et al. The Global Spine Care Initiative: World Spine Care executive summary on reducing spine-related disability in low- and middle-income communities. Eur Spine J. 2018;27(Suppl 6):776–85. https://doi.org/10.1007/s00586-018-5722-x. Epub 2018 Aug 27
25. Hartvigsen J, Hancock MJ, Kongsted A, Louw Q, Ferreira ML, Genevay S, et al. What low back pain is and why we need to pay attention. Lancet. 2018;391:2356–67.
26. Healy AT, Sundar SJ, Cardenas RJ, Mageswaran P, Benzel EC, Mroz TE, Francis TB. Zero-profile hybrid fusion construct versus 2-level plate fixation to treat adjacent-level disease in the cervical spine. J Neurosurg Spine. 2014;21(5):753–60. https://doi.org/10.3171/2014.7.SPINE131059. Epub 2014 Aug 29.PMID: 25170655
27. Hung W. Problem-based learning. In: Merrill PM, Elen J, Bishop MJ, editors. Spector Handbook of research on educational communications and technology. Springer; 2008. p. 485–506.
28. Hurwitz EL, Randhawa K, Torres P, Yu H, Verville L, Hartvigsen J, et al. The Global Spine Care Initiative: a systematic review of the individual and community-based burden of spinal disorder in rural populations in low- and middle-income communities. Eur Spine J. 2017; https://doi.org/10.1007/s00586-017-5393-z
29. Jackson D, Wall D. An evaluation of the use of the mini-CEX in the foundation programme. Br J Hosp Med (Lond). 2010;71(10):584–588.
30. Johnson C, Haldeman S, Chou R, et al. The Global Spine Care Initiative: model of care and implementation. Eur Spine J. 2018;27(S6):925–45.
31. Kato Y, Liew BS, Sufianov AA, et al. Review of global neurosurgery education: Horizon of Neurosurgery in the developing countries. Chinese Neurosurg J. 2020;6:1–13.
32. Kelly DC, Margules AC, Kundavaram CR, et al. Face, content, and construct validation of the daVinci skills simulator. Urology. 2012;79:1068–72.
33. Le CVan, Tromp JG, Puri V. Using 3D simulation in medical education: a comparative test of teaching anatomy using virtual reality. In: Emerging Technologies for Health and Medicine. Hoboken: Wiley; 2018. p. 21–33.

34. JFR L. The motivators to endoscopic spine surgery implementation in Latin America. J Spine Surg. 2020;6(Supplement 1):S45–S48. https://doi.org/10.21037/jss.2019.09.12.
35. Long DM. Assurance of competency in residency training: neurosurgical education in the 21$^{st}$ century. In: Bean JR, editor. Neurosurgery in transition. The socioeconomic transformation of neurological surgery, concepts in neurosurgery, vol. 9. Williams & Wilkins., Chap 10, 99; 1998. p. 147–156.
36. Masini M. Report president FLANC education Committee at Executive Committee Meeting. Cancún: Congreso Latinoamericano de Neurocirugía - CLAN; 2016.
37. Masini M. Residencia con Competencia: Bases para un proyecto. Péru. J Neurucirugía/Neurocirurgia FLANC. 2016;25:7–10.
38. Mello PA. Residents manual and neurosurgery – evaluation manual in neurosurgery. Joinville, Santa Catarina: Letra Médica; 2000.
39. Mixter SJ, Osgood RB. IV. Traumatic lesions of the atlas and axis. Ann Surg. 1910;51:193–207.
40. Mixter WJ, Barr JS. Rupture of the intervertebral disc with involvement of the spinal canal. N Engl J Med. 1934;211:210–5. https://doi.org/10.1056/NEJM193408022110506.
41. Murray MR, Wang T, Schroeder GD, Hsu WK. The 100 most cited spine articles. Eur Spine J. 2012;21:2059–69. https://doi.org/10.1007/s00586-012-2303-2.
42. Naderi S, Benzel EC. History of spine surgery. In: Steinmetz MP, Benzel EC, editors. Benzel's spine surgery techniques, complication avoidance and management. 4th ed. Elsevier; 2017.
43. NASS Guidelines. www.spine.org/Research-Clinical-Care/Quality-Improvement/Clinical-Guidelines
44. Nicolosi F, Rossini Z, Zaed I, Kolias AG, Fornari M, Servadei F. Neurosurgical digital teaching in low-middle income countries: beyond the frontiers of traditional education. Neurosurg Focus. 2018;45(4):E17. https://doi.org/10.3171/2018.7.FOCUS18288
45. Nordin M, Randhawa K, Torres P, et al. The Global Spine Care Initiative: a systematic review for the assessment of spine-related complaints in populations with limited resources and in low- and middle-income communities. Eur Spine J. 2018;27(Suppl 6):816–827. https://doi.org/10.1007/s00586-017-5446-3. Epub 2018 Feb 28.PMID: 29492717
46. Panjabi MM. The stabilizing system of the spine. Part I. function, dysfunction, adaptation, and enhancement. J Spinal Disord. 1992;5:383–9.
47. Parney IF, Allen PBR, Petruk KC. Howard H. Hepburn and the development of skull tongs for cervical spine traction. Neurosurgery. 2000;47(6):1430.
48. Perez-Cruet MJ, Foley KT, Isaacs RE, Rice-Wyllie L, Wellington R, Smith MM, et al. Microendoscopic lumbar discectomy: technical note. Neurosurgery. 2002;51(5 Suppl):S129–36.
49. Posadas G. Program for neurosurgery subspecializes. Vols. J Neurocirugía/ Neurocirurgia FLANC, by Germán Posadas. Perú. J Neurocirugía/Neurocirurgia FLANC. 2011;16:(pag. 24-38), 17 (pag. 46-60), 18 (pag. 28-43), 19 (pag. 34-52).
50. Schwender JD, Holly LT, Rouben DP, Foley KT. Minimally invasive transforaminal lumbar interbody fusion (TLIF): technical feasibility and initial results. J Spinal Disord Tech. 2005;18(Suppl):S1–6.
51. Scoville WB, Dohrmann GJ, Corkill G. Late results of cervical disc surgery. J Neurosurg. 1976;45:203–10.
52. Shrime MG, Bickler SW, Alkire BC, Mock C. Global burden of surgical disease: an estimation from the provider perspective. Lancet Glob Health. 2015;3:S8–9.
53. Spagnuolo E. Lecture unification project of the specialization and residency program in neurosurgery. Cancún: Congreso Latinoamericano de Neurocirugía - CLAN; 2016.
54. Tator CH, Fehlings MG. Review of the secondary injury theory of acute spinal cord trauma with emphasis on vascular mechanisms. J Neurosurg. 1991;75:15–26.
55. Traynelis VC, Andrews BT, Awad IA, et al. Resident curriculum guidelines for neurosurgery. Congress of Neurological Surgeons Education Committee. Clin Neurosurg. 2000;47:589–681.
56. Vishteh AG, Crawford NR, Chamberlain RH, Thramann JJ, Park SC, Craigo JB, Sonntag VK, Dickman CA. Biomechanical comparison of anterior versus posterior lumbar threaded

interbody fusion cages. Spine (Phila Pa 1976). 2005;30(3):302–10. https://doi.org/10.1097/01. brs.0000152155.96919.31. PMID: 15682011.

57. Waisbrod G, Mannion A, Fekete T, et al. Surgical training in spine surgery: safety and patient-rated outcome. Eur Spine J. 2019;28(4):807–16.
58. Walker CT, Kakarla UK, Chang SW, Sonntag VKH. History and advances in spinal neurosurgery. J Neurosurg Spine. 2019;31:775–85.
59. WFNS Spine Committee Recommendations. http://wfns-spine.org/recommendations
60. Yasargil MG. Microsurgical operation for herniated disc. In: Wüllenweber R, Brock M, Hamer J, et al., editors. Lumbar Disc Adult Hydrocephalus. Berlin: Springer-Verlag; 1977. p. 81.

# Chapter 8
# The Role of Neurosurgery in Global Health Epilepsy, Movement Disorders, and Psychiatric Diseases

**Ulrick Sidney Kanmounye, Lilyana Angelov, Susan C. Pannullo, Setthasorn Zhi Yang Ooi, Rosaline de Koning, Alexandre Jose Bourcier, Yvan Zolo, Edie Zusman, Yves Jordan Kenfack, Lorraine Sebopelo, Lucia Bederson, and Gail Rosseau**

U. S. Kanmounye
Research Department, Association of Future African Neurosurgeons, Yaounde, Cameroon

L. Angelov
Neurological Surgery, Cleveland Clinic Lerner College of Medicine of Case Western Reserve University, Section of Spinal Radiosurgery and Director of BBTC's Primary CNS Lymphoma Program, Brain Tumor and Neuro-Oncology Center, Cleveland Clinic, Cleveland, OH, USA

S. C. Pannullo
Department of Neurological Surgery, New York-Presbyterian Hospital and Weill Cornell Medicine, New York, NY, USA

S. Z. Y. Ooi
Centre for Medical Education (C4ME), Cardiff University School of Medicine, Cardiff, UK

R. de Koning
Medical Sciences Department, University of Oxford, Oxford, UK

A. J. Bourcier
David Geffen School of Medicine, The University of California, Los Angeles, CA, USA

Y. Zolo
Faculty of Health Sciences, University of Buea, Buea, Cameroon

E. Zusman
NorthBay Medical Center, Fairfield, CA, USA

Y. J. Kenfack
University of Texas Southwestern Medical School, Dallas, TX, USA

L. Sebopelo
Faculty of Medicine, University of Botswana, Gaborone, Botswana

L. Bederson
Icahn School of Medicine at Mount Sinai, New York, NY, USA

G. Rosseau (✉)
Department of Neurosurgery, George Washington University School of Medicine and Health Sciences, Washington, DC, USA

© The Author(s), under exclusive license to Springer Nature Switzerland AG 2022
I. M. Germano (ed.), *Neurosurgery and Global Health*,
https://doi.org/10.1007/978-3-030-86656-3_8

## Introduction

Health system strengthening is required in most countries around the world to adequately treat patients with neurosurgical conditions. Global neurosurgery is an emerging field at the interface of public health and contemporary clinical neurosurgery to provide access to safe, affordable, quality neurosurgical care for everyone, everywhere [1]. The field includes research, education, and advocacy for investments in the building blocks of neurosurgical systems, such as governance, funding, information management, infrastructure, workforce, and service delivery. As functional neurosurgery often requires some of the most sophisticated and costly devices in the neurosurgeon's armamentarium, this field is poorly developed in low- and middle-income countries (LMICs) [2].

There are geographical disparities in access to functional neurosurgery at the continental, national, and local levels. The specialist workforce deficit is also an important barrier to the global expansion of functional neurosurgical care. Most LMICs have less than the recommended neurosurgical workforce density of 1 neurosurgeon per 200,000 people [3], and few are trained to deliver specialty care in functional neurosurgery [4]. This report summarizes the current global situation for stereotactic radiosurgery (SRS), epilepsy, and neurosurgical psychiatric care.

## Global Stereotactic Radiosurgery

Since the initial development in the 1950s of radiosurgery for the treatment of intracranial lesions, the application of SRS has increased to the point where currently 66% of patients with CNS pathologies can be treated with this modality. Brain metastases account for the largest percentage of radiosurgery cases (47%), followed by meningiomas (17%) and vestibular schwannomas (12%) [5]. Moreover, SRS treatment has further been expanded to treat non-anatomically abnormal, functional targets such as in patients with trigeminal neuralgia, movement disorders, and neurobehavioral conditions. Unfortunately, geographical disparities in access to SRS are pronounced. For example, the number of people per SRS unit ranges from 1:0.8 million in North America to 1:1220 million in Africa [6]. These inequities are due to several factors, with the most significant barriers to increased access to SRS care thought to be infrastructure, capital equipment, and education. Infrastructure for SRS care has steep upfront costs, and multiple efforts to expand SRS care globally have been unsuccessful in the past. For example, the premature shutdown of boron neutron capture facilities on multiple continents created a negative narrative around the installment of SRS platforms [7]. Fortunately, LMIC success stories like the decade of success of the Gamma Knife Unit in Rabat, Morocco, have helped change this narrative [8]. Increased global access to radiosurgery in the future is anticipated and may result from the greater involvement of international organizations, such as the International Atomic Energy Agency (IAEA), which has offered technical and financial assistance to Uruguay via its Technical Cooperation Program [6]. In addition, private enterprises, such as Zap Surgical Systems, Inc. are actively developing lower-cost radiosurgery platforms for emerging markets [9].

The specialist workforce deficit is an equally important barrier to the global expansion of SRS care. Web-based platforms have emerged as a solution for education and capacity-building of radiation oncologists, medical oncologists, neurosurgeons, and medical physicists in LMICs, and remote dose planning is a current reality [10].

The World Society for Stereotactic and Functional Neurosurgery (WSSFN), founded in 1961, is one of the oldest and largest SRS professional societies [11]. It is composed of five continental societies: the American Society for Stereotactic and Functional Neurosurgery (ASSFN), Asian Society for Stereotactic, Functional and Computer-Assisted Neurosurgery (ASSFCAN), European Society for Stereotactic and Functional Neurosurgery (ESSFN), Middle Eastern Society for Stereotactic and Functional Neurosurgery (MSSFN), and Sociedad Latinoamericana de Neurocirugia Funcional y Estereotaxia (SLANFE) [11]. The WSSFN supports the expansion of SRS through its journal, conferences, outreach program, and SRS fellowships [12]. Furthermore, the Leksell Gamma Knife Society offers international observation fellowships [13]. The International Stereotactic Radiosurgery Society, the Radiosurgery Society, and the World Federation of Neurosurgical Societies are also excellent resources with global memberships [6].

There are a small number of international SRS databases. The International Radiosurgery Research Foundation (IRRF)/International Gamma Knife Research Foundation (IGKRF) is a consortium of academic and clinical SRS centers worldwide that researches, educates, and advocates regarding SRS-amenable diseases of public health interest. IRRF is composed of American, Canadian, Chinese, Czech, Spanish, and Taiwanese institutions [14]. This group pools data from its institutions to constitute larger patient cohorts and higher-quality evidence for SRS procedures.

Europe pioneered radiosurgery. Lars Leksell, Professor of Neurosurgery at the Karolinska Institute in Sweden, first described the technique in 1951, leading to his renown as the father of radiosurgery [15]. In 2016, there were 220 SRS units across the continent, with Brainlab having the highest number of devices (45%) [6]. The number of people per unit in each country ranged from 0.9 million in Belgium to 22.5 million in Ukraine, a large variance in SRS utilization within the continent, with greater access generally seen in Western Europe [6]. This is likely a reflection of high-quality structured training of neurosurgeons, radiation oncologists, and medical physicists incorporating a radiosurgical curriculum within the European Union countries.

To date, around 32,000 patients have been treated with Gamma Knife in the Middle East and Africa, the vast majority (69%) for benign disease, 10% vascular disorders, 13% malignant disease, and 8.8% functional disorders [5]. Access to SRS is limited across Africa, but this is gradually changing. First reports of SRS in Africa date back to 2004 when Attalla et al. [16] reported acquiring a Siemens PRIMUS M6/6ST linear accelerator by the National Cancer Institute (Cairo University, Cairo, Egypt). Until the late 2010s, the National Cancer Institute was Africa's only SRS center [6]. Egypt is set to boost access to SRS in the coming years, following a USD 1 million donation from the US Department of Energy's National Nuclear Security Administration via the International Atomic Energy Agency's (IAEA) Technical Cooperation Program [17]. In South Africa, the first Gamma Knife center was opened in 2017 by the Netcare Milpark Hospital (Johannesburg, South Africa) and Eurolab [18]. Two years later, the center reported that it had delivered care to more than 465 patients [18]. The majority of patients treated at Netcare Milpark Hospital were from Johannesburg and the surrounding area, confirming the need for health system strengthening and infrastructure support to increase access to SRS in Africa.

Egypt has built on its long SRS experience to build capacity in Africa and the Middle East. For example, African and Middle Eastern medical physicists train at Egyptian universities. These include Cairo University, Port Said University, and Suez Canal University, which all offer medical radiation physics master's and PhD degrees [19].

Khader et al. [20] described some of the challenges faced by patients in Jordan in accessing SRS, which include (1) the need to travel long distances to receive treatment; (2) high patient volume, which leads to frequent machine breakdown; and (3) insufficient support for staff members such as physicists, dosimetrists, and radiation therapists. These factors parallel the second and third delays described in the "Three Delays Model" (i.e., delays in reaching and getting care), explaining the poorer patient outcomes observed in LMICs. For stakeholders in surgical care and the health of underserved populations, it is key that focus is placed on the prevention of delays in treatment through investment in transport and medical education and facilities.

In Jordan, radiosurgery centers are led by three-member teams combining expertise in neurosurgery, radiation oncology, and radiation physics. The King Hussein Cancer Center has successfully implemented residency programs in these specialties that incorporate an externship in the USA and the UK and regular external examinations [20]. Similar efforts are underway in other countries in the region. Today, most Eastern Mediterranean countries have one or more SRS units [5, 21].

The first routine clinical use of SRS outside of Sweden began in North America in 1987 when L. Dade Lunsford installed a Gamma Knife (Elekta Instrument AB, Stockholm, Sweden) at the University of Pittsburgh, in the USA [22, 23]. There are now a reported 428 SRS systems in the USA, a 268% increase since 2003 [24]. Linear accelerator (LINAC)-based SRS systems are currently the most common SRS units in the USA (39%), followed by CyberKnife (35%) and Gamma Knife (26%) [24]. Canada has similarly experienced growth in SRS as the number of LINAC-based SRS systems increased from 169 in 2006 to 213 in 2010 [25]. With their lower cost and greater flexibility, LINAC systems are typically more commonly implemented in smaller North American community facilities and in Central America [24, 25]. However, perhaps the most significant expansion of radiosurgical treatments in recent years is seen in Mexico, with a growth rate outstripping that seen in the USA and Canada [26].

Pannullo et al. [6] estimated that there are 35.2 million people per SRS unit in South America. As in most regions, SRS units in South America tend to be located in large urban areas due to better access to healthcare funding, a specialist workforce, and infrastructure in urban settings. This geographical distribution leaves rural and small urban populations underserved. To increase access to SRS, Castromarin et al. [27] have proposed using surface-guided SRS with cone beam CT imaging to treat brain metastases. The use of SRS for functional conditions is limited to date.

SRS was introduced in Australia in the 1980s and was initially characterized by slow uptake of the technology. The number of LINACs has steadily grown to over 200 nationally [28, 29] paralleled by an increase in the number of facilities offering SRS to the current 76 treatment facilities, with 19 found in rural areas [28]. The financial accessibility of radiation therapy services in Australia has benefitted from contributions from the Health and Hospitals Fund, Regional Cancer Centres initiative, and the Better Access to Radiation Oncology program [28].

The WSSFN and ASSFCAN have benefited greatly from the involvement of Southeast Asian national member societies. These include the Chinese Society of Stereotactic and Functional Neurosurgery (CSSFN), Japan Society for Stereotactic and Functional Neurosurgery (JSSFN), Korean Functional and Stereotactic Society (KFSS), and Indian Society of Stereotactic and Functional Neurosurgery (ISSFN). The JSSFN, KFSS, and ISSFN are prominent national member organizations within the WSSFN [11]. The CSSFN, founded in 1963, is one of the oldest and most effective LMIC national subspecialty societies. Between 1986 and 2000, the CSSFN created a journal (the *Chinese Journal of Stereotactic and Functional Neurosurgery*), trained more than 80% of functional neurosurgeons in China, and facilitated the creation of 50 SRS centers [30]. The CSSFN organizes annual national meetings, which it hosts at the first Chinese Institute of Stereotactic and Functional Neurosurgery [30]. The other Asian national societies have also achieved success developing clinical guidelines, training SRS specialists, and advocating for increased access to SRS care [31–33].

The global burden of SRS-amenable diseases is compounded by limited access to SRS care. Acceptance and access to SRS have increased globally (Fig. 8.1);

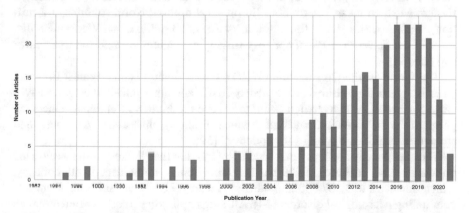

**Fig. 8.1** Stereotactic radiosurgery publications out of low- and middle-income countries. (Medline and Global Index Medicus were searched from inception to April 16, 2021)

however, many countries still lack access to SRS units. The recent increases in global access have been made possible by the work of professional SRS societies, multilateral civil society organizations, high-income country (HIC) governments, and HIC and LMIC SRS institution dyads. More research, education, and advocacy are needed to reduce global SRS health disparities. The value of this highly effective, minimally invasive outpatient procedure cannot be underestimated. Global SRS research should focus on mapping and tracking the global burden of SRS-amenable diseases, including functional diseases and conditions and exploration of opportunities to enhance delivery of this treatment paradigm to underserved patients.

## Global Epilepsy Surgery

Around 46 million people worldwide live with epilepsy, and over 125,000 epilepsy-related deaths are recorded annually [34]. Comorbidities and financial distress further compound the burden of epilepsy. The most common comorbidities occurring with epilepsy are psychiatric, with prevalence ranging between 6% and 55% [35]. All comorbidities diminish the quality of life for these individuals and their families, impact the management and prognosis of epilepsy negatively, and increase the cost of epilepsy care [35]. In addition, approximately 50% of patients with epilepsy experience impoverishing or catastrophic health expenditures due to direct and indirect out-of-pocket expenditures [36]. This is especially true in LMICs. The combination of high epilepsy prevalence, limited access to care, and epilepsy care-related financial distress has led to inferior outcomes. At least 22 LMICs recorded increased mortality rates between 1990 and 2016 [34].

Although epilepsy surgery can reduce morbidity and mortality in the right patient population, only a handful of LMIC patients have access to safe and affordable epilepsy surgery. There are more than ten million potential candidates for epilepsy surgery worldwide [37], distributed by regions as follows: Africa, 1.8 million; Eastern Mediterranean, 0.8 million; Europe, 1.0 million; North America, 1.2 million; South America, 1.1 million; Southeast Asia, 2.3 million; and Western Pacific, 1.7 million. Fewer than 1% of epilepsy surgery candidates are referred to a neurosurgeon [38].

The World Health Organization (WHO), International League Against Epilepsy (ILAE), International Bureau for Epilepsy (IBE), and other stakeholders have advocated for health system strengthening to reduce the burden of epilepsy. One such program is the Global Campaign Against Epilepsy that aims "to assess and strengthen health care systems for epilepsy" [39].

The prevalence of epilepsy in Africa is 26% higher than the rest of the worldwide population [34]. In Africa, 11.29 per 1000 individuals are burdened with epilepsy, which translates to 3,367,000 individuals on a single continent suffering from this debilitating neurological disorder [34]. Although epilepsy surgery is often curative, its usage in African countries is sparse for multiple reasons, including lack of technology, limited training in epilepsy, shortage of anesthetists, limited access to MRI and EEG facilities, and persistent superstitious beliefs [40]. The current state of epilepsy surgery in Africa can be stratified into three levels. Countries in the first level use epilepsy surgery with invasive presurgical evaluation. South Africa is the only one in this category. Those countries in the second level use epilepsy surgery without invasive presurgical evaluation and include Morocco, Uganda, Kenya, Tunisia, Algeria, and Mali. Countries in the third level do not generally have routine access to epilepsy surgery. This group includes Nigeria, the Democratic Republic of the Congo, Burkina Faso, Benin, and Gambia [40]. Collaboration between HICs and African countries has shown promise in promoting the use of epilepsy surgery. For example, Morocco started an epilepsy surgery program in 2005 in association with colleagues in France and reported on operations on 51 patients from 2005 to 2011 [40]. Epilepsy surgery was also performed on ten patients in Uganda in 2009, in collaboration with an American team based in Virginia [40].

Similarly, the creation of epilepsy surgery centers in Asia has benefitted from North American and regional input. The first records of epilepsy surgery in Asia were in South Korea and dated back to the 1940s [41]. Ten years later, Yi-Cheng Zhao, a trainee of Wilder Penfield, performed epilepsy surgery in Tianjin and Beijing [42]. South Korean and Chinese epilepsy surgery has since evolved to become the largest service providers in the region. South Korea has at least 17 epilepsy centers of excellence (ECOEs), while all 23 Chinese provinces have one or more ECOEs [41, 42]. Jacob Chandy, another trainee of Wilder Penfield, performed a left hemispherectomy at the Christian Medical College in Vellore, India, in 1952 [43]. By 1995, epilepsy surgery became widely available in India, and currently, nearly 40 centers offer such treatment [43]. The first epilepsy surgery in Thailand was performed in 1992; 4 years later, neighboring Malaysia and the Philippines recorded their first surgeries [41, 44, 45]. In 2002, Nepal performed its first epilepsy surgery at Kathmandu Model Hospital under Japanese functional neurosurgeons Tomokatsu Hori and Katsuhori Arita [46]. Japanese neurosurgeons equally helped develop an epilepsy surgery center in Indonesia (Kariadi General Hospital, 1999) [47].

The first reports of epilepsy surgery in Europe date to early in the twentieth century. Pioneers of epilepsy surgery in Europe included Victor Horsley in the UK, Fedor Krause in Germany, Johan Guldenarm in the Netherlands, and Theodor Kocher in Switzerland [48]. These outstanding surgeons helped promote the development and acceptance of epilepsy surgery in Europe, further developed in North America. Mexican neurosurgeons performed the first epilepsy surgeries in that country at Juarez Hospital in the early 1950s [26]. Over the years, access to epilepsy surgery increased as Mexican neurosurgeons returned from the USA, where they had trained in functional neurosurgery. Today, surgical epilepsy care in Mexico is delivered by 15 neurosurgeons working at 11 functional neurosurgery centers [26]. Of note, five of the centers are ECOEs: Children's Hospital of Mexico, General Hospital of Mexico, Epilepsy and Brain Damage Center, National Institute of Neurology and Neurosurgery, and Zambrano Hellion Medical Center [26]. The growth of epilepsy care in North America has benefited South American countries, such as Peru. In Peru, the first ECOE was founded in 2008 at the National

Neurological Sciences Institute in Lima, with support from the Partnering Epilepsy Centers in America (PECA) program of the North American Commission of the ILAE [49]. The ECOE's neurosurgeon and neuropsychologist had completed their fellowship training in Mexico [49].

The history of epilepsy surgical care tells a story of interconnectedness. It highlights the potential of collaborations between HICs and LMICs, as well as those between LMICs. These global epilepsy surgery collaborations have accelerated the development of workforce and service delivery globally.

Access to epilepsy surgery is unevenly distributed globally. Few LMICs have access to epilepsy surgery; however, Watila et al. [50] estimate LMICs that perform epilepsy surgery do so at lower costs with outputs comparable to HICs. They also report that most LMICs offer open surgery, while only a handful offer minimally invasive epilepsy surgery (MIES) [50].

Vagal nerve stimulation (VNS) therapy is a neuromodulation treatment introduced in the 1990s that stimulates electrodes connected to the vagus nerve. It was developed based on the finding that vagal stimulation desynchronizes the EEG and can therefore rectify the hypersynchronization characteristic of epileptic episodes [51]. Although its precise mode of action is still unclear, VNS therapy has been approved by the Food and Drug Administration and the European community for over 20 years. It has become an established treatment method [52].

Other than North American and European HICs, VNS therapy is a less common treatment. A comprehensive search of the literature identified a small number of studies investigating VNS therapy as a treatment method for epilepsy [53]. The majority of studies were conducted in Asia, with three papers published in Saudi Arabia, two in South Korea and China, and one in each Iran and Jordan; three studies were published from Brazil and one each in Puerto Rico, Mexico, Slovakia, Slovenia, Turkey, and the Czech Republic; and there were no outcome studies from Africa [53].

The indications for VNS therapy are relatively uniform across the literature, being offered to patients with medically refractory epilepsy, for whom resective surgery is not an option. A consensus statement on the indications for VNS therapy has been published in both Saudi Arabia and Brazil [54, 55]. In Brazil, for example, the consensus statement stipulates that, for patients to be referred for the treatment, they must have failed to achieve seizure control following at least two first-generation antiepileptic drugs and the patient needs to agree to the risks and benefits of the surgery [55].

A major challenge that VNS therapy faces in LMICs is the lack of access due to both policy and cost. The opportunity to receive VNS therapy in LMICs where it is not yet standard practice and widely available is limited. There are often administrative hurdles for patients to overcome. In Brazil, for example, fulfilling the above requirements requires an in-depth consultation, following which they need for surgery must be agreed upon by at least two epilepsy center teams [56]. It can be very difficult for low-income populations to arrange the transport and the time away from work to attend these multiple appointments, even before receiving treatment. The second major issue hindering access is cost, which was emphasized by several studies conducted in LMICs [57]. Fan-Gang et al. [58] in China emphasized that this new brain stimulation treatment is not covered by medical insurance in many developing countries and that patients need to pay around USD 30,000 out of pocket for the treatment.

Similarly, Alonzo-Vanegas et al. in Mexico stated that the device itself – disregarding surgical expenses and recovery – costs about USD 20,000. They suggest that the long-term benefits in seizure reduction and quality of life might justify this, although longer-term studies are needed [59].

SRS, stereotactic radiofrequency thermocoagulation (SRT), laser-induced thermal therapy (LITT), and MRI-guided focused ultrasound ablation (MRgFUS) have lower morbidity rates, can be repeated if necessary, and are more cost-efficient per procedure than open epilepsy surgery [60]. However, they have higher upfront costs than open surgery and are not widely available. To circumvent these challenges, Mansouri et al. [61] propose engaging charitable organizations to crowdfund the creation and maintenance of regional ECOEs in LMICs.

Despite continuous evidence highlighting the effectiveness of epilepsy surgery, it is still widely underutilized. Underutilization is partly attributed to hesitancy from patients and the perception of healthcare providers. Patients with lower economic income and lower levels of education have been documented to have the most misconceptions about this surgical treatment [62]. A large proportion of LMIC patients are unaware of the availability of epilepsy surgery [62]. Public health education measures should be increased to raise epilepsy (surgery) awareness and educate patients [63].

The perception of healthcare workers toward epilepsy surgery is more positive than those of patients [64]. More than half of practitioners surveyed in one study had positive attitudes toward epilepsy surgery, and practitioners who trained abroad were most likely to have positive attitudes [64]. Healthcare workers need to be knowledgeable about epilepsy surgery because trust in local providers can be instrumental in helping patients understand the potential benefits of epilepsy surgery [65].

In Oceania, there has been a decline in the total number of epilepsy surgeries [66]. A survey involving nine epilepsy centers revealed a rise in non-lesional surgical cases and a significant decline in mesial temporal sclerosis-related surgeries in the past 30 years [66]. A study from the region that compared epileptic surgery to medical treatment in children found surgical intervention was more expensive but improved the overall outcome of patients with epilepsy [67]. An online platform, EpiNet, was developed in 2009 in New Zealand and was designed to enable doctors and patients with epilepsy to work hand in hand in developing clinical research as a way of optimizing treatment [68].

## Functional and Stereotactic Neurosurgery for Movement Disorders

The increasing burden of non-communicable diseases follows epidemiologic transition and population aging occurring in all nations. It is estimated that by 2030 the prevalence of movement disorders (MD) will increase to double in most countries [69] with even a more significant increase to ≥178% in sub-Sahara Africa [70]. The belief that treatment of movement disorders required interruption of pathological signals in the pyramidal tract led to the use of primary cortex ablative surgery, with the first reported cortical ablation for the treatment of Parkinson's disease (PD) tremor in 1937 by Bucy and Case [71]. In 1952, Cooper inadvertently injured the anterior choroidal artery of a patient with PD during a pedunculotomy [72]. The patient emerged from anesthesia with resolution of his tremor and rigidity and with no motor deficit despite infarction of the globus pallidus [72]. This serendipitous discovery, along with the advent of human stereotactic surgery using a modified Horsley-Clarke frame, which reduced operative mortality to 2%, resulted in the development of exploratory procedures on various subcortical targets [73]. In the 1960s, the introduction and success of levodopa resulted in a dramatic decline in the use of surgery for movement disorders. However, the realization that long-term levodopa therapy is associated with troublesome adverse effects (motor fluctuations and dyskinesia), along with an improved understanding of functional neuroanatomy, resulted in a resurgence of surgery for MD. Chronic deep brain stimulation (DBS) was first reported as a therapeutic intervention for movement disorders in the 1980s [74, 75]. DBS has since gained popularity because of excellent clinical efficacy, its reversibility, and adjustability [76]. DBS is now a well-established treatment for movement disorders such as PD, ET, and dystonia. Other techniques such as thermal ablation, magnetic resonance-focused ultrasound, and Gamma Knife lesioning are also commonly used. Neurorestorative procedures for PD, such as gene therapy and fetal and stem cell transplantation, are promising but are currently experimental.

A recent study highlights the global use of DBS for surgical treatment of MD [77]. Data from respondents in 59 countries across 5 continents revealed high variability on the best approaches for DBS candidate selection, brain target selection, procedure type, and postoperative practices. Cognitive and mood assessments were underutilized. There were small but significant differences in practice across global regions, especially regarding multidisciplinary teams. These data highlight the importance of continuing global collaboration to decrease the variability in the multiple facets of DBS surgery and the need for prospective studies to inform global evidence-based guidelines.

## Functional and Stereotactic Neurosurgery for Psychiatric Disorders

The neurosurgical treatment of psychiatric diseases or "psychosurgery" can be traced back to prehistory with a resurgent interest in the nineteenth century. Gottlieb Burckhardt, a Swiss psychiatrist, first reported the results of cortical excisions for psychiatric patients in 1891 [78] and is considered the founder of psychosurgery. Inspired by the effects of frontal cortical ablation on primate behavior reported in 1935 [79], Egas Moniz (neurologist) and Almeida Lima (neurosurgeon) performed the first prefrontal leukotomies (severing of white matter tracts) for psychiatric patients in Portugal [80]. Their results served as a stimulus for similar operations in the USA, first carried out by Walter Freeman (neurologist) and James Watts (neurosurgeon) [81]. The main indications for frontal lobotomy or leukotomy were schizophrenia, depression, anxiety, and obsessive-compulsive disorders (OCD). The rationale for the procedure was based on the disruption/ablation of the Papez circuit [82].

The unacceptable side effects of these ablative procedures, such as apathy, impulsivity, and labile affect, as well as the advent of psychotropic drugs in the early 1950s, led to waning enthusiasm for psychosurgery. In the following decades, growing public concern about such procedures being performed indiscriminately on minors, prisoners, or patients incapable of giving informed consent further contributed to a decline in psychosurgery [83].

Despite remarkable advances in pharmacotherapy, the side effects of many psychotropic drugs can be debilitating, and a substantial number of patients treated with drugs and behavioral therapy either do not improve or relapse. More than one billion people suffer from psychiatric diseases, and at least 10% of them have treatment-resistant disorders [84, 85].

Over the past 20 years, a greater understanding of the pathophysiology and functional anatomy involved, coupled with advances in neurosurgical techniques, stereotactic frames, and image guidance, contributed to a resurgence of this field. In particular, the concurrent use of MRI with fMRI and DTI sequences has provided high-resolution depictions of brain structures and their functional and structural connectivity. These advanced imaging techniques created a new focus on non-ablative surgical procedures to modulate pathways involved in such diseases. For these procedures, deep brain stimulation (DBS) technology is utilized with new electrodes to deliver stimulation and provide recording [86].

DBS for psychiatric disorders stemmed from and paralleled this treatment for movement disorders. The observation that, during thalamotomy, the tremor was consistently and suppressed at 100 Hz in a fully reversible manner made neurosurgeons realize that stereotactically implanted electrodes could be used for this purpose [75, 76]. Such electrodes were already in use to treat pain by stimulation of the periaqueductal gray and other areas.

Interest in neurosurgery for psychiatric disorders has grown globally over recent decades. An international survey documented that 35% of the functional neurosurgery centers surveyed reported neurosurgical treatment of psychiatric disorders as the most frequent procedure in their practice, with OCD and depression as the two most frequently treated disorders [84]. Notwithstanding the ubiquity of DBS in HIC, a significant proportion of such treatment is ablative (41.2%, 21/51) in much of the world. Although this choice is multifaceted, cost-effectiveness likely plays a role since the cost of DBS remains prohibitive in most LMIC.

A deeper understanding of the circuitry involved in psychiatric disorders results in enlarging the arena of surgical interventions to other disorders. For example, the understating of the Alarm, Belief, Coping (ABC) theory circuit of anxiety allows its centers to be targeted with neuromodulation in patients affected by anxiety and refractory to serotonin reuptake inhibitors and cognitive behavioral therapy [87]. Current barriers to optimizing treatment success include the heterogeneity of symptom presentation and pathologic networks in OCD, coupled with suboptimal tools that can be scaled to quantify treatment responses. Incorporating functional MRI (fMRI) diffusion tensor imaging (DTI) with routine MR images may increase targeting precision.

The field of neurosurgery for psychiatric disorders is poised to advance as neurosurgeons globally address some of the issues currently hindering its progress. Similar to other neurological disorders like epilepsy, there is still a cultural stigma surrounding psychiatric disorders. This stigma is globally perceived as an obstacle in providing psychiatric treatment, including neurosurgical treatment. The ethical boundaries of defining the scope of surgical intervention for psychiatric surgery are still under debate.

A global constraint to further provide surgical care of psychiatric disease is the current cost of implantable devices needed for DBS surgery. A new technology that does not require implantable devices is emerging, including magnetic resonance-guided focused ultrasound (MRgFUS) [88]. Although this technology is still cost-prohibitive in most regions, if proven beneficial, its lack of implantables may make it more cost-effective in the long run and possibly more broadly geographically applicable.

## Conclusion

Functional neurosurgery often requires sophisticated and costly imaging and devices and subspecialty training and multidisciplinary teams. As a result, this field is highly developed in technologically advanced countries and poorly developed in LMICs. The geographical disparities in access to functional neurosurgery can be overcome by health system strengthening and training. Through dedication to education, research, and advocacy, global neurosurgery is working to advance access to neurosurgical care worldwide, including care for functional diagnoses.

## References

1. Esene I, Park KB. The Journal of Global Neurosurgery. J Global Neurosurg. 2021;1(1):10–2.
2. Fezeu F, Ramesh A, Melmer PD, Moosa S, Larson PS, Henderson F. Challenges and solutions for functional neurosurgery in developing countries. Cureus. 10(9) https://doi.org/10.7759/cureus.3314.
3. Kanmounye US, Lartigue JW, Sadler S, et al. Emerging trends in the neurosurgical workforce of low- and middle-income countries: a cross-sectional study. World Neurosurg. Published online July 17. 2020; https://doi.org/10.1016/j.wneu.2020.07.067.
4. Robertson FC, Gnanakumar S, Karekezi C, et al. The WFNS young neurosurgeons survey (Part II): barriers to professional development and service delivery in neurosurgery. World Neurosurgery: X. Published online May 11, 2020:100084. https://doi.org/10.1016/j.wnsx.2020.100084.

5. Team EW. Leksell Gamma Knife Treatment Centers. Elekta AB. Accessed 28 April 2021. https://www.elekta.com/patients/gammaknife-treatment-process/
6. Pannullo SC, Julie DAR, Chidambaram S, et al. Worldwide access to stereotactic radiosurgery. World Neurosurg. 2019;130:608–14. https://doi.org/10.1016/j.wneu.2019.04.031.
7. Kiyanagi Y, Sakurai Y, Kumada H, Tanaka H. Status of accelerator-based BNCT projects worldwide, vol. 050012; 2019. https://doi.org/10.1063/1.5127704.
8. Khamlichi AE, Melhaoui A, Arkha Y, Jiddane M, Gueddari BKE. Role of gamma knife radiosurgery in the management of pituitary adenomas and craniopharyngiomas. Acta Neurochir Suppl. 2013;116:49–54. https://doi.org/10.1007/978-3-7091-1376-9_8.
9. Weidlich GA, Schneider MB, Adler JR. Characterization of a novel revolving radiation collimator. Cureus. 10(2) https://doi.org/10.7759/cureus.2146.
10. Balogun O, Ball A, Simonds H, et al. Implementation of a web-based platform to improve radiation oncology education and quality in African nations. Int J Radiat Oncol Biol Phys. 2020;108(3):e432–3. https://doi.org/10.1016/j.ijrobp.2020.07.2516.
11. World Society for Stereotactic and Functional Neurosurgery. World Society for Stereotactic and Functional Neurosurgery (WSSFN) | History. wssfn. Accessed 28 April 2021. https://www.wssfn.org/history
12. World Society for Stereotactic and Functional Neurosurgery. World Society for Stereotactic and Functional Neurosurgery (WSSFN) | Fellowship. wssfn. Accessed 28 April 2021. https://www.wssfn.org/fellowship
13. Lars Leksell Radiosurgery Fellowships. LGK Society. Accessed 30 April 2021. https://www.lgksociety.com/events-education/lars-leksell-radiosurgery-fellowships
14. Langlois A-M, Iorio-Morin C, Faramand A, et al. Outcomes after stereotactic radiosurgery for schwannomas of the oculomotor, trochlear, and abducens nerves. J Neurosurg. Published online January 22. 2021:1–7. https://doi.org/10.3171/2020.8.JNS20887.
15. Leksell L. The stereotaxic method and radiosurgery of the brain. Acta Chir Scand. 1951;102(4):316–9.
16. Attalla EM, Deiab NA, Elawady RA. Physical properties of a linear accelerator-based Stereotactic Installed at National Cancer Institute. Published online 2004:11.
17. U.S. funding to IAEA Supports Cancer Treatment in Egypt. U.S. Embassy in Egypt. Published September 23, 2020. Accessed 28 April 2021. https://eg.usembassy.gov/u-s-funding-to-iaea-supports-cancer-treatment-in-egypt/
18. Gamma Knife successes give hope to South Africans with brain diseases, cancers and abnormalities – Eurolab. Accessed 28 April 2021. https://eurolab.co.za/gamma-knife-sa-successes-give-new-hope-to-south-africans-with-brain-diseases-cancers-and-abnormalities/
19. Deiab N, Shahat K, Attalla E. Medical physics education and training in Egypt. Published online December 1, 2019.
20. Khader J, Al Mousa A, Al-Kayed S, et al. History and current state of radiation oncology services and practice in Jordan. JCO Glob Oncol. 2020;6:852–8. https://doi.org/10.1200/GO.20.00074.
21. Location Finder - Brainlab. Brainlab.org. Accessed 28 April 2021. https://www.brainlab.org/brain-metastases-treatment/
22. Yang I, Udawatta M, Prashant GN, et al. Stereotactic radiosurgery for neurosurgical patients: a historical review and current perspectives. World Neurosurg. 2019;122:522–31. https://doi.org/10.1016/j.wneu.2018.10.193.
23. Gamma Knife at the University of Pittsburgh | University of Pittsburgh. Accessed 30 April 2021. https://www.neurosurgery.pitt.edu/centers/image-guided-neurosurgery/gamma-knife
24. Dean MK, Ahmed AA, Johnson P, Elsayyad N. Distribution of dedicated stereotactic radiosurgery systems in the United States. Appl Rad Oncol. 2019;8(1):26–30.
25. AlDuhaiby EZ, Breen S, Bissonnette J-P, et al. A national survey of the availability of intensity-modulated radiation therapy and stereotactic radiosurgery in Canada. Radiat Oncol. 2012;7:18. https://doi.org/10.1186/1748-717X-7-18.

26. Beltrán JQ, Carrillo-Ruiz JD. Neurological functional surgery in Mexico: from pre-Columbian cranial surgery to functional neurosurgery in the 21st century. World Neurosurg. 2019;122:549–58. https://doi.org/10.1016/j.wneu.2018.11.165.

27. Castromarin J, Perez AAM, Albarracin ER, et al. Implementing Surface Guided Stereotactic Radiotherapy (SG-SRT) at one institution in Colombia: experience of the first year of a new paradigm of radiotherapy in a developing country. Int J Radiat Oncol Biol Phys. 2020;108(3):e431–2. https://doi.org/10.1016/j.ijrobp.2020.07.2514.

28. Hobbs K. Administration of the Radiation Oncology Health Program Grants Scheme. Published February 9, 2016. Accessed 28 April 2021. https://www.anao.gov.au/work/performance-audit/administration-radiation-oncology-health-program-grants-scheme

29. Radiation Oncology Services in Australia – Key Issues | Planning for the Best. Accessed 28 April 2021. http://www.radiationoncology.com.au/executive-summary/radiation-oncology-services-in-australian-key-issues/

30. Sun B, Lang LQ, Cong PY, Liu KY, Pan L. History of Chinese stereotactic and functional neurosurgery. Stereotact Funct Neurosurg. 2001;77(1–4):17–9. https://doi.org/10.1159/000064588.

31. Chung SS. History of stereotactic surgery in Korea. In: Lozano AM, Gildenberg PL, Tasker RR, editors. Textbook of stereotactic and functional neurosurgery. Springer; 2009. p. 171–8. https://doi.org/10.1007/978-3-540-69960-6_13.

32. Doshi PK. History of stereotactic surgery in India. In: Lozano AM, Gildenberg PL, Tasker RR, editors. Textbook of stereotactic and functional neurosurgery. Springer; 2009. p. 155–69. https://doi.org/10.1007/978-3-540-69960-6_12.

33. Ohye C. History of stereotactic surgery in Japan. In: Lozano AM, Gildenberg PL, Tasker RR, editors. Textbook of stereotactic and functional neurosurgery. Springer; 2009. p. 59–63. https://doi.org/10.1007/978-3-540-69960-6_5.

34. Beghi E, Giussani G, Nichols E, et al. Global, regional, and national burden of epilepsy, 1990–2016: a systematic analysis for the Global Burden of Disease Study 2016. Lancet Neurol. 2019;18(4):357–75. https://doi.org/10.1016/S1474-4422(18)30454-X.

35. Srinivas HV, Shah U. Comorbidities of epilepsy. Neurol India. 2017;65(7):18. https://doi.org/10.4103/neuroindia.NI_922_16.

36. Allers K, Essue BM, Hackett ML, et al. The economic impact of epilepsy: a systematic review. BMC Neurol. 2015;15(1):245. https://doi.org/10.1186/s12883-015-0494-y.

37. Vaughan KA, Lopez Ramos C, Buch VP, et al. An estimation of global volume of surgically treatable epilepsy based on a systematic review and meta-analysis of epilepsy. J Neurosurg. Published online September 1, 2018:1–15. https://doi.org/10.3171/2018.3.JNS171722.

38. Engel J. The current place of epilepsy surgery. Curr Opin Neurol. 2018;31(2):192–7. https://doi.org/10.1097/WCO.0000000000000528.

39. World Health Organization, International Bureau for Epilepsy, International League Against Epilepsy. Global Campaign Against Epilepsy: Out of the Shadows. Accessed April 28, 2021. https://www.who.int/mental_health/management/en/GcaeBroEn.pdf

40. Kissani N, Nafia S, El Khiat A, et al. Epilepsy surgery in Africa: state of the art and challenges. Epilepsy Behav. 2021;118:107910. https://doi.org/10.1016/j.yebeh.2021.107910.

41. Phi JH, Chung CK. Development and future of epilepsy surgery in Korea. Neurol Asia.:4. 12:13.

42. Xu L, Xu M. Epilepsy surgery in China: past, present, and future. Eur J Neurol. 2010;17(2):189–93. https://doi.org/10.1111/j.1468-1331.2009.02871.x.

43. Rathore C, Radhakrishnan K. Epidemiology of epilepsy surgery in India. Neurol India. 2017;65(7):52. https://doi.org/10.4103/neuroindia.NI_924_16.

44. Yee AS, Tharakan J, Idris Z, et al. Epilepsy surgery in Hospital Universiti Sains Malaysia: our experiences since 2004. Malays J Med Sci. 2017;24(6):97–102. https://doi.org/10.21315/mjms2017.24.6.12.

45. Chua A. Epilepsy surgery in the Philippines. Neurol Asia. 3:45.

46. Pant B, Shrestha P, Dhakal S, Sainju RK. Current status of epilepsy surgery in Nepal. Neurol Asia.:5. 12:29.

47. Thohar Arifin M, Hanaya R, Bakhtiar Y, et al. Initiating an epilepsy surgery program with limited resources in Indonesia. Sci Rep. 2021;11 https://doi.org/10.1038/s41598-021-84404-5.

48. Schijns OEMG, Hoogland G, Kubben PL, Koehler PJ. The start and development of epilepsy surgery in Europe: a historical review. Neurosurg Rev. 2015;38(3):447–61. https://doi.org/10.1007/s10143-015-0641-3.
49. Steven DA, Vasquez CM, Delgado JC, et al. Establishment of epilepsy surgery in Peru. Neurology. 2018;91(8):368–70. https://doi.org/10.1212/WNL.0000000000006029.
50. Watila MM, Xiao F, Keezer MR, et al. Epilepsy surgery in low- and middle-income countries: a scoping review. Epilepsy Behav. 2019;92:311–26. https://doi.org/10.1016/j.yebeh.2019.01.001.
51. Binnie CD. Vagus nerve stimulation for epilepsy: a review. Seizure. 2000;9(3):161–9. https://doi.org/10.1053/seiz.1999.0354.
52. Krahl SE. Vagus nerve stimulation for epilepsy: a review of the peripheral mechanisms. Surg Neurol Int. 2012;3(Suppl 1):S47–52. https://doi.org/10.4103/2152-7806.91610.
53. Timárová G, Ramos Rivera GA, Kolníková M, et al. Vagal nerve stimulation for drug-resistant epilepsy: efficacy and adverse events in an epilepsy centre with long-term follow-up. J Neurol Sci. 2017;381:691. https://doi.org/10.1016/j.jns.2017.08.1945.
54. Youssef A-S, Saleh B, Muhammad K, Mohamed A, Kayyali Husam R. Vagus nerve stimulation for refractory epilepsy: experience from Saudi Arabia. Ann Saudi Med. 2015;35(1):41–5. https://doi.org/10.5144/0256-4947.2015.41.
55. Terra VC, D'Andrea-Meira I, Amorim R, et al. Neuromodulation in refractory epilepsy: Brazilian specialists consensus. Arq Neuropsiquiatr. 2016;74(12):1031–4. https://doi.org/10.1590/0004-282x20160158.
56. Terra VC, Amorim R, Silvado C, et al. Vagus nerve stimulator in patients with epilepsy: indications and recommendations for use. Arq Neuropsiquiatr. 2013;71(11):902–6. https://doi.org/10.1590/0004-282X20130116.
57. Arhan E, Serdaroglu A, Kurt G, et al. The efficacy of vagal nerve stimulation in children with pharmacoresistant epilepsy: practical experience at a Turkish tertiary referral center. Eur J Paediatr Neurol. 2010;14(4):334–9. https://doi.org/10.1016/j.ejpn.2009.09.010.
58. Meng F-G, Jia F-M, Ren X-H, et al. Vagus nerve stimulation for pediatric and adult patients with Pharmaco-resistant epilepsy. Chin Med J. 2015;128(19):2599–604. https://doi.org/10.4103/0366-6999.166023.
59. Alonso Vanegas M, Austria-Velásquez J, López-Gómez M, Brust-Mascher E. Chronic intermittent vagal nerve stimulation in the treatment of refractory epilepsy: the experience in Mexico in 35 cases. Cir Cir. 2009;78:15–23. 24
60. Quigg M, Harden C. Minimally invasive techniques for epilepsy surgery: stereotactic radiosurgery and other technologies. J Neurosurg. 2014;121(Suppl):232–40. https://doi.org/10.3171/2014.8.GKS141608.
61. Mansouri A, Ibrahim GM. Providing surgery for medically intractable epilepsy in low- and middle-income countries: shifting the focus from if to how. JAMA Neurol. 2018;75(9):1041–2. https://doi.org/10.1001/jamaneurol.2018.1318.
62. Ladino LD, Benjumea-Cuartas V, Diaz-Marin DM, et al. Patients' perceptions of and attitudes towards epilepsy surgery: mistaken concepts in Colombia. Rev Neurol. 2018;67(1):6–14.
63. Alaqeel A, Sabbagh AJ. Epilepsy; what do Saudi's living in Riyadh know? Seizure. 2013;22(3):205–9. https://doi.org/10.1016/j.seizure.2012.12.010.
64. Aljafen B, Alomar M, Abohamra N, et al. Knowledge of and attitudes toward epilepsy surgery among neurologists in Saudi Arabia. Neurosci J. 2020;25(1):43–49. https://doi.org/10.17712/nsj.2020.1.20190051.
65. Natesan D, Ravindran P, Saminathan P. Awareness and attitudes of general physicians' toward epilepsy surgery. In: International Journal of Epilepsy, vol. 05. Thieme Medical and Scientific Publishers Private Ltd; 2018. p. A0030. https://doi.org/10.1055/s-0039-1694886.
66. Jehi L, Friedman D, Carlson C, et al. The evolution of epilepsy surgery between 1991 and 2011 in nine major epilepsy centers across the United States, Germany, and Australia. Epilepsia. 2015;56(10):1526–33. https://doi.org/10.1111/epi.13116.
67. Catchpool M, Dalziel K, Mahardya RTK, Harvey AS. Cost-effectiveness of epileptic surgery compared with medical treatment in children with drug-resistant epilepsy. Epilepsy Behav. 2019;97:253–9. https://doi.org/10.1016/j.yebeh.2019.04.004.

68. Bergin PS, Beghi E, Sadleir LG, et al. EpiNet as a way of involving more physicians and patients in epilepsy research: validation study and accreditation process. Epilepsia Open. 2017;2(1):20–31. https://doi.org/10.1002/epi4.12033.

69. Bach JP, Ziegler U, Deuschl G, Didel R. Doblhammer-ReiterG. Projected numbers of people with movement disorders in the years 2030 and 2050. Mov Disord. 2011 Oct;26(12):2286–90.

70. Dotchin C, Jusabani A, Gray WK, Walker R. Projected numbers of people with movement disorders in the years 2030 and 2050: implications for sub-Saharan Africa, using essential tremor and Parkinson's disease in Tanzania as an example. Mov Disord. 2012;27(9):1204–5.

71. Bucy PC, Case JT. Tremor: physiological mechanism and abolition by surgical means. Arch Neurol Psychiatr. 1939;41:721–46.

72. Cooper IS. Ligation of the anterior choroidal artery for involuntary movements; parkinsonism. Psychiatry Q. 1953;27:317–9.

73. Spiegel EA, Wycis HT, Marks M, et al. Stereotaxic apparatus for operations on the human brain. Science. 1947;106:349–50.

74. Benabid AL, Caparros-Lefebvre D, Pollak P. History of surgery for movement disorders. In: Germano IM, editor. Neurosurgical treatment of movement disorders. AANS Publisher; 1998. p. 19–36.

75. Benabid AL, Pollak P, Louveau A, et al. Combined (thalamotomy and stimulation) stereotactic surgery of the VIM thalamic nucleus for bilateral Parkinson's disease. Appl Neurophysiol. 1987;50:344–6.

76. Germano IM, Gracies JM, Weisz DJ, Tse W, Koller WC, Olanow CW. Unilateral stimulation of the subthalamic nucleus in Parkinson's disease- a double blind 12-month evaluation study. J Neurosurg. 2004;101:36–42.

77. Mahajan A, Butala A, Okun M, Mari Z, Mills K. Global variability in deep brain stimulation practices for Parkinson's disease Front Hum Neurosci 15:667035.

78. Stone JL. Dr. Gottlieb Burckhardt--the pioneer of psychosurgery. J Hist Neurosci. 2001;10(1):79–92. https://doi.org/10.1076/jhin.10.1.79.5634.

79. Fulton JF. The functions of the frontal lobes: a comparative study in monkeys, chimpanzees, and man. In: Abstracts of the second international neurological congress; 1935. p. 70–1.

80. Moniz E. Essai d'un Traitement Chirurgical de Certaines Psychoses. Masson; 1936.

81. Freeman W, Watts JW. Waco VA Medical Center. Psychosurgery: in the treatment of mental disorders and intractable pain. Charles C. Thomas; 1950.

82. Papez JW. A proposed mechanism of emotion. Arch Neurol Psychiatr. 1937;38(4):725–43. https://doi.org/10.1001/archneurpsyc.1937.02260220069003.

83. Diering SL, Bell WO. Functional neurosurgery for psychiatric disorders: a historical perspective. SFN. 1991;57(4):175–94. https://doi.org/10.1159/000099570.

84. Mendelsohn D, Lipsman N, Lozano AM, Taira T, Bernstein M. The contemporary practice of psychiatric surgery: results from a global survey of functional neurosurgeons. SFN. 2013;91(5):306–13. https://doi.org/10.1159/000348323.

85. Rehm J, Shield KD. Global burden of disease and the impact of mental and addictive disorders. Curr Psychiatry Rep. 2019;21(2):10. https://doi.org/10.1007/s11920-019-0997-0.

86. Mayberg H. Deep Brain Stimulation (DBS) for treatment resistant depression: exploration of Local Field Potentials (LFPs) with the medtronic summit RC+S "Brain Radio" system. clinicaltrials.gov; 2020. Accessed 27 April 2021. https://clinicaltrials.gov/ct2/show/NCT04106466

87. Bystritsky A, Spivak N, Dang B, et al. Brain circuitry underlying the ABC model of anxiety. J Psychiatr Res. 2021;138:3–14. https://doi.org/10.1016/j.jpsychires.2021.03.030.

88. Davidson B, Hamani C, Meng Y, et al. Examining cognitive change in magnetic resonance-guided focused ultrasound capsulotomy for psychiatric illness. Transl Psychiatry. 2020;10(1):1–10. https://doi.org/10.1038/s41398-020-01072-1.

# Chapter 9
# The Role of Neurosurgery in Global Health Integrating Mass Casuality Disaster Response

**Leonidas M. Quintana, Nigel Crisp, Annette Kennedy, Rifat Latifi, Laura Lippa, Jeffrey V. Rosenfeld, and Russell J. Andrews**

L. M. Quintana
World Federation of Neurosurgical Societies, Nyon, Switzerland

Valparaiso University School of Medicine, Valparaiso, Chile

N. Crisp
Independent Member, House of Lords, London, UK

All-Party Parliamentary Group on Global Health, London, UK

A. Kennedy
International Council of Nurses, Geneva, Switzerland

R. Latifi
Department of Surgery, Westchester Medical Center, Valhalla, NY, USA

New York Medical College School of Medicine, Valhalla, NY, USA

L. Lippa
Department of Neurosurgery, Ospedali Riuniti, Livorno, Italy

J. V. Rosenfeld
Monash University, Melbourne, VIC, Australia

Alfred Hospital, Melbourne, VIC, Australia

R. J. Andrews (✉)
World Federation of Neurosurgical Societies, Nyon, Switzerland

Nanotechnology & Smart Systems, NASA Ames Research Center, Moffett Field, CA, USA
e-mail: rja@russelljandrews.org

© The Author(s), under exclusive license to Springer Nature Switzerland AG 2022
I. M. Germano (ed.), *Neurosurgery and Global Health*,
https://doi.org/10.1007/978-3-030-86656-3_9

# Introduction

## *The United Nations (UN) and Disaster Mitigation*

The Third UN World Conference on Disaster Risk Reduction was held in Sendai, Japan, in March 2015. The product of this conference was the *Sendai Framework for Disaster Risk Reduction 2015–2030* [1]. The overall goal is [1]:

> Prevent new and reduce existing disaster risk through the implementation of integrated and inclusive economic, structural, legal, social, health, cultural, educational, environmental, technological, political and institutional measures that prevent and reduce hazard exposure and vulnerability to disaster, increase preparedness for response and recovery, and thus strengthen resilience.

In order to achieve this goal for 2030, the Sendai Framework identified four priorities (Table 9.1) [1].

## *What Constitutes a Disaster?*

The World Health Organization (WHO) defines a "disaster" as follows [2]:

> A disaster is an occurrence disrupting the normal conditions of existence and causing a level of suffering that exceeds the capacity of adjustment of the affected community.

"Disaster" typically evokes images of a natural event – earthquake, hurricane, volcanic eruption, tsunami, wildfire, and severe flooding. Other events include epidemics resulting from communicable diseases such as Ebola or COVID-19. However, disasters can be "unnatural" (man-made), either infrastructure failures (transportation accidents, building collapse) or terrorist events (bombing, shootings, biochemical attacks). The common thread among disasters is the resultant mass casualty situation.

Since a disaster is typically abrupt and "exceeds the capacity" of the "affected community," assistance from beyond the local community has been required. A response by an outside agency can be effective if there has been sufficient preparation (i.e., coordination between local and outside emergency response agencies) and the disaster is relatively slow in evolution, e.g., environmental stresses resulting from climate change, refugee situations resulting from prolonged conflicts, or pandemics where spread is in terms of days to weeks.

**Table 9.1** Sendai Framework for Disaster Risk Reduction 2015–2030

| |
|---|
| 1. Mitigation/prevention: understanding disaster risk |
| 2. Preparedness: strengthening disaster risk governance to manage disaster risk |
| 3. Response: investing in disaster risk reduction for resilience |
| 4. Recovery/rehabilitation: enhancing disaster preparedness for effective response and to "Build Back Better" in recovery, rehabilitation, and reconstruction |

The role of neurosurgery in mass casualty disaster response is primarily that of managing trauma (although in a pandemic, for example, treatment of nervous system infections may be encountered). Mass casualty disaster trauma victims need medical/surgical/neurosurgical care in hours, not the days to a week or more typically required by outside agencies to reach the disaster site. Enhancing the trauma care resources in the region of the disaster appears to be the optimal way to address the temporal and geographic challenges of mass casualty disasters.

The importance of a robust local response in disasters that result in emergent trauma situations has been recognized by the WHO [3]:

> ...the most timely and cost effective response to trauma is the one mobilized by the affected country itself...

## How Can We Improve Mass Casualty Disaster Response?

Since the role of neurosurgery in mass casualty disaster response is primarily the management of traumatic injuries, we can build on concepts and programs that have been shown to be effective on a worldwide scale. Three themes are particularly relevant:

1. The *trauma/stroke center* model is well-documented to improve outcomes in trauma and stroke at the "non-mass casualty" level, i.e., where the number of victims does not reach a disaster level.
2. *Integration* of healthcare resources at both the *country/regional level* and the *international level*. At the country/regional level, this entails integration of the public and private healthcare sectors, as well as the military and nongovernmental (NGO) organizations. At the international level, this entails integration methods such as the ongoing "twinning" or "dyad" programs between low- and middle-income countries (LMICs) and high-income countries (HICs), as well as coordinating with local and country/regional-level healthcare the resources of NGOs (e.g., Red Cross) and international agencies (e.g., WHO, UN).
3. The benefits of the trauma/stroke center and integrated healthcare resources will be realized as *improvement in day-to-day healthcare as well as disaster response in the region served.*

The four priorities of the Sendai Framework can be addressed using the following three themes:

1. Trauma/stroke centers include the gamut of healthcare for emergencies: from prevention programs to pre-hospital care to acute hospital treatment – operating room (OR) and intensive care unit (ICU) – to rehabilitation to long-term follow-up and research.
2. Integration optimizes the local and global resources for both emergency and day-to-day care as well as for the education and training of all healthcare personnel (clinical and administrative). Global standards for care and training can be

established and verified by quality assurance metrics. Integration maximizes efficacy and efficiency of care and minimizes duplication of services – resulting in long-term healthcare (and societal) benefits that far outweigh the initial costs (in terms of both establishing collaborations and economic investments).

3. Since trauma/stroke centers include 24/7/365 resources such as radiology, blood bank, and pathology – in addition to emergency department, OR, and ICU capabilities – the level of care for the region served is greatly enhanced around the clock.

## Chapter Outline

After briefly discussing the current status of disaster response, the primary disaster response agencies worldwide are presented. The limitations of the current global disaster response are noted. The considerable resources established to date are reviewed, e.g., the WHO's Emergency Medical Team (EMT) certification program and Joint External Evaluation (JEE) tool and the International Council of Nurses (ICN) Core Competencies in Disaster Nursing program. Examples of countries that have relatively high levels of mass casualty disaster response capabilities are described.

The resources available to improve mass casualty disaster response are considered next. The benefits of the trauma/stroke center model are detailed. On the personnel side, examples of twinning or dyad programs that integrate LMIC and HIC education, training, clinical care, and research are described. Examples of equipment for resilient acute care delivery – during both mass casualty disasters and day-to-day "disasters" (e.g., power outages) – are noted, e.g., portable operating rooms (ORs) and battery-powered mobile computerized tomography (CT) scanners. Most importantly, digital information technology (IT) is streamlining all aspects of both disaster and day-to-day healthcare. From drones that can detect the living buried in the rubble of a collapsed building and can optimize disaster scene triage to telemedicine that can save both lives and expense by optimizing referrals for tertiary care to smartphones that can reduce pre-hospital transport times, IT is revolutionizing healthcare. The benefit is greatest in LMICs, where the lack of legacy infrastructure allows "leapfrogging" directly to much more efficient and resilient healthcare delivery.

The chapter concludes with a summary of how the three themes – the trauma/stroke center model, the integration of healthcare resources both locally and internationally, and the enhancement not only of mass casualty disaster response but also day-to-day healthcare – can address the four priorities set by the Sendai Framework for 2030. In addition to facilitating the global sharing of training techniques for clinical care (both emergent and routine care), these themes can bring about worldwide standards for medical training and licensure. Moreover, a global network of mass casualty centers presents the opportunity for a worldwide network of research facilities, together with the improvement in communication and camaraderie among healthcare personnel (clinical and administrative) – across medical disciplines, governmental agencies (civilian and military), and international organizations – that is sorely needed given the current world situation.

## Current Status of Mass Casualty Disaster Response

### *Evolution of Disasters Worldwide*

Global deaths from natural disasters frequently reached into the millions of persons annually until the 1970s. The vast majority of these deaths were due to droughts and floods – catastrophes rarely causing mass casualty situations that require extensive neurosurgical support. However, the number of deaths due to earthquakes – resulting in trauma that frequently requires neurosurgical attention – has remained relatively constant from 1900 to 2016, in some years approaching 300,000 deaths worldwide (Fig. 9.1a) [4].

In contrast, the number of deaths due to terrorist incidents and conflicts overall has increased dramatically in recent decades [5–8]. Since 1970, the number of terrorist incidents annually has increased from a few hundred to 10,000 to 15,000, and the number of deaths and injuries both have exceeded 25,000 routinely since 2010 (Fig. 9.1b) [5]. Although no "World War" has occurred for over 70 years, the number of deaths due to military/paramilitary conflicts has increased in recent years: in 2005, deaths in the top 5 countries totaled less than 23,000 (from 16,583 in Iraq to 330 in Sri Lanka); in 2015, deaths in the top 5 countries totaled 135,000 (from 55,219 in Syria to 8122 in Mexico) [6].

Although the number of fatalities from natural disasters (droughts and floods) worldwide has decreased over the past century, the increasing need for effective neurosurgical mass casualty disaster response is evident from the twin facts that (1) deaths and injuries from earthquakes have remained significant at tens to hundreds of thousands annually and (2) deaths and injuries from terrorist events and conflicts have been increasing to the point where the annual death toll worldwide exceeds 200,000.

### *Current Status of Disaster Response Worldwide*

The lack of resources in most LMICs to effectively manage even day-to-day health conditions requiring either emergency or elective surgical service has been well-documented recently [9]. The most robust emergency response resources are typically in the military rather than the civilian healthcare sector; these military resources are usually not available for immediate response to a civilian mass casualty disaster due to the need for bureaucratic approvals and lack of experience in cooperation

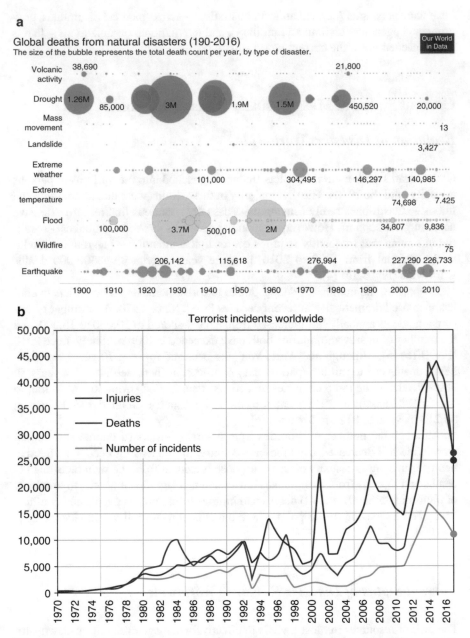

**Fig. 9.1** (**a**) Global deaths from natural disasters (1900–2016). The size of the bubble represents the total death count per year, by type of disaster (Ref. (4)). (**b**) The number of deaths and injuries due to terrorist incidents (1970–2016) (Ref. (5))

between civilian and military healthcare agencies and personnel [10, 11]. The benefit of reducing the time between injury and definitive treatment in hospital (the "golden hour" of trauma care [12]) has been debated, but evidence from the US military experience in Afghanistan is compelling: reduction in the transport time from battlefield to hospital from 90 to 43 minutes resulted in a case fatality rate reduction from 13.7 to 7.6 [13]. A recent presentation has reviewed the literature on earthquake-related injuries, with special reference to head injury as the primary cause of morbidity and mortality – supporting the importance of rapid response in earthquake-related trauma [14].

There are numerous agencies that can respond to requests for disaster assistance, both international organizations (e.g., WHO and UN) and NGOs such as the Red Cross/Red Crescent, Médecins Sans Frontières (MSF), International Medical Corps (IMC), and faith-based groups. However, all of these responders – because they are not integrated into the healthcare system of the region or country served – require both an invitation to respond and the time to mobilize and transport their resources to the disaster site. Arrival several days to a week or more is of little benefit to a trauma victim; sanitation workers and grave diggers are more useful than neurosurgeons and trauma surgeons at that point. As an example, it is estimated that 20,000 people died daily the first few days following the 2010 Haiti earthquake due to lack of basic surgical care [15].

## Examples of Disaster Response at the Country Level

There have been efforts to improve mass casualty disaster care in particular and trauma care in general, both at the national and international levels. In the USA, more than 45 years ago (1984), the National Disaster Medical System (NDMS) was established [16, 17]. At present, however, fewer than 6000 medical professionals have joined the voluntary NDMS program [17].

Other countries have had greater – if still relatively modest – success in establishing disaster response programs. Chile has a ministry for emergency response – Oficina Nacional de Emergencia del Ministerio del Interior y Seguridad Publica (ONEMI) – that facilitates coordination between civilian and military emergency response resources [18]. There is not, however, complete integration of the civilian and military emergency response resources – although the joint response time is significantly reduced in comparison with countries without such an emergency response ministry.

Australia formed the National Critical Care and Trauma Response Centre (NCCTRC), located in Darwin, following the Bali bombings in 2002 [19]. An essential aspect of Australia's mass casualty disaster response capabilities is the Australian Medical Assistance Team (AUSMAT): personnel ranging from physicians and nurses to firefighters and pharmacists who are specifically trained for mass casualty disaster response [19]. These teams respond not only to mass casualty disasters in Australia but also deploy teams to disasters throughout the Asia Pacific region.

Israel likely has the most well-developed national program for mass casualty disaster response. The Israeli Trauma/Mass Casualty Management System has significantly integrated civilian and military emergency response resources, including injury prevention, pre-hospital care, acute care, and rehabilitation [20]. In recognition of this level of mass casualty disaster response capability, the Israeli Defense Forces Field Hospital (IDF-FH) was the first foreign medical team (FMT) to be awarded FMT type 3 designation (the highest level of emergency care) by WHO in 2016 [21].

## Examples of Disaster Response at the International Level

At the university level, several training and certification programs for emergency medicine and disaster response have been established. One example is the European Master in Disaster Medicine (EMDM) program, awarding the Advanced Master of Science in Disaster Medicine degree [22]. It is based primarily at Università del Piemonte Orientale (Italy) and Vrije Universiteit Brussel (Belgium), in collaboration with other universities in Ireland, Turkey, Sweden, Switzerland, and the USA as well as organizations including WHO, MSF, and the European Society for Emergency Medicine (EuSEM). Università del Piemonte Orientale and Vrije Universiteit Brussel have also initiated the International Doctoral Program in Global Health, Humanitarian Aid, and Disaster Medicine [23].

In 2018–2019, the ICN brought together nursing experts from organizations around the world (including WHO) to develop version 2.0 of "Core Competencies in Disaster Nursing" – the goal being to set standards for effective disaster response nursing worldwide [24]. The competencies are composed of four areas and eight domains, the four competencies following the four priorities of the Sendai Framework (Table 9.1).

WHO has recognized the need for training and certification for mass casualty disaster response [3, 25, 26]. The WHO EMT (Emergency Medical Team) initiative is a program for healthcare professionals who desire to respond rapidly to global healthcare disasters – from earthquakes to Ebola outbreaks [25]:

> The mission of the EMT initiative is to enhance preparedness and promote the rapid deployment and efficient coordination of Emergency Medical Teams adhering to minimum standards in order to reduce the loss of life, alleviate suffering, and prevent long-term disability as a result of disasters, outbreaks and/or other emergencies...

Although in principle ready for rapid deployment to a disaster site anywhere globally, a WHO EMT has no integration with the local or in-country healthcare system and is intended to function independently [26]:

> [EMTs] come from governments, charities (NGOs), militaries and international organisations such as the International Red Cross/Red Crescent movement. They work to comply with the classification and minimum standards set by WHO and its partners, and come trained and self-sufficient so as not to burden the national system.

The need to establish and maintain quality healthcare for true progress in global health has recently been documented [27, 28]. At the 2005 World Health Assembly (WHA), the International Health Regulations (IHR) were adopted as a reporting mechanism for countries to certify their "capacity to respond promptly and effectively to public health risks and public health emergencies of international concern" [29]. In 2016, WHO published the first edition of the Joint External Evaluation (JEE) tool to enhance quality healthcare reporting by countries worldwide, a key aspect of the JEE being that "rapid and effective response requires multisectoral, national and international coordination and communication" [29]. In the JEE second edition, the indicators most relevant to mass casualty disaster response (assessed through site visits to the country undergoing JEE by international experts) are the following (R = respond phase) [29]:

R.1.1: Strategic emergency risk assessments conducted and emergency resources identified and mapped.
R.1.2: National multisectoral multihazard emergency preparedness measures, including emergency response plans, are developed, implemented, and tested.
R.2.1: Emergency response coordination.
R.2.2: Emergency operations center (EOC) capacities, procedures, and plans.
R.2.3: Emergency exercise management program.
R.4.1: System in place for activating and coordinating medical countermeasures during a public health emergency.
R.4.2: System in place for activating and coordinating health personnel during a public health emergency.
R.4.3: Case management procedures implemented for IHR relevant hazards.
R.5.1: Risk communication systems for unusual/unexpected events and emergencies.
R.5.2: Internal and partner coordination for emergency risk communication.
R.5.3: Public communication for emergencies.
R.5.4: Communication engagement with affected communities.
R.5.5: Addressing perceptions, risky behaviors, and misinformation.

The goal of the JEE is for countries to achieve a score of "5" ("sustainable capacity") in all indicators for the major categories of "Prevent," "Detect," and "Respond." To achieve a score of "5," innovative and ambitious programs must be developed and implemented. The proposals offered in this chapter (expansion of the trauma/stroke center model, collaboration of healthcare personnel across borders, and incorporation of progressive technologies on a global scale) can help achieve JEE scores of "5" worldwide.

## Current Status of Mass Casualty Disaster Response: Summary

Integrated mass casualty disaster response has made modest progress on the country level – Israel likely being the most progressive example. On the global level, there are exemplary training and certification programs – thanks to international organizations such as WHO and ICN – but integration (or even coordination) with local healthcare resources in the country of the disaster site is markedly inadequate.

From the trauma aspect, mass casualty disasters result in fractures and internal bleeding that require emergency care by orthopedic surgeons and general surgeons, respectively. Intracranial bleeding (e.g., epidural and subdural hematomas) and spinal trauma require emergency care by a neurosurgeon. To reduce morbidity and mortality in mass casualty disasters globally, the care must be available in minutes to hours, not the many days to a week or more that is the current standard.

## Resources for Mass Casualty Disaster Response

### *Trauma/Stroke Centers*

World War II was a major impetus for trauma treatment as a special aspect of healthcare delivery. Dedicated trauma teams appeared in several English hospitals following World War II; similar teams appeared in the USA in the 1950s and 1960s [30, 31]. The trauma center concept became formalized in the USA in the past 20 to 30 years, and the value of the Level 1 (the highest certification) trauma center in reducing mortality has been established [32]. The stroke center concept has become formalized somewhat more recently in the USA (in the past 10 to 15 years), and Comprehensive Stroke Centers (the highest certification) have also been shown to reduce mortality [33]. In the UK, there are approximately 30 trauma centers; in the USA, there are approximately 200 each of Level 1 trauma centers and Comprehensive Stroke Centers.

The benefits of the trauma/stroke center go far beyond acute care. Not only are a full complement of surgical and medical subspecialties required but also services such as extensive radiology, pathology, and laboratory (including blood bank) resources. Enhanced pre-hospital care (i.e., ambulance service) and rehabilitation facilities are necessary; ancillary programs such as community education on injury prevention and lifestyle optimization are common.

The value of the resources a trauma/stroke center provides for day-to-day non-trauma/non-stroke emergency care should not be underestimated. One only needs to consider the thousands of women worldwide who die each year in childbirth because of lack of basic surgical and blood bank resources. A less obvious example comes from a nationwide study in India regarding deaths from acute abdomen [34]. Across India, low-mortality clusters from acute abdomen were more likely than high-mortality clusters to be closer to well-resourced district hospitals (i.e., those with 24/7/365 surgery/critical care), but not for district hospital with only basic resources. The authors concluded [34]:

> Full access to well-resourced hospitals within 50 km by all of India's population could have avoided about 50,000 deaths from acute abdominal conditions, and probably more from other emergency surgical conditions.

The trauma/stroke center model has significant benefits not only for mass casualty disasters but also for day-to-day events requiring critical care and/or surgery.

## Personnel for Mass Casualty Disaster Response

Two aspects of mass casualty disaster response are particularly relevant for neurosurgeons. The first has been made clear by the COVID-19 pandemic: neurosurgeons, frequently subspecialty-trained, may need to become generalist physicians to meet the specific requirements of the type of disaster. For the COVID-19 pandemic, pulmonary and intensive care management may overshadow neurosurgical conditions; measures to minimize the spread of a pandemic may render non-life-threatening neurosurgical procedures of secondary importance.

The second aspect is the possible need – in overwhelming mass casualty events – for "negative triage," i.e., rationing emergency care to those who are most likely to survive. Negative triage is a grim concept familiar to wartime military surgeons, but much less so to civilian surgeons. Establishing mass casualty centers will make the occurrence of situations requiring negative triage much less frequent.

Several programs to train personnel for expertise in mass casualty disaster response – at both the national and international levels – have been noted above. At the international level in particular, however, such highly trained personnel will not have the benefit of having worked previously (i.e. prior to the disaster) with the local healthcare personnel when a disaster strikes. There is no better training for the coordinated response a disaster requires than working side by side on day-to-day healthcare delivery for an extended period of time prior to the disaster. That is one of the keys to the success of the trauma/stroke center – the integrated team approach.

Over the past several decades, in many medical/surgical specialties (including neurosurgery), the concept of "twinning" or "dyads" between medical centers in HICs and LMICs has been developed. In neurosurgery, the concept grew out of individual neurosurgeons from a HIC neurosurgical program making repeated visits to the same LMIC neurosurgical program. Typically the twinning program would expand with the personnel going in both directions for several months at a time – HIC to LMIC and LMIC to HIC – and additional personnel (residents, nurses, anesthesiologists, etc.) would be incorporated in the exchange. The many issues that need to be addressed to make an LMIC neurosurgical program viable – for both disaster response and day-to-day care – have been documented; it is "a time-consuming endeavor and requires both horizontal and vertical integration within the local health system" [35].

Examples of twinning programs in neurosurgery that have developed over the past decade include medical centers in the following countries: Uganda-USA, Ukraine-Canada, and Myanmar-Switzerland [36–38]. In general surgery, the American College of Surgeons Operation Giving Back program has partnered 13 training programs in the USA with Hawassa University in Ethiopia, a twinning effort that is improving the number and quality of general surgeons throughout sub-Saharan Africa [39].

Twinning programs not only provide an ongoing platform to develop quality medical/surgical training and care in LMICs for both emergency and non-emergency conditions but also establish long-standing collaborations between healthcare providers in HICs and LMICs. Enduring relationships and interactions that twinning programs foster can enhance the benefit of training and certification programs for disaster response such as the WHO EMT initiative and the ICN competencies for disaster nursing. Coordination among both twinning programs and disaster response programs worldwide can result in truly rapid and effective mass casualty disaster response as well as improved day-to-day healthcare.

## *Resilient and Mobile Equipment*

Although the need for resilient and mobile medical/surgical equipment is obvious during disasters such as earthquakes, storms, and terrorist events that disrupt the healthcare infrastructure, in many LMICs, events such as power outages are still routine occurrences. Thus, resilient and mobile equipment can benefit day-to-day care as well as mass casualty disasters. Examples relevant to surgical care include portable ORs and mobile, battery-powered CT scanners (Fig. 9.2) [40, 41]. Together

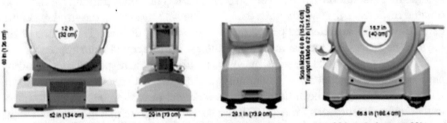

Left - Mobile head CT scanner (438 kg), Right - Mobile body Ct scanner (726 kg). (reference 32)

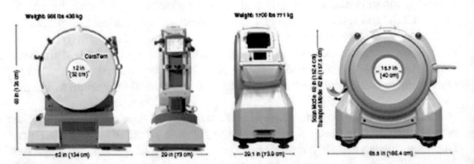

**Fig. 9.2** (**a**) Left – mobile head CT scanner (438 kg). Right – mobile body CT scanner (Ref. (34)). (**b**) Left – portable CT-equipped operating room. Right – mobile CT-equipped clinic (Refs. (40, 41))

with devices such as portable oxygen generators, this equipment allows both surgical procedures and critical care to be performed virtually anywhere (i.e., a surgical field hospital) – with delivery either by surface (road) transport or by helicopter transport of containerized facilities and equipment.

## Telemedicine and Telepresence

The benefits of telemedicine have been especially apparent during the COVID-19 pandemic [42, 43]. However, telemedicine has been an increasingly essential part of improved healthcare for LMICs for years, as evidenced by organizations such as the International Virtual e-Hospital Foundation and the Apollo Telemedicine Network Foundation [44, 45]. Not only does a robust country-wide telemedicine program benefit daily consultations between remote facilities and specialists in a tertiary hospital – as documented in Albania and Cabo Verde [44] – but it can be extremely cost-effective due to the reduction in transfers of patients who prior to telemedicine evaluation would be unnecessarily transported to a higher level of care, as has been documented for neurotrauma patients in Albania as well as other disciplines in both Albania and Cabo Verde [44, 46].

A recent pilot study in Malaysia has integrated smart glasses (worn by a physician or other healthcare providers) with telemedicine to provide a more interactive exchange of information between a remote provider (e.g., a specialist) and personnel (wearing smart glasses) in an ICU setting [47]. Telementoring is another application that can improve the quality of both emergency and routine care. A further example of cost-effective technology to enhance telemedicine is teleultrasound: healthcare providers can be quickly trained to use ultrasound in the ICU setting to provide patient information rapidly to a specialist who may be remotely located [48]. The benefits of a robust telemedicine system have been noted not only for regional security organization such as the North Atlantic Treaty Organization (NATO) but also detailed for disaster response in particular [42, 49].

## Information Technology (IT)

Documentation of healthcare quality is key to improvement in healthcare outcomes [27, 28]. In the previous section, we saw examples of how telemedicine can improve emergency and acute patient evaluation. One of the recommendations of *The Lancet Global Health Commission* to improve healthcare in LMICs (and globally) is "measure better" [27]:

> Quality measurement should be parsimonious, timely, and transparent...The high-quality health systems toolkit should include...real-time health system intelligence systems...Investing in national institutions and expertise for measurement and translation of evidence to policy is crucial for making use of the data.

To "measure better," not only is a user-friendly, standardized electronic health record (EHR) necessary, but the effects of interventions and technologies need to be tracked. The benefits of telemedicine on ICU mortality have been documented recently [50]. Furthermore, digitization of information with IT allows artificial intelligence (AI) to improve care, as discussed recently in regard to neurocritical care [51]. To quote the authors' summary [51]:

> AI has the potential to reduce healthcare costs, minimize delays in patient management, and reduce medical errors.

Smartphone availability globally (i.e., sales to end users) has surged in the past decade: from approximately 300 million per year in 2010 to 1.5 billion per year since 2016 [52]. The accelerometer (to detect falls or significant trauma) and global positioning system (GPS) make smartphones invaluable in day-to-day emergency care as well as mass casualty disaster response. Perhaps the most extensive use of smartphones for emergency response has been developed by GoodSAM [53]. From dispatching emergency response personnel to the site of an emergency to alerting a "good Samaritan" witness to a cardiac arrest of the nearest automated external defibrillator (AED) – or delivering an AED immediately by drone – GoodSAM's use of smartphone capabilities has led to partnering with numerous ambulance and emergency response organizations throughout the UK. In western Kenya, a mobile phone-based Uber-like transport system (mostly motorcycle taxis) has been developed to lessen maternal mortality by reducing transport time for in-hospital delivery as well as by increasing participation in antenatal and postnatal care visits [54].

The Kenya maternal health program is an example of HIC IT pairing with LMIC practical ingenuity. The key to effective and efficient global mass casualty disaster response – like global healthcare in general – is collaborative innovation [55]. Our collective imagination is limitless!

## Drones and Robots

Drones and robots, like smartphones, have myriad potential applications in mass casualty disaster response. Their use in transporting cardiac defibrillators to heart attack victims (with simple directions so a passerby can administer the device) and items like blood products, medications, and lab specimens to remote sites is well-documented [56–58]. The company Zipline has a drone that can carry a payload of 1.75 kg up to 80 km at 100 km/h; such drones have been in daily use for medical supplies transport in Ghana and Rwanda, where difficult terrain makes ground transport impractical [58].

For mass casualty disaster response, multiple drones with high-resolution cameras can provide triage personnel (through smart glasses) with constantly updated images of the disaster site. Sophisticated thermal imaging can identify living persons at night, under rubble, and in terrain inaccessible by ground-based search teams. As with smartphones, the combination of HIC and LMIC ingenuity can optimize the role of drones and robots in both day-to-day healthcare and mass casualty disaster response.

## Mass Casualty Disaster Response: Improving Global Health Daily

### *The Cost of "Routine" (I.E., Non-disaster) Care: Trauma and Otherwise*

The global economic burden of failure to treat surgical conditions in general – and mass casualty conditions in particular – is enormous. In 2015, *The Lancet Commission on Global Surgery* projected the loss in gross domestic product (GDP) in LMICs from the failure to treat surgical conditions for the years 2015 through 2030 (Fig. 9.3) [9]. In 2020 alone, the loss in LMIC GDP from the two major conditions – trauma and neoplasia – will likely exceed US$500 billion; by 2030, the cumulative loss will likely exceed US$12 trillion.

We cannot afford *not* to address this huge global economic burden. By establishing resilient and integrated mass casualty response centers worldwide, the benefit is not only improvement in mass casualty disaster response – but also a remarkable "return on investment" for day-to-day healthcare. The former lead of the WHO's Emergency and Essential Surgical Care Program – Walter Johnson – and his colleagues estimated the cost of improving the surgical resources in the 88 lowest-income countries over the 15 years 2015–2030 would be US$420 billion; the cost in

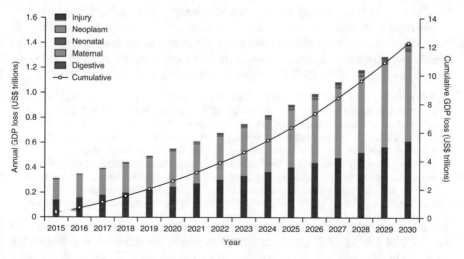

**Fig. 9.3** Annual and cumulative GDP lost in LMICs from five surgical conditions (2010 US$, purchasing power parity). Data are based on WHO's Projecting the Economic Cost of Ill Health (EPIC) model (Ref. (9))

terms of disability and lost productivity over the same period if that investment is *not* made would be over US$12 trillion [59]. For every dollar invested, 25 dollars are saved!

## Integration for Global Health: Across Specialties, Across Countries, and Across Continents

For decades, the trauma/stroke center model has integrated medical/surgical disciplines across the entire spectrum of healthcare personnel: from prevention programs to pre-hospital care to emergency surgery and ICU care to rehabilitation to medical/surgical research and from physicians to nurses to administrators to the support staff essential for 24/7/365 full-service healthcare. Recently, innovations from smartphones to telemedicine to drones – increasingly available in LMICs thanks to technological progress and economies of scale – have made "standard-of-care" health in HICs potentially available in LMICs worldwide.

The world's countries have agreed on international standards that make possible phone calls to the most remote villages, wireless money transfer to an impoverished family member anywhere, and – for the more well-to-do – air travel to any community with an airport. The pervasiveness of the Internet worldwide over the past several decades has made communication among healthcare professionals everywhere something we now take for granted.

Perhaps the best example of global integration specifically in healthcare is the Digital Imaging and Communications in Medicine (DICOM) standard that defines the formats for the exchange of medical images [60]. It was realized over 35 years ago that images generated by CT and magnetic resonance imaging (MRI) scanners would need a standard format for communication. It was about 20 years later, in 2004, that web access to DICOM objects (WADO) was added to exchange DICOM images over hypertext transfer protocol (HTTP) connections. A quote from the scope and purpose of the DICOM standards committee is informative [60]:

> The mission of the DICOM Standards Committee ("DSC") is to create and maintain an international standard for the communication of biomedical, diagnostic and therapeutic information in those medical disciplines that use digital images and associated data…
>
> The Standard is cooperatively developed. Its governance has been designed to ensure a balanced representation of stakeholders worldwide who share the vision. The overwhelming majority of diagnostic medical-imaging manufacturers including every major vendor in the world has incorporated the standard into its product design, and most are actively participating in the enhancement of the standard. Most biomedical professional societies throughout the world support and participate in the enhancement of this standard.

Where would global healthcare be today – from webinars to telemedicine – without the DICOM standard? Certainly a shared platform for the exchange healthcare information worldwide, e.g., a standard for medical data collection for quality assurance and research purposes, is technically a modest challenge in comparison with that faced by the founders of DICOM.

The ability to share medical information worldwide goes far beyond collaborations between healthcare institutions in HICs and LMICs. Quality assurance and determination of "best practices" (in terms of both outcomes and cost-effectiveness) are benefits of the sharing of evidence-based medicine globally. Research platforms from Berlin to Bujumbura (Burundi) can share protocols. Standardization of medical education – with input from both LMICs and HICs – is another benefit of a global network of mass casualty centers sharing a common data collection and communication platform.

Integration of the various healthcare providers within a country has extensive benefits. Military emergency response resources augment the capabilities during mass casualties; the same military emergency response resources (e.g., ambulances and helicopters) can maintain proficiency by providing day-to-day emergency care for the population as a whole (and thus reducing the exercises needed in order for emergency response personnel to "stay current"). Military healthcare facilities such as clinics and hospitals tend to be underutilized when the military is not involved in warfare (i.e., the majority of the time), providing additional medical resources for the underserved civilian sector.

Integration at the worldwide level can take programs such as the WHO and ICN certification standards for emergency response and expand those standards to day-to-day healthcare delivery as well. The distinction between a trauma nurse or surgeon and a disaster response nurse or surgeon becomes moot when centers are established that are sufficiently resilient and comprehensively equipped to address both day-to-day healthcare and mass casualty occurrences.

Following the Lancet Commission on Global Surgery 2030 report [9], the National Surgical, Obstetric, and Anesthesia Plan (NSOAP) was developed for countries to have a framework to develop surgery in LMICs in order to meet the four priorities of the Sendai Framework for Disaster Risk Reduction (Table 9.2) [61]. It has been argued recently that resilient healthcare systems are essential for both surgical improvement and disaster planning – and that there have been parallels in disaster management and global surgery policy development over the past 50 years (Fig. 9.4) [61]. Integrating the development of both surgery and mass casualty disaster response is an important step in realizing the healthcare-related UN Sustainable Development Goals (SDGs) for 2030 [62].

**Table 9.2** National Surgical, Obstetric, and Anesthesia Plan (NSOAP) domains

| |
|---|
| 1. Infrastructure |
| 2. Workforce |
| 3. Service delivery |
| 4. Financing |
| 5. Information management |
| 6. Governance |

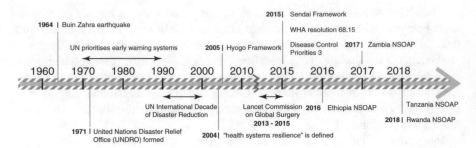

**Fig. 9.4** Timeline of key events in disaster management and global surgery policy since 1960. NSOAP, National Surgical, Obstetric, and Anesthesia Plans; UN, United Nations; WHA, World Health Assembly (Ref. (61))

## Never Let a Disaster Go to Waste

In 1976, Myron F. Weiner published an article entitled "Don't Waste a Crisis – Your Patient's or Your Own" in *Medical Economics* [63]. Various others have expressed a similar sentiment since, i.e., that a crisis or a disaster should be viewed as an opportunity for improvement (for Weiner, the message was using a medical crisis to improve one's personality, mental health, or lifestyle).

The same can be applied to mass casualty disasters. We can take the challenge of mass casualty disasters worldwide to improve day-to-day healthcare globally. Not only will mass casualty morbidity and mortality be reduced, but day-to-day morbidity and mortality will also be markedly reduced.

The economics clearly favor a modest investment at present to avoid an expense that is orders of magnitude greater in the future – not to mention the humanitarian benefits.

The only thing standing in the way of this improvement is a collective lack of common sense!

## References

1. Sendai Framework for Disaster Risk Reduction 2015–2030. UN, 2015, p37.
2. Disasters & Emergencies: Definitions. WHO/EHA Training Package, 2002, p. 26.
3. Norton I, von Schreeb J, Aitken P, et al. Classification and minimum standards for foreign medical teams in sudden onset disasters. Geneva: WHO Press; 2013. p. 104.
4. Global deaths from natural disasters (1900–2016). www.ourworldindata.com. Accessed 7 Aug 2020.
5. List of terrorist incidents. www.wikipedia.com. Accessed 7 Aug 2020.
6. List of number of conflicts per year. www.wikipedia.com. Accessed 7 Aug 2020.
7. Center for Systemic Peace/Integrated Network for Societal Conflict Research. High casualty terrorist bombings (HCTB) 1989–2020. www.systemicpeace.org. Accessed 16 Sept 2020.
8. National Consortium for the Study of Terrorism and Responses to Terrorism (START). Trends in Global Terrorism – Global Terrorism Database. www.start.umd.edu/gtd. Accessed 16 Sept 2020.

9. Meara JG, Leather AJM, Hagander L, et al. Global surgery 2030: evidence and solutions for achieving health, welfare, and economic development. Lancet. 2015;386:569–624.
10. Michaud J, Moss K, Licina D, et al. Militaries and global health: peace, conflict, and disaster response. Lancet. 2019;393:276–86.
11. Thomson N, Littlejohn M, Strathdee SA, et al. Harnessing synergies at the interface of public health and the security sector. Lancet. 2019;393:207–9.
12. Lerner EB, Moscati RM. The golden hour: scientific fact or medical "urban legend"? Acad Emerg Med. 2001;8:758–60.
13. Berwick D, Downey A, Cornett E, et al. A national trauma care system: integrating military and civilian trauma systems to achieve zero preventable deaths after injury. Washington DC: The National Academies Press; 2016: pp530.
14. Iagarshi Y, Matsumoto N, Kubo T, et al. A systematic review of earthquake-related head injuries. Presented at the WADEM Congress on Disaster and Emergency Medicine, Brisbane, Australia, May, 2019.
15. CBS News. @katiecouric: Disaster in Haiti. Available: http://www.cbsnews.com/videos/katiecouric-disaster-in-haiti/. Accessed 30 Mar 2014.
16. Reardon JD, Sandwall S. National disaster medical system: medical manpower establishment. Fed Regist. 1988;53:12994–5.
17. National Disaster Medical System. www.phe.gov/preparedness/responders/ndms. Accessed 7 Aug 2020.
18. Oficina Nacional de Emergencia del Ministerio del Interior y Seguridad Publica (ONEMI). Plan Nacional de Emergencia. Santiago: ONEMI; 2017. p. 41.
19. National Critical Care and Trauma Research Centre. www.nationaltraumacentre.nt.gov.au. Accessed 7 Aug 2020.
20. Borgohain B, Khonglah T. Developing and organizing a trauma system and mass casualty management: some useful observations from the Israeli trauma model. Ann Med Health Sci Res. 2013;3:85–9.
21. Alpert EA, Weiser G, Kobliner D, et al. Challenges in implementing international standards for the field hospital emergency department in a disaster zone: the Israeli experience. J Emerg Med. 2018;55:682–7.
22. European Master Disaster Medicine, Advanced Master of Science in Disaster Medicine. www.dismedmaster.com. Accessed 16 Sept 2020.
23. The International Doctoral Program in Global Health, Humanitarian Aid, and Disaster Medicine. www.crimedim.uniupo.it/new-phd/. Accessed 16 Sept 2020.
24. Maaitah R, Conlan L, Gebbie K, et al. Core competencies in disaster nursing version 2.0. Geneva: International Council of Nurses; 2019.
25. World Health Organization. Emergency medical teams strategic Advisory group meeting No. 8; 2018: 20.
26. World Health Organization. Emergency medical teams; 2019. Available: https://www.who.int/hac/techguidance/preparedness/emergency_medical_teams/en/. Accessed 15 Dec 2018.
27. Kruk ME, Gage AD, Arsenault C, et al. High-quality health systems in the sustainable development goals era: time for a revolution. Lancet Global Health. 2018;6:e1196–252.
28. Kruk ME, Gage AD, Joseph NT, et al. Mortality due to low- quality health systems in the universal health coverage era: a systematic analysis of amenable deaths in 137 countries. Lancet. 2018;392:2203–12.
29. Joint external evaluation tool: International Health Regulations (2005), second edition. Geneva: World Health Organization; 2018.
30. Wilson WC, Grande CM, Hoyt DB, editors. Trauma: emergency resuscitation, perioperative anesthesia, surgical management. CRC Press; 2007. p. 912.
31. Trunkey DD. History and development of trauma care in the United States. Clin Orthop Relat Res. 2000;374:36–46.
32. MacKenzie EJ, Rivara FP, Jurkovich GJ, et al. A national evaluation of the effect of trauma-center care on mortality. N Engl J Med. 2006;354:366–78.

33. Gorelick PB. Primary and comprehensive stroke centers: history, value and certification criteria. J Stroke. 2013;15:78–89.
34. Dare AJ, Ng-Kamstra JS, Patra J, et al. Deaths from acute abdominal conditions and geographic access to surgical care in India: a nationally representative spatial analysis. Lancet Glob Health. 2015;3:e646–53.
35. Dempsey RJ. Neurosurgery in the developing world: specialty service and global health. World Neurosurg. 2018;112:325–7.
36. Haglund MM, Warf B, Fuller A. Past, present, and future of neurosurgery in Uganda. Neurosurgery. 2017;80:656–61.
37. Romach MK, Rutka JT. Building healthcare capacity in pediatric neurosurgery and psychiatry in a post-Soviet system: Ukraine. World Neurosurg. 2018;111:166–74.
38. Schucht P, Zubak I, Kuhlen D. Assisted education for specialized medicine: a sustainable development plan for neurosurgery in Myanmar. World Neurosurg. 2019;130:e854–61.
39. Boeck MA, Goodman LF, Lin Y, et al. American College of Surgeons member involvement in global surgery: results from the 2015 Operation Giving Back Survey. World J Surg. 2018;42:2018–27.
40. Product information, NeuroLogica/Samsung. Available: https://neurologica.com. Accessed 27 Apr 2019.
41. Product information, Forts Medical. Available: https://fortsmedical.com. Accessed 27 Apr 2019.
42. Latifi R, Doarn CR. Perspective on COVID-19: finally, telemedicine at center stage. Telemed J E Health. 2020; https://doi.org/10.1089/tmj.2020.0132.
43. Ganapathy K. How telemedicine can help fight coronavirus better. The Times of India, March 18, 2020.
44. Latifi R, Azevedo V, BOci A, Parsikia A, Latifi F, Merrell RC. Telemedicine consultation as an indicator of local telemedicine champions' contributions, health care system needs or both: tales from two continents. Telemed J E Health. 2020; https://doi.org/10.1089/tmj.2020.0132.
45. ATNF – Apollo Telemedicine Networking Foundation. www.atnf.org. Accessed 7 Aug 2020.
46. Olldashi F, Latifi R, Parsikia A, et al. Telemedicine for neurotrauma prevents unnecessary transfers: an update from a nationwide program in Albania and analysis of 590 patients. World Neurosurg. 2019;128:e340–6.
47. Munusamy T, Karuppiah R, Bahuri NFA, et al. Telemedicine via smart glasses in critical of the neurosurgical patient – a COVID-19 pandemic preparedness and response in neurosurgery. World Neurosurg. 2020. (accepted).
48. Becker C, Fusaro M, Patel D, et al. The utility of teleultrasound to guide acute patient management. Cardiol Rev. 2017;25:97–101.
49. Doarn CR, Latifi R, Poropatich RK, et al. Development and validation of telemedicine for disaster response: the North Atlantic Treaty Organization multinational system. Telemed J E Health. 2018; https://doi.org/10.1089/tmj.2017.0237.
50. Fusaro MV, Becker C, Scurlock C. Evaluating tele-ICU implementation based on observed and predicted ICU mortality: a systematic review and meta-analysis. Crit Care Med. 2019;47:501–7.
51. Al-Mufti F, Kim M, Dodson V, et al. Machine learning and artificial intelligence in neurocritical care: a specialty-wide disruptive transformation or a strategy for success. Curr Neurol Neurosci Rep. 2019;19:89.
52. Number of smartphones sold to end users worldwide from 2007 to 2020. www.statista.com/statistics/263437/global-smartphone-sales-to-end-users-since-2007/. Accessed 15 Aug 2020.
53. GoodSAM Cardiac, Pro, AED Static + Dynamic Registry & Drone delivery. www.goodsamapp.org. Accessed 16 Sept 2020.
54. Onono MA, Wahome S, Wekesa P, et al. Effects of an expanded Uber-like transport system on access to and use of maternal and newborn health services: findings of a prospective cohort study in Homa Bay, Kenya. BMJ Glob Health. 2019;4:e001254.

55. Crisp N. Turning the world upside down: the search for global health in the 21st century. Boca Raton, FL: CRC Press; 2010. p. 228.
56. Boutilier JJ, Brooks SC, Janmohamed A, et al. Optimizing a drone network to deliver automated external defibrillators. Circulation. 2017;135:2454–65.
57. Murphy RR. Disaster robotics. Cambridge, MA: MIT Press; 2014. p. 240.
58. Provide every human on earth with instant access to vital medical supplies. www.flyzipline.com. Accessed 15 Aug 2020.
59. Park KB, Johnson WD, Dempsey RJ. Global neurosurgery: the unmet need. World Neurosurg. 2016;88:32–5. https://doi.org/10.1016/j.wneu.2015.12.048.
60. DICOM – history, key concepts, governance. www.dicomstandard.org. Accessed 29 Aug 2020.
61. Pyda J, Patterson RH, Caddell L, et al. Towards resilient health systems: opportunities to align surgical and disaster planning. BMJ Glob Health. 2019;4:e001493.
62. World Health Organization (WHO). Health in 2015: from MDGs, millennium development goals to SDGs, sustainable development goals. Geneva: WHO; 2015. p. 216.
63. Weiner MF. Don't waste a crisis – your patient's or your own. Med Econ. 1976;53:227.

# Chapter 10

# The Role of Neurosurgery Quality of Care and Patients Safety in Global Health

Souhil Tliba, Abdulrahman Al-Shudifat, Maria M. Bederson, and Teresa Somma

## Quality of Care and Patient Safety in Medicine: Historical Background

Since the days of Hippocrates, the general population has been attentive to issues regarding the characteristics of patient care in terms of quality and safety. This can be implied from Hippocrates' (460–370 BC) writing "ἀσκέειν, περὶ τὰ νουσήματα, δύο, ὠφελέειν, ἢ μὴ βλάπτειν," translated "To work around the diseases in two ways, do good and do no harm," where the do good stands for quality and the do no harm stands for safety. Later in history, only the second part of the sentence was passed along and changed to "first, do no harm." It took centuries to translate these concerns into local policies. Clinical hazards and patients' safety were acknowledged by most countries as significant concerns within the workplace in the early 1990s and eventually turned into an international priority in the early 2000s.

S. Tliba (✉)
Bejaia University Hospital Center, Bejaia University, Research Laboratory "Biological Engineering of Cancers", Bejaia, Algeria

A. Al-Shudifat
Neurosurgery Department, Faculty of Medicine, University of Jordan, Amman, Jordan
e-mail: A.shudifat@ju.edu.jo

M. M. Bederson
Carl Illinois College of Medicine, Champaign, IL, USA

T. Somma
Department of Neurosciences and Reproductive and Odontostomatological Sciences, Division of Neurosurgery, Università degli Studi di Napoli Federico II, Naples, Italy
e-mail: https://www.neurochirurgia.unina.it

© The Author(s), under exclusive license to Springer Nature Switzerland AG 2022
I. M. Germano (ed.), *Neurosurgery and Global Health*,
https://doi.org/10.1007/978-3-030-86656-3_10

The first references to medicine belong to the Egyptian world (2700 BC) where Imhotep describes the diagnosis and treatment of 200 diseases. In these descriptions, sickness is connected to a magical concept. Later, there was the birth of Mesopotamian medicine, whose main written testimony is the Code of Hammurabi (about 1772 BC). Medicine assumes the value of an autonomous science in its first form of medical science. With Hippocrates, ancient Greek medicine transitioned from the pre-scientific phase – linked to magical and religious practices and beliefs – and organized around a decidedly rational, rigorous, and empirical methodology. In the Middle Ages, surgical practices inherited from the ancient masters were improved and then systematized in Rogerius's *The Practice of Surgery*. During the later centuries of the Renaissance came an increase in experimental investigation, particularly in the field of dissection and body examination, thus advancing our knowledge of human anatomy. The development of modern neurology began in the sixteenth century. Public health measures started being developed in the nineteenth century.

Neurosurgery, or premeditated incision in the head to relieve pain, has been around for thousands of years. The Incas practiced a procedure known as trepanation since the Late Stone Age. During the Middle Ages in Al-Andalus from 936 to 1013 AD, Al-Zahrawi performed surgical treatments of head injuries, skull fractures, spinal injuries, hydrocephalus, subdural effusions, and headaches. There was not much progress in neurosurgery until the late nineteenth and early twentieth centuries. The final establishment of modern neurosurgery has been linked to the development of clinical neurology, neuropathology, neurophysiology, and neuro-anesthesiology. Great improvements occurred with the creation of extremely precise tools.

## Concepts and Definitions: Quality, Complication, Incident, and Error

The word *quality* remains standard and yet its meaning varied, obeying constraints of space, time, and matter, that is to say that although the soul aim of quality of care is to serve the patient and to ease his suffering by devoting all the means present (technical platforms, human skills) and planned (training, mobility, comprehensiveness) to serve him, the ways in which such improvements of quality are achieved must be contextualized. Quality of care is understood differently in various parts of the world, for example, the Institute of Medicine (IOM) defines healthcare quality as "the degree to which health care services for individuals and populations increase the likelihood of desired health outcomes and are consistent with current professional knowledge."

Quality measurements typically focus on structures or processes of care that have a demonstrated relationship to positive health outcomes and are under the control of the healthcare system. Even in antiquity, the ancient philosophers such as Aristotle and Plato contemplated the concept of quality of care. Harteloh [1] considered multiple interpretations of quality and concluded with a very abstract definition: "Quality is an optimal balance between possibilities realized and a framework of norms and values." In the modern era of evidence-based medicine, the improvements in quality are measured in clinical outcome metrics such as length of survival, disease-free survival, and quality of life.

In the 1950s, American statistician, William Edwards Deming [2], introduced and influenced the concept of continuous quality improvement with a cyclical method that changed the world of management. Indeed, today we are talking about the Deming wheel or the Plan, Do, Check, Act or Adjust (PDCA) method that can be adapted to all areas (Fig. 10.1). The health sector, which has experienced very important scientific advances, quickly adopted this concept of continuous quality improvement and has since generalized it to different disciplines and procedures. Neurosurgery has adhered to this dynamic because it has orchestrated its technical, training, and research activities in flexible and evolving protocols and guidelines over time.

Any divergence from the common preoperative course is defined as a *complication*. The definition of complications fails to consider sequelae or curative failure into its proper academic description. A myriad of scales was formulated to quantify the severity of a complication within the neurosurgical field. Based on the characteristics of therapeutic complications, grading systems were proposed and validated in the field of general surgery, such as the Clavien-Dindo classification system [3].

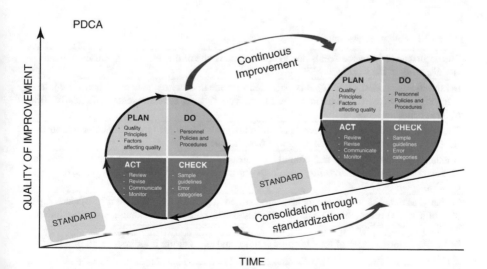

**Fig. 10.1** The Plan, Do, Check, Act or Adjust (PDCA) method

The WHO describes healthcare incidents as any event or occurrence which resulted or could have resulted in patient harm [4]. Healthcare incidents are characterized by either being harmful (i.e., resulting in adverse effects) or non-harmful (i.e., results in near misses or zero harm occurrences). Presently, the term "adverse effects" commonly corresponds to harmful incidents. The reporting of incidents, whether they are harmful or not, is actively encouraged throughout the health sectors of various countries.

Patient safety must therefore also be considered as an aspect of quality of care. Patient safety was defined by the Institute of Medicine (IOM) as "the prevention of harm to patients." Emphasis is placed on the system of care delivery that must prevent errors – learn from the errors that do occur – and built on a culture of safety that involves healthcare professionals, organizations, and patients.

In neurosurgery, the rate of complication and mortality remains significant, due to the complexity of the procedures and the high risk of errors that can lead to lifelong disabilities and fatalities. The complex nature of neurosurgery is deeply associated with slim margins for errors and potential of life adverse events. This has driven a continuous innovation within the field since the earliest times. New ideas, new technologies, or new surgical techniques have therefore remained a cornerstone of the specialty. However, such innovations are expensive and can only be maintained by instituting an equity/quality value-based healthcare systems in which effectiveness and cost of care are both taken into consideration. The ultimate goal of neurosurgery is to implement innovations that provide maximal improvement in quality at minimal cost. Furthermore, novel techniques or technologies should be assessed in an ethical manner to adequately care for the millions of world inhabitants without

**Table 10.1** Patient safety key facts

| |
|---|
| The occurrence of adverse events due to unsafe care is one of the ten leading causes of death and disability in the world |
| In high-income countries (HIC), it is estimated that one in every ten patients is harmed while receiving hospital care. The harm can be caused by a range of adverse events, with nearly 50% of them being preventable |
| Each year, 134 million adverse events occur in hospitals in low- and middle-income countries (LMICs), due to unsafe care, resulting in 2.6 million deaths |
| Another study has estimated that around two-thirds of all adverse events resulting from unsafe care and the years lost to disability and death (known as disability-adjusted life years, or DALYs) occur in LMICs |
| Globally, as many as four in ten patients are harmed in primary and outpatient healthcare. Up to 80% of harm is preventable. The most detrimental errors are related to diagnosis, prescription, and the use of medicines |
| In OECD countries, 15% of total hospital activity and expenditure is a direct result of adverse events |
| Investments in reducing patient harm can lead to significant financial savings and more importantly better patient outcomes. An example of prevention is engaging patients; if done well, it can reduce the burden of harm by up to 15% |

*OECD* Organisation for Economic Co-operation and Development (https://www.oecd.org)

access to neurosurgical care. Table 10.1 summarizes a few important key facts about patient's safety [5–8].

## Access to Healthcare Inequality and Socioeconomic Disparities

Access to healthcare is an important point of quality of care across the globe with differences among nations and within each nation. Maria Punchak et al. [9] had qualified for the first time the timing access to healthcare in low- and middle-income countries (LMICs) using algorithms using a satellite geolocation software (Table 10.2). In this work, the delay of 02 hours regardless of the means of transport was taken as a benchmark.

Additional socioeconomic disparities can affect the availability of infrastructure necessary to perform successful neurosurgery, such as availability of anesthesia and nurses, prolonged wait time, and insufficient training [10]. The lack of access to safe, timely, affordable surgical and anesthesia care are nearly universal. However, these barriers affect only 5% of the population in high-income countries (North America, Western Europe), while 95% of the population in low-income countries (South Asia, sub-Saharan Africa) is affected. In the latter areas, 143 million additional surgical procedures, among which 15% are neurosurgical, are needed each year to save lives and prevent disability [11]. Table 10.3 summarizes a classification system proposed by the WFNS used to stratify establishments according to the level of neurosurgical care provided [10].

## Global Health Non-governmental Efforts in Quality of Care and Safety Policies

Over the past two decades, the concept of "Global Health" has emerged in the field. An ideal Global Health system would be one in which physicians can provide healthcare to patients rapidly, in some cases instantaneously. Globalism mandates an effort to achieve equality both between different continents and nations and between different categories within the same country, requiring technical-scientific

**Table 10.2** Timing access to neurosurgery units in 68 LMICs

| No access to neurosurgery | 11 countries |
|---|---|
| Access in less than 02 hours | Sub Saharan Africa: 25.26% |
| | Latin America and the Caribbean: 62.3% |
| | East Asia and the Pacific: 29.64% |
| | South Asia: 52.83% |
| | Middle East and North Africa: 79.65% |
| | Eastern Europe and Central Asia: 93.3% |

**Table 10.3** Stratification of hospital and city levels according to the WFNS

|         | Establishments                     | Cities                                                                                      |
|---------|------------------------------------|---------------------------------------------------------------------------------------------|
| Level 0 | No neurosurgery                    | No neurosurgeon                                                                             |
| Level 1 | Macro-neurosurgery (trauma)        | At least one neurosurgeon                                                                   |
| Level 2 | Basic micro-neurosurgery           | At least one neurosurgeon + CT or MRI imaging and bipolar cautery                          |
| Level 3 | Micro-neurosurgery (high level)    | At least one neurosurgeon + CT or MRI imaging, bipolar cautery, microscope, and a high-speed drill |

adaptations as well as economic, political, moral, or ethical adaptations. However, such a system implies a shift in mentality and behavior that are likely to be slower than the speed at which telemedicine may allow our world to adopt such a health-care system.

The theory and practice of policymaking has advanced through a concomitant wave of research, which was conducted in parallel to the development of the field. The importance of safety, its slow progress, and its dire need for future improvements through creative ideas were demonstrated in landmark reports, published at the turn of the twentieth century. Such reports include but are not limited to "To Err is Human" (IOM, 1999) [12], "An Organization with a Memory" (Donaldson, 2000), and "Crossing the Quality Chasm" (IOM, 2001). Around this period, high-resource countries started creating and promoting specialized agencies dedicated to the improvement of patient's care quality and patient's safety programs across their healthcare organizations. Such specialized organizations include the National Patient Safety Agency in Britain (2001), the Agency for Healthcare Research and Quality in the USA (1999), and the Australian Council on Safety and Quality in Healthcare (2000).

One example of health policy assessment in developed countries is a review of a decade worth of safety-related activities throughout the health sector of North Carolina. The review demonstrates that 18% of patients exhibited harmful incidents during their hospital stays. Sixty-three percent of these injuries were preventable. Moreover, the report shows that 2.4% of medical errors have resulted in death, while 2.9% of patients exhibited permanent injury. The results of such observation hold much significance since North Carolina has been the most involved state in improving its patient's safety program more than any of its state counterparts [13].

The World Federation of Neurosurgical Societies (WFNS) along with other international neurosurgical societies has been particularly active on the subject of quality of care and patients' safety and collaborates officially with World Health Organization (WHO). WFNS representatives attend the annual meeting of the World Health Assembly (WHA) with an active and growing number of neurosurgeons. This strong presence led to the creation of a WFNS-WHO Liaison Committee, hence offering a key position to neurosurgery representatives to debate and make proposals for the quality and safety of care in health systems, including a fundamental place for training programs.

WHO has prioritized improving the quality of patient care for the past two decades. Their efforts are demonstrated through their published manual and global program for the development and promotion of healthcare policies of acceptable quality at the national level [14–16]. The development of healthcare policies evolved at a very rapid pace. Such policies leapt from the national level, and many have now been adopted globally such that the health and safety of patients is at the core of all developed mandates and regulations.

With the introduction of the Lancet Commission on Global Surgery (LCGS) and the WHO resolution (WHA68.15) in 2015, global surgery has reached its goals in terms of healthcare policy development. Once considered an overly complex field, neurosurgery has integrated itself into mainstay global health discussions due to several improvements. These improvements were in the form of planned directives that emphasized the need for neurosurgical expansion, which led the WHO to place neurosurgery as a top priority in their Emergency and Essential Surgical Care program.

Subsequently, neurosurgical input regarding healthcare was assimilated into the Bogota Declaration on Global Neurosurgery on 2016 at the International Conference on Recent Advances in Neuro-traumatology in Bogota, Colombia. The declaration addressed a variety of neurosurgical related concerns such as the non-optimal global delivery of neurosurgical care, prehospital care, training, education, research, equipment, and initiatives for neurosurgical innovation. As of late, the Global Neurosurgery Initiative (GNI) of the Program in Global Surgery and Social Change (PGSSC) demonstrated that each year five million emergency and neurosurgical operations are in deficit. Consequently, the availability of neurosurgical services was geospatially mapped by the WFNS and PGSSC. Such mapping allows for the adjudication of policymakers on both the national and international levels since they can visualize which areas need critical neurosurgical services.

The lack of patient safety is mostly found in preventable errors, which the WHO estimates to be around 10%. These have direct consequences on the state of health of patients including mortality, disability, pain, and physical and psychological trauma with economic consequences also estimated at a loss of 10% of total health spending in the countries.

According to the Organisation for Economic Co-operation and Development (OECD), "one of the most important developments of the last decade is the general awareness of quality issues in health care. In OECD countries, signs of serious quality deficiencies are increasing, resulting in deaths, disabilities or health consequences which should not have occurred, and increased the health care costs."

# Quality of Care and Patients' Safety Initiatives in Neurosurgery

In 1999, the American College of Surgeons validated the start of a quality improvement project called the National Surgical Quality Improvement Program (NSQIP). The integration of this program allowed hospitals to voluntarily report the outcomes of surgical operations up to 30 days of postoperative care in an open-access manner. Since then, the NSQIP has been utilized as a vital source for the examination of worldwide trends in neurosurgical outcomes (3–7). Nonetheless, the NSQIP's data was faced with various skepticisms due to its systematic inaccuracies and lack of validity [17]. In response, the American Association of Neurological Surgeons launched the Cerebrovascular Module of the National Neurosurgery Quality and Outcomes Database (N2QOD) in 2014. The database's primary goal is to present and report on the quality of neurosurgical care, with a special focus on clinically significant data. In April 2014, the Society of British Neurological Surgeons started the Neurosurgical National Audit Programme (NNAP). The aim of the NNAP is to publish reports about the 30-day mortality rates associated with neurosurgical care as seen appropriate by neurosurgeons and surgical units all over the nation.

Overall, public registries of reliable and clinically significant data on surgical outcomes are always appreciated by the body of medical practitioners. Patient satisfaction has recently emerged as a popular predictor of quality of care, despite being a poor proxy for general quality of care and postoperative morbidity. The use of such predictor ranges from hospital reimbursements in the USA to inter-treatment center comparisons in Australia [18, 19].

By integrating healthcare policies and strengthening health system projects and multilevel advocacy, neurosurgical groups have expanded their scope in the last 5–10 years. Nonetheless, a strong perception dominates, that is, the unfeasibility of neurosurgical care development in the developing world. This perception must be challenged using smart, cost-effective, and efficient innovations in order to help the neurosurgical communities in such areas. Valuable data such as large studies, predictive models, and machine learning decision-based programs could be the initiators of change on such a global scale.

Surgical checklists improved perioperative outcomes such as mortality and morbidity [19]. Moreover, these improvements were associated with a polished image of teamwork and safety culture within the context of multidisciplinary surgical work and among its active members. Such implementation was directly supported by the WHO Safe Surgery Saves Lives campaign. Unfortunately, the neurosurgical literature lacks any published reports on the beneficial outcomes of improved teamwork and communication and standardized checklists on standardized clinical care and neurosurgical safety culture.

Despite the limited amount of evidence, checklist use in neurosurgery has been found to reduce complications related to hospital-acquired infections, enhance safety culture within the operating room, and improve patient safety in general.

Irrespective of their shortcomings, checklists will still be relevant and shall be improved with advancing research that seeks to mend the gaps within such checklists [20].

For example, a study has shown that the use of intraoperative electrical stimulation (IES) can reduce healthcare-related costs and improve patient outcomes in patients with WHO grade II gliomas, if used in eloquent areas of the brain. The study demonstrated that the mean cost per QALY for IES-assisted resection is 12,222 US$, while conventional craniotomy costed 31,927 US$. Moreover, the IES-treated group has shown decreased morbidity and better preservation of advanced function. Despite its huge upfront costs, such studies should be focused on, as they provide evidence for the advantages of innovative technology usage in terms of patient outcomes and economic costs.

Outcome measures are of increasing importance due to the rise of "pay for performance" phenomenon. Quality initiatives were started in 2007 due to poor ranking performances such as the University HealthSystem Consortium (UHC) report card. However, common challenges persist such as how to engage providers, how to ensure the validity of data, how to individualize data, and how to ensure significant improvements. Post analysis, a strategy was developed to include three metrics including 1) (mortality, infection rates and complications), 2) neurosurgical leadership qualities, predictors of protocol development and adherence, 3) and subspecialization. In addition, these metrics were altered as to apply them for entire teams and not only neurosurgeons. More metrics were added (to a current total of 48) as the program developed and outcomes improved. Such improved metrics involve a decrease of UHC mortality ratios by 75% and an 80% decrease in infection rates. The UHC paper provides a practical guideline that could be used among other groups undertaking similar initiatives.

## Future Opportunities to Improve Quality of Care and Patients' Safety

### Simulation-Based Training Medicine

Modern medical simulation bridges the gamut of sophistication from the simple anatomic models of individual organs through complex computer-based high-fidelity human simulators that accurately replicate anatomic and physiological parameters and allow interaction with medical learners in biologically reproducible and meaningful ways [21]. Clinical trainees like all physicians occasionally make errors with some errors likely based on inexperience.

In a simulated neurosurgical environment, the freedom to make errors is a key component of experiential learning. Errors in a simulation can be allowed to progress to a simulated bad outcome, allowing the trainee to understand the implications of the error and, retrospectively, how it could have been detected, prevented, and rectified, ultimately improving the quality of care and the safety of patients.

To improve the quality of neurosurgical procedure, the European Union of Medical Specialists (UEMS) (Section of Neurosurgery) decided to implement the quality of neurosurgical training. It is the UEMS's conviction that the quality of medical care and expertise is directly linked to the quality of training provided to the medical professionals, with the development of European standards in the different medical disciplines. Adopting this principle, no matter where in Europe the young neurosurgeons train, they should receive the same core competencies.

## New Therapeutic Frontiers and Artificial Intelligence

Healthcare and neurosurgery have already entered their next phase of rapid advancements. By using precision medicine technologies, genetic vulnerabilities to chronic and deadly diseases at the individual level can now be identified, potentially preempting disease decades later. Gene therapy has been under development for more than 30 years, but several recent major advances have tipped the scales toward clinical feasibility, including improved delivery methods and the development of robust molecular technologies for gene editing in human cells. As an example, CAR T cells are used in the treatment of monogenic diseases, as a possible therapeutic strategy for the treatment of glioblastomas.

Another important frontier is the development of cancer vaccines. Vaccines that target the causative agents or tumor antigen have already been shown to be effective. With these technologies and the wealth of data that will become available as precision medicine becomes more routine, new discoveries can be expected that identify the first genetic and inflammatory changes that occur within a pre-cancerous cell. Thus, opportunities will grow to develop vaccine approaches to prevent cancer initiation/progression.

The big hope is that 25 years from now, medical sciences will have progressed enough to enable people to have healthier and more active lives almost up until their eventual death. Going forward, the direct targeting of mechanisms of aging, including with existing drugs, presents an opportunity to reduce disability and illness in late life. Geroprotective drugs, which target the underlying molecular mechanisms of aging, are coming over the scientific and clinical horizons and may help to prevent the most intractable age-related disease, that is, dementia.

*Artificial intelligence (AI)* in neurosurgery can provide individualized guidance for the prevention and optimal management of medical conditions, acting as a virtual medical coach for patients and a platform for clinicians to review a patient's real-time, real-world, extensive, and cumulative dataset [21].

In neurosurgery, AI is used, for example, in the context of deep brain stimulation, with a device that uses software for processing and analysis of brain signals in real time, allowing the stimulation to be modulated based on the recorded data. Applying techniques in algorithm development and machine learning to multimodal sensing will extend these technologies to the prediction of affective states and to use feedforward and feedback control to deliver therapies to prevent and to stabilize clinical manifestations.

The idea is that technical objects extend the human organism by repairing, replicating, or amplifying bodily and mental abilities such as exoskeleton used to help a tetraplegic to walk.

This new current of thought, which has become more real in recent years in the field of medicine, is called *transhumanism*. It is possible, and desirable, to use technology to push the boundaries of what it means to be human and to transcend our biological condition. The enhancement of technology is leading humanity to a state in which more perfect beings can be artificially created out of the human species.

## Telemedicine and Global Access to Care

It is great to benefit from technological progress, but it is equally important to ensure access to care worldwide. To achieve the goal, during the last decades, the focus has been moved on *high-quality care*, through a reduction of sanitary costs and a better distribution of economic resources in order to ensure the best quality and holistic patient management.

In order to ensure access to care, telemedicine has become more important, to bring crucial medical expertise to more patients everywhere. The World Health Organization has adopted the following broad description: "The delivery of health care services, where distance is a critical factor, by all health care professionals using information and communication technologies for the exchange of valid information for diagnosis, treatment and prevention of disease and injuries, research and evaluation, and for the continuing education of health care providers, all in the interests of advancing the health of individuals and their communities.".

We are entering a new chapter of medicine, one which may realistically offer the combination of greater safety, truly individualized personalization of therapy, and substantially reduced morbidity and mortality.

## References

1. Harteloh PPM. The meaning of quality in health care: a conceptual analysis. HCA J Health Philos Policy. 2003;11(3):259–67. https://doi.org/10.1023/B:HCAN.0000005497.53458.ef.
2. Tague NR. The quality toolbox. 2nd ed. Milwaukee, WI: ASQ Quality Press; 2005.
3. AssesSurgery GmbH, The Clavien-Dindo Classification, AssesSurgery GmbH. Accessed 8 Dec 2020. https://www.assessurgery.com/clavien-dindo-classification/.
4. Cooper J, et al. Classification of patient-safety incidents in primary care. Bull World Health Organ. 2018;96(7):498–505. https://doi.org/10.2471/BLT.17.199802.

5. Slawomirski L, Auraaen A, Klazinga NS. The economics of patient safety: strengthening a value-based approach to reducing patient harm at National Level; 2017. https://doi.org/10.1787/5a9858cd-en.
6. de Vries EN, et al. The incidence and nature of in-hospital adverse events: a systematic review. Qual Saf Health Care. 2008;17(3):216–23. https://doi.org/10.1136/qshc.2007.023622.
7. Institute of Medicine (US) Committee on Quality of Health Care in America. Crossing the quality chasm: a new health system for the 21st century. Washington, DC: National Academies Press (US); 2001. http://www.ncbi.nlm.nih.gov/books/NBK222274/.
8. Jha AK, et al. The global burden of unsafe medical care: analytic modelling of observational studies. BMJ Qual Saf. 2013;22(10):809–15. https://doi.org/10.1136/bmjqs-2012-001748.
9. Cost-Effectiveness of Short-Term Neurosurgical Missions Relative to Other Surgical Specialties, Surgical Neurology International. Aaccessed 8 Dec 2020. https://surgicalneurologyint.com/surgicalint-articles/cost-effectiveness-of-short-term-neurosurgical-missions-relative-to-other-surgical-specialties/.
10. Adler NE, Newman K. Socioeconomic disparities in health: pathways and policies. Health Aff. 2002;21(2):60–76. https://doi.org/10.1377/hlthaff.21.2.60.
11. Meara JG, et al. Global surgery 2030: evidence and solutions for achieving health, welfare, and economic development. Lancet (London, England). 2015;386(9993):569–624. https://doi.org/10.1016/S0140-6736(15)60160-X.
12. Donaldson L. An organisation with a memory. Clin Med (London, England). 2002;2(5):452–7. https://doi.org/10.7861/clinmedicine.2-5-452.
13. Rolston JD, et al. Frequency and predictors of complications in neurological surgery: national trends from 2006 to 2011. J Neurosurg. 2014;120(3):736–45. https://doi.org/10.3171/2013.10.JNS122419.
14. Committee for Assessing Progress on Implementing the Recommendations of the Institute of Medicine Report The Future of Nursing: Leading Change, Advancing Health, Institute of Medicine, and National Academies of Sciences, Engineering, and Medicine, Assessing Progress on the Institute of Medicine Report The Future of Nursing, ed. Stuart H. Altman, Adrienne Stith Butler, and Lauren Shern. Washington, DC: National Academies Press (US), 2016, http://www.ncbi.nlm.nih.gov/books/NBK350166/.
15. Cohen FL, Mendelsohn D, Bernstein M. Wrong-site craniotomy: analysis of 35 cases and systems for prevention. J Neurosurg. 2010;113(3):461–73. https://doi.org/10.3171/2009.10.JNS091282.
16. Alkire BC, et al. Global access to surgical care: a modelling study. Lancet Glob Health. 2015;3(6):e316–23. https://doi.org/10.1016/S2214-109X(15)70115-4.
17. Rolston JD, Han SJ, Chang EF. Systemic inaccuracies in the National Surgical Quality Improvement Program database: Implications for accuracy and validity for neurosurgery outcomes research. Journal of clinical neuroscience : official journal of the Neurosurgical Society of Australasia. 2017;37:44–47. https://doi.org/10.1016/j.jocn.2016.10.045.
18. Rutka JT. Editorial. Global neurosurgery and our social responsibility. J Neurosurg. 2019;130(4):1050–2. https://doi.org/10.3171/2019.1.JNS19189.
19. Haynes AB, et al. A surgical safety checklist to reduce morbidity and mortality in a global population. N Engl J Med. 2009;360(5):491–9. https://doi.org/10.1056/NEJMsa0810119.
20. Weiser TG, et al. Effect of a 19-item surgical safety checklist during urgent operations in a global patient population. Ann Surg. 2010;251(5):976–80. https://doi.org/10.1097/SLA.0b013e3181d970e3.
21. Al-Elq AH. Simulation-based medical teaching and learning. J Fam Community Med. 2010;17(1):35–40. https://doi.org/10.4103/1319-1683.68787.

# Chapter 11
# Ethical and Legal Consideration in Global Neurosurgery

**Ahmed Ammar, Stephen Honeybul, Cameron Stewart, Alejandra Rabadán, and Marike Broekkman**

## Introduction

Over the past 50 years, the field of neurosurgery has seen the introduction and acceptance into everyday practice of a wide range of diagnostic and therapeutic technologies. Many of these advances have significantly increased the capability of neurosurgeons to solve complex problems and in many circumstances considerably extend a patient's lifespan. However, paradoxically as each clinical problem is resolved, there have arisen new difficult and increasingly complicated ethical and legal issues.

The ultimate goal of any healthcare system is to provide the best possible care for its patients. There is evidence showing that patients may get better satisfaction, more benefit, and respond more positively to roles of management if their cultures, values and beliefs are respected. Respecting and understanding patients' values will also improve the communication, and gain patient trust and

A. Ammar (✉)
Department of Neurosurgery, King Fahd University Hospital, Al Khobar, Saudi Arabia
e-mail: ahmed@ahmedammar.com

S. Honeybul
Department of Neurosurgery at Royal Perth Hospital Neurological Surgery,
Perth, WA, Australia

C. Stewart
Faculty of Law, Sydney, NSW, Australia

A. Rabadán
Department of Neurosurgery, Faculty of Medicine, Buenos Aires University,
Buenos Aires, Argentina

M. Broekkman
Department of Neurosurgery, Leiden University, Medical Center, Utret Area, the Netherlands

© The Author(s), under exclusive license to Springer Nature Switzerland AG 2022   157
I. M. Germano (ed.), *Neurosurgery and Global Health*,
https://doi.org/10.1007/978-3-030-86656-3_11

satisfaction, thereby enhancing management alternatives, better compliance, and definitely better outcome. The ethics and bioethics traditionally were written and studied by philosophers. However, the need to implement the ethics in daily practice challenged neurosurgeons and physicians to study, research, and bring the ethical principles down from bookshelves to patients' beds and hospital facilities. As medicine and neurosurgery successfully crossed the geographical borders, it has become necessary to understand and appreciate the cultures, ethics, and values of different nations. The ethical principles are universal; however, the implementation and understanding may be differing between different societies.

## Ethics, Clinical Ethics, and Values-Based Medicine

### A Basic Introduction to Ethics

Ethics is primarily informed by moral philosophy, an enormous field that includes approaches such as *deontology*, which focuses on the question of how to develop universal rules of behavior. It presumes that it is possible to discover right ways of action and that such judgments should be made on the basis of principles, without necessarily referring to outcomes. Many deontological approaches are religiously based, such as in the Abrahamic traditions, but there have also been nonreligious systems, based on human reason. For example, Immanuel Kant's (1724–1804) work was based on a model of universal rules discoverable via "pure" reason. It was Kant who argued that it was a universal rule that it was unethical to treat a person solely as means [1, 2].

A second major movement is the consequentialist philosophy of *utilitarianism*, which competes most directly with deontology in the way that it focuses on consequences of decision-making as providing reasons for action. For Jeremy Bentham (1748–1832), the only universal rule was to maximize pleasure and minimize pain. Each act should be judged on the basis of its consequences and whether they minimized pain and maximized pleasure (*act utilitarianism*). Other utilitarians, like JS Mill (1806–1873), argued that rules are important and central to moral decision-making, but they need to be formulated on the basis of how they maximize pleasure and minimize pain (*rule utilitarianism*) [3].

*Virtue theory* is a third ethical stream that challenges the primacy of both deontology and utilitarianism by arguing that morality should be determined by questions of what personal attributes we consider to be virtuous or morally excellent. Aristotle (384 BCE–322 BCE) is the father of virtue theory, but it is also found in the work of Thomas Aquinas (1225–1274), Philippa Foot (1920), and Alasdair MacIntyre (1929). This notion has particular resonance for many medical practitioners who find the language of seeking virtue through experience and *practical wisdom* similar to their professional philosophies.

The *feminist theory* has also made an enormous contribution to our understanding of the role of sex gender in moral and ethical choices. Carol Gilligan (1936), argued that women approach ethical decision-making in a way that focuses on people and relationships whereas men have a tendency to look for impartiality and objectivity with a focus on rules and principles. Radical feminists, like Catharine MacKinnon (1946), melded Marxist ideas of ideology and class structure with feminist ideas and argued that relationship and power structures between men and women are inevitably based on the domination of men in society.

*Postmodern ethics* directly challenges the values of reason, autonomy, and freedom. For example, Foucault (1926–1984) argued that professionalization of health and the emergence of new health sciences, like psychiatry and psychology, transferred power away from the traditional state-based forms and dispersed it into new system of power/knowledge or *bio-power*. For Foucault, society has become less free, more controlling, and more disciplined even while it constantly promotes itself as being the opposite.

## Clinical Ethics and Principle-Based Approaches

Clinical ethics attempts to employ ethical theories into specific healthcare contexts and apply them to particular clinical problems. The most often cited approach to clinical ethics is that of Beauchamp and Childress, called the *Principles of Biomedical Ethics* (2001). Beauchamp and Childress created an ethical framework made of four clusters of moral principles, namely [4], the following:

- *Respect for autonomy* (a norm of respecting the decision-making autonomy of an autonomous person).
- *Non-maleficence* (avoiding causing harm).
- *Beneficence* (providing benefits and balancing benefits against risks and costs).
- *Justice* (distributing benefits, risks, and costs fairly).

The framework then creates a common structure upon which to test the ethics of any given bioethical problem that can be employed by people coming from different ethical traditions.

## Evidence-Based Medicine and Values-Based Medicine

Evidence-based medicine is an approach to medicine that requires that medical practitioners carefully weigh the best scientific evidence available regarding the conditions affecting patients in order to decide how best to treat them. Because of its weighting toward best scientific evidence, information generated through a rigorous scientific process is preferred over other forms of knowledge. Criticisms of evidence-based medicine point out that very little of the research currently being generated is useful for application in medicine due to its poor design and construction. The bulk of everyday medical practice has no evidence base or is at least not based on evidence generated according to the high standards required by evidence-based medicine [5].

The emergence of values-based medicine (VsBM) emergence as an approach to implementing the medical ethics in daily medical practice in some way is a direct response to these shortcomings in evidence-based medicine. Values-based medicine can be defined as "medical practice that aims at maximizing value, specifically desirable or positive value in every step of a patient's medical management" (Ammar, 2018: 2) [6, 7]. VsBM stresses the need to place patient care and well-being at the center of modern medicine. Advocates for VsBM argue that VsBM and evidence-based medicine approaches should be integrated and complement each other. It is argued that the combination of the best available medical evidence and its conversion into usable data for individual patients, based on the patient's own wishes and desires for treatment, should deliver higher-quality patient care than a purely evidence-based approach [8].

## The Definition of Law

Laws can be defined as norms generated by a person, or a political body, who has been given the authority to make law. This approach to defining law is referred to as *positivism* because it defines a law purely by reference to whether it was made or *posited* by someone with law-making power. According to positivism, there is no necessary connection between law and morality. Law is defined solely by its origins.

Another way to define law is by examining its content. In natural law theory, law has a necessary minimum content, so that some commands are not lawful, even if they come from the sovereign. The minimum content of law requires that there is some connection between law and morality. This can be seen in some religious traditions such as Judaism, Christianity, and Islam, but it can also be seen in modern international laws like the *International Covenants of Civil and Political Rights*. In practice, most laws in modern societies come from multiple sources. Some societies rely primarily on legislation or codes created by parliamentary bodies or councils. Other laws might originate from custom or from judgments handed down by learned decision-makers.

## Implementation of Ethics in Daily Neurosurgical Practice

We are hereby presenting different real cases, highlighting the impact of ethics on the decision-making, clinical management, research, innovation, learning curve, and conflict of interest.

## Mental Capacity and Substitute Decision-Making for Informed Consent

### Illustrative Case

*A 14-year-old girl was involved in a high-speed motor vehicle accident. Her initial Glasgow coma score (GCS) was recorded as 4 (E1, M2, V1). She was intubated and ventilated in the emergency department and taken to the CT scanner, which confirmed the presence of multiple parenchymal contusions. The attending neurosurgeon was reluctant to proceed to surgery given the likelihood of a poor neurological outcome. She met with the family to discuss the situation and mentioned nonoperative management. The family insisted that all measures be taken to prevent her death and asserted that she is strong enough to make a good recovery. The attending neurosurgeon somewhat reluctantly agrees to proceed. Just before she leaves, the father states that they are Jehovah's Witnesses and he refuses point blank to provide consent for a blood transfusion.*

### Ethical and Legal Perspective on Consent and Consent Without Patient's Capacity

In Western societies, particularly those based on common law traditions, mentally competent adults have the right to exercise autonomy and refuse any form of treatment that infringes their beliefs, even though it may result in death or serious injury. Nearly all Western societies recognize the religious rights of Jehovah's Witnesses to refuse blood transfusions.

However, our scenario involves a child. Children lack the same legal rights as adults in most societies, and in common law counties they tend to lack the power to refuse treatment that is necessary to preserve their health and well-being, even when they have the capacity to do so. In our situation, the child is incapacitated and unable to communicate her preferences, but even if she refused a blood transfusion, doctors in most jurisdictions would be able to do so as children lack the legal right to refuse.

Parents also have the right to refuse consent to treatment, but most societies place limits around decisions that fail to safeguard the best interests of the child. For example, in the United States, the United Kingdom, Canada, New Zealand, and Australia, parents who refuse blood transfusions may have their decisions overridden by doctors when that decision is not concordant with the best interests of the child (normally after a process of notification and assessment, such as a judicial review).

Ethically, the respect for autonomy requires the surgeon to emphasize that every effort will be made to minimize the need for transfusion; however, because of concerns for beneficence and non-maleficence, it must also be clearly stated that the surgeon would not allow the child to die from lack of blood transfusion. In such circumstances, and respecting justice, the surgeon should also be able to explain the local processes involved in providing blood against the families' wishes and any avenues they may have to appeal to decision to transfuse.

# Withdrawal and/or Withholding of Futile Treatment

## Illustrative Case

*The patient is taken to the operating room and a decompressive craniectomy is performed. An ICP monitor is inserted, and she is taken back to the intensive care unit. Over the following days, she remained stable and her postoperative CT scan confirmed adequate decompression. A week postoperatively her sedation was reduced. Her pupils remained midpoint and fixed, her best motor response was bilateral flexion, and she consistently triggers the ventilator. Over the following 8 weeks, she remains clinically unchanged. There are numerous family meetings to discuss treatment withdrawal because the clinical staff feel that ongoing cardiorespiratory support is futile. However, the family refuse to accept this as the clinical staff could not state that they were "certain" that she would not make any further recovery, no matter how small. The patient's family continues to want "everything to be done" and accuses the clinical staff of euthanasia.*

## Ethical and Legal Perspective on Clinical Decision-Making and Withdrawal of Treatment

In many clinical situations, withdrawing treatment that is providing no clinical benefit should be relatively straightforward; however, the ethical tension rises considerably when the most likely result of treatment withdrawal is the death of a patient. While some have argued that there is no ethical difference between withholding and withdrawal of treatment, others have stated that withdrawing treatment is more problematic once it has been started as withdrawal may involve some active steps, which might be seen as contributing to the patient's death. Legally, all higher court decisions (at least from common law courts in the United Kingdom, Ireland, the United States, and Canada) appear to adopt the view that withholding and withdrawing have the same legal status.

It is important that clinicians recognize that these types of decisions are difficult and may lead to feelings of guilt and responsibility for the eventual death of the patient [9, 10]. However, the ultimate principle to be adhered to is to act according to the patient's wishes (or will and preference) and, in cases where those preferences are unknown, like the present one, doctors must follow the patient's best interests. The importance of will and preference to the best interest's test means that doctors should consult with family members to determine what they think is in the patient's best interest. But their views are not determinative, and ultimately the doctor must make an assessment based on the mix of objective and subjective factors, relating to the individual patient.

In the present case, the clinicians are considering withdrawal because they believe that ongoing ventilatory support is "futile." However, as demonstrated, one of the overriding limitations when considering the concept of futility is that it seems to imply a level of a certainty that in clinical practice is not only unrealistic but would appear to provide little room for discussion [11]. Further problems are encountered when attempting to define why ongoing treatment is futile. Physiologically, all clinical parameters seem to indicate that she has sustained a devastating injury, but it is not *certain* that she will not make some recovery. Quantitatively, there is perhaps a very small chance that she can recover, as has been highlighted in a few, highly publicized cases. Qualitatively, it is not possible to assess the degree to which the patient and family feel the clinical outcome is acceptable or that the treatment is overly burdensome. Finally, from a contextual viewpoint, continuing to ventilate a patient in these circumstances may deny treatment to other, arguably more deserving patients, especially where healthcare resources are limited.

In these circumstances, a more practical approach is to consider the therapeutic options as either "proportionate" and "disproportionate." This allows stakeholders to acknowledge that a specific treatment may not necessarily be futile but may have progressively declining benefit and therefore increasing burden in any one particular clinical situation. In the illustrative case, it could be argued that the initial surgical intervention was proportionate in that, notwithstanding the neurosurgeon's initial concerns, there may be a small chance of a good outcome and people can learn to adapt to disability, especially in the case of a young individual. However, as time goes by it becomes increasingly apparent that continued therapy is becoming disproportionate not only from an outcome perspective but also from the viewpoint of equitable resource allocation. Maintaining patients with poor neurological outcome on prolonged cardiorespiratory support at the request of the family may mitigate conflict; however, resources are always finite and need to be allocated reasonably and fairly [12].

Legally, it is important that doctors know the legal requirements for treatment withholding and withdrawal in the jurisdiction in which they operate. Some jurisdictions like Texas (USA) provide for treatment withdrawal via an internal hospital process of futility determination. Other jurisdictions may require court or tribunal review. Courts are often called upon to decide these issues when disputes become intractable.

## Unconventional Interventions and Patient's Best Interests

### Illustrative Case

*The dispute between the family and the treatment team led to media interest in the case of the child. A practitioner from another country heard about the case and proposed an experimental use of thalamic deep brain stimulation. This treatment has proven efficacy in Parkinson's disease; however, there is limited evidence for its use in TBI. While the surgeon has the support of the surgical safety committee in his own hospital, no health professional supports the safety of moving the child overseas to be given this experimental intervention. A multidisciplinary treatment team decides that the best interests for the child would be served by withdrawing treatment and palliating the patient. Nevertheless, the parents wish to try this "treatment," and they raise sufficient funds to transport the child overseas and to have the procedure.*

Clinical innovations may occur without the benefit of evidence that would satisfy the evidence-based medicine approach [13]. Evidence supporting such interventions is often based purely on case reports. It is difficult a priori to know if the success of the intervention reported in a few cases might escalate to be proven beneficial for the entire population and have an evidence-based clinical benefit in the future. In such cases, it may be difficult to assess the best interests of the patient. In *Great Ormond Street Hospital for Children NHS Foundation Trust v Yates* [2017] EWCA Civ 410 ("Charlie Gard's case"), the English courts rejected the request of the parents of a terminally ill child to take him overseas for experimental treatment on the basis that the child was too ill and the chance of benefit so remote that it was not in his best interests to travel. In other cases, the balance of best interests falls the other way and courts allow the child to go and seek treatment. For example, in *Raqeeb v Barts NHS Foundation Trust* [2019] EWHC 2531 (Admin) and [2019] EWHC 2530 (Fam), the courts approved the parental decision to take a brain-damaged child to Italy for treatment. The judge was swayed by the quality of the Italian institution, the fact that the child could not feel pain and discomfort, and the fact that the child's family was highly religious and believed fervently in trying all options for treatment.

Claims that a procedure is innovative does not automatically mean that they are in any sense "good" or in the patients' best interests [14]. To some degree, it might be said that surgery (and neurosurgery in particular) is always innovative because every patient is anatomically different, and surgeons usually have to adopt slight modifications of current techniques every time surgery is performed. This has meant that it has been difficult to define innovation in neurosurgery. Different interpretations of what constitutes innovation result in a lack of standardization in the evaluation of novel procedures. Even if there is consensus about what constitutes innovation, there might be disagreement about whether some form of oversight is necessary. Some argue that innovation should not be subjected to oversight as too strict oversight might stifle innovation and the continual advancement of surgery; however, appropriate oversight that balances patient safety and the surgeon's autonomy should be the goal [13].

It might be argued by some that an informed consent process would be sufficient to ensure that the child's best interests are being served. However, this ignores the reality that parents in such cases are often desperate and are willing to take any chance in the hope of an improved outcome. Neurosurgeons in such cases should not rely solely on consent but should seek the critical review of their peers (such as through a surgical safety committee), or they should demonstrate a commitment to sharing information about the procedure and report the results widely. Nor should the practitioners charge fees beyond that which is necessary to recover the costs of the treatment.

In our illustrative case, the court agrees that, on balance, the best interests of the child would be served by going overseas to have the implant procedure. The child has the procedure and dies. After the procedure, an investigative journalist uncovers proof that the medical evidence that supported performing the procedure was fraudulently created. The doctor pocketed a large sum of money from the parents and now refuses to speak with them. He also applies for a patent over the implanted technology. Conflict of interests (CoIs) describe a situation where an action or judgment determined by primary values arising from the doctor–patient relationship such as beneficence and distributive justice is influenced by secondary interests, such as economic benefits or the desire for prestige. In such cases, the conflict of interests and duties may adversely affect neurosurgical performance, and in extreme cases, it may be fraudulent.

## Innovation and Clinical Research

### Illustrative Case

*In 2013, two California neurosurgeons inoculated bacteria into the resection cavity of patients with recurrent GBM. The rationale rested on reports suggesting that bacterial infection in patients with GBM could stimulate an immune response resulting in improved survival.*

*Since the prognosis of patients with recurrent GBM is dire, with most patients surviving only a few months, the doctors wanted to provide an alternative. They discussed this with their patients and obtained informed consent. The ethics board in their hospital had given permission to treat the first patient as it was considered compassionate use. However, the neurosurgeons did not have approval from their institutions, medical boards, or government regulatory agency to conduct research on this topic.*

### Ethical and Legal Perspective About the Fine Line between Innovation and Clinical Research

Surgical innovation is fundamentally different from medical innovation and has historically received less focus in ethical discussions. To a certain extent, this can be explained by the "exceptional" status of surgery. The argument that surgery is exceptional makes both regulation of and innovation in surgical procedures different from those of medical treatments. Indeed, it is often in hindsight that one recognizes innovation in (neuro) surgery. Slight modifications of (an indication for) a current technique could result in an altogether new technique. Rarely are these innovations subject to the traditional regulatory structures of a randomized, controlled clinical trial (RCT). This contrasts with medical innovation, which generally follows the structure and oversight of prospective trials.

Because of the nature of innovation in neurosurgery, a clear definition is currently lacking.

Indeed, great heterogeneity exists in what surgeons consider innovative. For example, an international survey showed that 47% of neurosurgeons consider a new high-speed drill innovative – nearly an equal divide in opinion among the approximately 350 respondents [13]. Different interpretations of what constitutes innovation result in a lack of standardization in evaluating novel procedures. Even if there is consensus about what constitutes innovation, there might be disagreement about whether some form of oversight is necessary. Some argue that innovation should not be subjected to oversight as too strict oversight might stifle innovation and the continual advancement of surgery; however, appropriate oversight that balances patient safety and advancement of our field is the goal.

When proposing a novel treatment, it is important to establish the clinical benefit before the treatment becomes available to the public. Furthermore, it is important that such treatment has oversight to eliminate a potential conflict of interest with the surgeons(s) proposing it and to avoid the exploitation of vulnerable patient groups [15]. The form and amount of oversight should be based on the potential risk for patients and could vary from no oversight to full ethics review.

In the example provided above, one could argue that after the first procedure the goal was no longer just to provide care for an individual patient, but also to generate generalizable knowledge. It was at that point unclear if the specific technique would be superior to another technique (equipoise). For this reason, in combination with the potential risks for patients, the procedure should have been considered research. The question then arises what constitutes ethically sound research. In their 2000 article, Emanuel et al. [16] formulated seven requirements that must be fulfilled for research to be considered ethical. When reviewing research proposals, most ethics committees will evaluate if these seven criteria have been met (Table 11.1).

## Transparency in Obtaining Informed Consent

### Illustrative Case

*A 66-year-old man was admitted due to confusion and right-sided weakness. The brain MRI showed large (4.4 × 6.6 × 5.7 cm) left parietal–occipital tumor causing significant mass effect. The decision was to perform a craniotomy for tumor resection. The young neurosurgeon who admitted the patient asked the senior neurosurgeon who does most of such cases if he could proceed with the surgery and was granted permission. During the process of taking the consent for surgery, the patient and his eldest son asked who was going to perform the surgery, and the young neurosurgeon replied that the senior neurosurgeon would perform the surgery and he would assist in the surgery.*

*Question: Were the patient and his son deceived?*

**Table 11.1** Seven requirements to determine if a research trial is ethical (Adapted from [16])

| Requirement | Description |
| --- | --- |
| Intrinsic value | The research aims to result in improvement in health or knowledge |
| Scientific validity | The research must be methodologically rigorous |
| Fair subject selection | The inclusion criteria for individual subjects should be based strictly on scientific criteria and on distribution of risks and benefits |
| Favorable risk–benefit ratio | The risks must be minimized and potential benefits enhanced |
| Independent review of the protocol | It must be done by unaffiliated individuals to avoid potential conflict of interest |
| Informed consent | It must be obtained for each subject |
| Respect for enrolled subjects | Including patients' privacy and confidentiality |

## Ethical and Legal Perspective on Transparency Obtaining Informed Consent

Deceiving patients or patients' family is unethical and should not occur.

If the young neurosurgeon had made clear that he was the one performing the surgery, would the patient and his family agreed and signed the consent? This is even more important in countries/geographical areas where trainees might be allowed to operate independently. We suggest that precautions should be taken to secure the patient's safety. First, the consultant/senior neurosurgeon/attending should review all the details of surgery preparation, position, incision, etc., in detail with the trainee before surgery. Second, prior to the surgery, the senior neurosurgeon and trainee should discuss and find solutions for any anticipated surgical problems that may occur during surgery such as bleeding, brain edema, high ICP, not identifying lesions, and other pertinent scenarios. Finally, the consultant should be in the operating theater, scrubbed, and assisting the trainee, as well as observing the procedure, technique, and handling of instruments and brain tissue, ready to intervene at any time where necessary and available to provide feedback necessary for the trainee to improve in future surgeries.

## Ethical Considerations for the Neurosurgery Trainer and Trainee

The first surgery is a first step in the career development of every neurosurgeon. It is usual to see the trainee eager and anxious to successfully preform the first operation. In that status and mode of thinking, the concerned trainee is focusing mainly on the performance of surgery. During that mental and physical process, some ethical principles may be breached; therefore, it is fundamentally important to observe them and implement the ethical principle to secure patient's safety and enhance the core and central principle of values-based medicine in which the patient is the center of care. There are several ethical questions that should be clearly considered including patient's safety, ethics of learning, and accountability for any undesirable outcome.

One of the main goals of every training program is to train a safe surgeon. No doubt that the trainees should be provided with the opportunity to perform surgery under supervision, not only to gain confidence and successfully fulfill the requirement of their training programs. The patient's safety and well-being should be considered first before any other consideration and should be implemented as early in the training program as possible ideally to focus the trainee on patient safety over their first surgery, new instruments, and techniques.

## Conflict of Interest: Incentives, Gifts, and Presents "Does the End Justify the Means?"

### Illustrative Case

*Mary A. is a 30-year-old neurosurgeon at a university hospital in an LMIC. She has a reliable personality and has always shown devotion to her patients, technical excellence, as well as good communication with colleagues and patients. She also participates in scientific and research activities. A medical representative visited her and suggested that she should share her experience in an international congress and attend the advanced training course provided at the meeting. Their company will fund all expenses. Mary is having second thoughts about accepting the offer and opts to consult her Program Director.*

*This subject was analyzed institutionally in a Bioethical Committee session, which included residents and medical students. Questions were raised on whether the acceptance of the "gift or favor" could condition the use of a determined material, or whether it could affect the confidence of patients in their doctor's prescriptions, or whether it could become a negative example for the trainees.*

### Ethical and Legal Perspective on Conflict of Interest

Conflict of interest (CoI) describes a situation where an action or a judgment is determined by primary values arising from the doctor–patient relationship such as beneficence and distributive justice. It is influenced by secondary interests such as economic benefits or the search for prestige. These personal benefits may affect the objectivity of results and even foster fraud. It also is a potential source of distortion that may encompass all medical roles, assistance, management, teaching, and investigation [17, 18].

CoI is frequent and inherent to human nature for the mere existence of economic reward, rivalry among colleagues and institutions, competition for power or fame, and the need of recognition; moreover, since medicine is an intense activity with multiple and intricate economic interests, CoI might seem inevitable.

Marketing teams in the industry are aware of how beneficial it is to have direct relationships with physicians. The longer they interact with them, the more likely they are to prescribe their products. The giving of gifts and favors such as travel fees, invitations to conferences, and edition of books/videos by business companies might influence the choice of products, thus affecting the credibility of the professional [19, 20].

That is, even without direct or explicit complicity, influence exists. Any discordant situation produced by incentives may undermine professional ethics and should be adequately recognized by the physician [21].

## Public and Private Industry Agreements

It is clear that medicine and the related industry need each other in the development of new drugs and/or medical devices [22]. To this effect, the public–private alliances may offer a solution to avoid the possibility of conflicts. It is very important to be aware of what the rules and regulations in the country we practice are before closing a public or private agreement with a company. For example, in Argentina, an official path can be followed to sign a cooperation between the Ministry of Science, Technology and Productive Innovation (MINCYT) and companies and institutions. It is accepted that relations with companies are lawful and contribute to scientific progress, but these relations should not influence medical decisions and the patient should be aware of it. For other countries, any financial agreement between the neurosurgeon (physician) and industry must be publicly disclosed online to allow patients and others to be aware.

## Conclusion

The ultimate goal of any healthcare service is patient benefit, satisfaction, and well-being. The availability of healthcare resources varies widely across the globe; however, many of the moral and ethical imperatives are universal. Clinical decision-making should be guided by the resources available, the best available evidence, and the skills and experience of the surgical practitioner. At all times, it is important to recognize that patients and their families have different values based on culture and religion, and every attempt must be made to respect these values when making clinical decisions. Across all aspects of neurosurgery, the decision-making paradigm will continue to evolve in concert with advances in medical technology and a clear understanding of issues such as consent, treatment withdrawal, and conflict of interest, to name but a few, will become increasingly important in order to navigate the complex neurosurgery bioethical landscape.

# References

1. Hare J. Kant, the passions, and the structure of moral motivation. Faith Philos. 2011;28(1):54–70.
2. Harris D. Ethics in health services and policy: a global approach. Wiley; 2011. ISBN 9780470531068.
3. Driver J. Pleasure as the standard of virtue in Hume's moral philosophy. Pac Philos Q. 2004;85:173–94.
4. Rauprich O. Common morality: comment on Beauchamp and Childress. Theor Med Bioeth. 2008;29(1):43–71.
5. Szajewska H. Evidence-based medicine and clinical research: both are needed, neither is perfect. Ann Nutr Metab. 2018;72(suppl 3):13–23.
6. Ammar A. Value based medicine. In: Ammar A, Bernstein M, editors. Neurosurgical ethics in practice: value based medicine. Berlin, Germany and New York: Springer; 2014. p. 7–9.
7. Ammar A. Values-Based Medicine (VsBM) and Evidence-Based Medicine (EBM), vol. 1. IntechOpen; 2019. p. 13.
8. Brown MM, Brown GC. Update on value-based medicine. Curr Opin Ophthalmol. 2013;24:183–9.
9. Welie JV, Ten Have HA. The ethics of forgoing life-sustaining treatment: theoretical considerations and clinical decision making. Multidiscip Respir Med. 2014;9:14.
10. Wilkinson D, Savulescu J. A costly separation between withdrawing and withholding treatment in intensive care. Bioethics. 2014;28:127–37.
11. Honeybul S, Gillett GR, Ho, Janzen C, Kruger K. Long-term survival with unfavorable outcome: a qualitative and ethical analysis. J Med Ethics.
12. Honeybul S, Gillett GR, Ho K. Futility in neurosurgery: a patient-centered approach. Neurosurgery. 2013;73:917–22.
13. Zaki MM, Cote DJ, Muskens IS, Smith TR, Broekman ML. Defining innovation in neurosurgery: results from an International Survey. World Neurosurg. 2018;114:e1038–48. https://doi.org/10.1016/j.wneu.2018.03.142. Epub 2018 Mar 29. PMID: 29604357.
14. Broekman ML, Carriere ME, Bredenoord AL. Surgical innovation: the ethical agenda: a systematic review. Medicine (Baltimore). 2016;95:e3790.
15. Gupta S, Muskens IS, Fandino LB, Hulsbergen AFC, Broekman MLD. Oversight in surgical innovation: a response to ethical challenges. World J Surg. 2018;42(9):2773–80.
16. Emanuel EJ, Wendler D, Grady C. What makes clinical research ethical? JAMA. 2000;283(20):2701–11.
17. Barcat JA, Del Bosco CG. Conflicto de intereses. Medicina (BsAs). 2003;63:87–9.
18. Foster RS. Conflicts of interest: recognition, disclosure and management. J Am Coll Surg. 2003;196:505–17.
19. Abbasi K, Smith R. No more free lunches. BMJ. 2003;326:1155–6.
20. Madhavan S, Amonkar M, Elliot D, Burke K, Gore P. The gift relationship between pharmaceutical companies and physicians: an exploratory survey of physicians. J Clin Pharm Ther. 1997;22:207–15.
21. Martin JB, Reynolds TP. Academic-industrial relationships: opportunities and pitfalls. Sci Eng Ethics. 2002;8:443–54.
22. Rabadán AT, Tripodoro V. When to consult the institutional bioethics committee? The deliberative method for resolving possible dilemmas. Medicina (B Aires). 2017;77(6):486–90.

# Chapter 12
# The Role of Neurosurgery in Global Health: Future Directions

David P. Bray and Nelson M. Oyesiku

## Brief Historical Background

The idea and subject of "global neurosurgery" has only recently gained traction in academic neurosurgical journals over the last decade [1]. However, practitioners within neurosurgery have inculcated a global view within their specialty since its inception. As the breadth of neurosurgery developed over the nineteenth and twentieth centuries, so did its influence on global health.

As neurosurgery developed, its founding members traveled around the world to share ideas and inform their own future directions. Often considered the patriarch of neurosurgery in the United States, Dr. Harvey Cushing was a key member in the founding of modern neurosurgical practice. Soon after his graduation surgical residency at the Johns Hopkins Hospital, Dr. Cushing traveled to Switzerland and Italy to study blood pressure variability in animals with compressed brains, undoubtedly contributing to his description of the "Cushing's Triad" [2, 3]. Dr. Cushing valued sharing experiences internationally; he helped found the Society of Clinical Surgery, a group dedicated to the general advancement of worldwide surgery [4]. Famously, Dr. Cushing volunteered to assist his European colleagues in the First World War [5]. From the genesis of modern neurosurgery, founders of the field have stressed a global worldview and engagement.

Support: Dr. David P. Bray is partially supported by the *Nell W. and William S. Elkin Research Fellowship in Oncology*, Winship Cancer Institute, Emory University Hospital, Atlanta, GA.

D. P. Bray (✉) · N. M. Oyesiku
Department of Neurosurgery, Emory University School of Medicine, Atlanta, GA, USA
e-mail: dbray3@emory.edu; david.painton.bray@emory.edu

# Current Status

After the dawn of the inception of modern neurosurgery, neurosurgeons from developed countries have attempted to assist in the fight against neurosurgical diseases across the world. In these efforts, neurosurgeons from high-income countries have employed cost-effective strategies to combat more common neurosurgical diseases. Dr. Benjamin Warf's implementation of the CURE protocol for hydrocephalus treatment in Africa is a good example. The CURE protocol emphasizes the use of endoscopic third ventriculostomy with choroid plexus cauterization for the primary treatment of hydrocephalus, which reduces the need for expensive hardware and iterative shunt repair surgeries [6, 7]. By performing cost-effective surgeries, neurosurgeons such as Dr. Warf have created fruitful enterprises in the treatment of neurosurgical disease in less-developed countries.

In the later twentieth century and early twenty-first century, the emphasis of global neurosurgery has broadened from consultation to proactive participation of wealthy nations in the development of neurosurgical care in low-to-middle-income countries (LMICs). International societies have prosecuted this effort across the globe. The Foundation for International Education in Neurological Surgery (FIENS) was established in 1969 to create durable neurosurgical training programs in LMICs. FIENS was instrumental in the implementation of resident training programs in Ghana, Ethiopia, Kenya, Tanzania, and Uganda. The College of Surgeons of East, Central, and Southern Africa (COSECA) approved the neurosurgical residency training program, which is a major step in helping LMICs increase access to neurosurgical care, while maintaining national preferences and autonomy [8, 9].

Founded in 1955, the World Federation of Neurosurgical Societies (WFNS) is a professional, scientific, nongovernmental organization comprising 130 member societies, consisting of 5 Continental Associations, 119 National Neurosurgical Societies, and 6 Affiliate Societies, representing over 50,000 neurosurgeons worldwide. The WFNS promotes education training programs, unifies international neurosurgical societies, and assists LMIC distribute neurosurgical care [10].

# Future Opportunities and Unmet Needs

By the beginning of the twenty-first century, it was clear that there were major discrepancies in global surgical care. It was estimated that almost three-quarters of all major surgery in the world was completed in wealthy countries [11]. Meanwhile, global health efforts to date had emphasized communicable and infectious diseases such as HIV/AIDS, malaria, and tuberculosis [12]. In 2013, the Lancet Commission on Global Surgery set out to define the state of surgery worldwide.

The Lancet Commission report revealed the large gap in access to basic surgical care in LMICs. They found that 90% of persons living in LMICs have no access to basic surgical care. The Commission estimated that 18.6 million people die every year due to basic surgical disease; more than three times the number that die from infectious disease such as HIV/AIDS and malaria. Thirty-three million people faced catastrophic health expenditure for the surgical procedures that they did obtain. The Commission estimated that there was a need for 2.2 million more surgeons, obstetricians, and anesthetists worldwide [13]. In sum, there is dire need for promulgation of surgical specialty care across the world, especially in LMICs.

The 2015 Lancet Commission exhibited the necessity for an increase in surgical care across the world; they stated that basic surgical care was an "indivisible, indispensable" aspect of universal health rights [13, 14]. The global awareness of inequality in access to basic surgical care is growing; however, it is unclear where neurosurgical care will fit in the worldwide surgical "call-to-arms." We depend on our international neurosurgical societies such as the WFNS to inject neurosurgery into the global push for access to surgical care.

In 2019, the first annual Global Neurosurgery Symposium (GNS), sponsored by international delegates as well as members in the FIENS and WFNS, was held in New York City [14]. Among the many goals of the meeting was to take stock of the state of global surgical care and consolidate resources so that neurosurgical care could increase in step with the worldwide effort. The GNS defined the advances of global surgery inequity becoming part of the global health consciousness. The World Bank Group and Bill and Melinda Gates foundation coauthored the third edition of *Disease Control Priorities*, which newly included "essential surgery" as a volume [14]. Of the United Nations Sustainable Development Goals, 8 of the 13 targets within the "Good Health and Well-Being" goal were related to essential surgical care; a marked increase from the Millennium Development Goals [14, 15]. In 2015, the World Health Assembly passed a new resolution solidifying essential surgical care as an important aspect of global health care [14, 16].

An important step in responding to the discrepancies of access to neurosurgical care across the world is to define the state of neurological disease in LMICs. A good example of this is the effort of categorizing the incidence and effect of traumatic brain injury (TBI) across the globe. In the last 15 years, experts have begun to recognize the severe, but unreported and insidious impact of TBI in global health, naming it the "silent epidemic" [17]. A recent meta-analysis found that approximately 69 million people suffer a TBI each year [18]. In response, international delegations such as the National Institute for Health Research (NIHR) Global Health Research Group on Neurotrauma aim to enumerate the need for TBI work in LMIC. This group recently launched the first observational study of patients receiving neurosurgery for TBI and has created a global TBI registry. In order to increase access to neurosurgical care, we will first need to categorize the prevalence of neurological disease worldwide as well as encourage continuing neurosurgical research in LMIC [12, 19].

Another effort for global neurosurgery in the twenty-first century will be creating sustainable training programs and self-sufficient neurosurgical hospitals. Volunteerism and mission work, while helpful, are difficult to maintain throughout generations. Through various international groups, neurosurgeons have helped LMICs develop postgraduate neurosurgical training programs. By 2018, there were

23 neurosurgeons that graduated via the COSECA program; all of which practice in East Africa [20]. Key to the success of this program was partnering with COSECA, so the program had institutional support and national "buy-in." Global neurosurgery efforts like those from the Duke Neurosurgery program in Uganda have also allied with global surgical and anesthesia teams to develop hospital networks in LMICs [9]. All of these strategies help to build sustainable training programs and LMIC neurosurgical hospitals.

Additionally, international neurosurgical societies provide support to training and development of neurosurgeons in LMIC by creating guidelines for neurosurgical practice and mentoring. International neurosurgical societies help direct and unify standard practices for neurosurgeons in LMICs by creating accessible consensus statements and guidelines for them to follow. An example is the WFNS Spine Committee recommendations for management of lumbar spinal stenosis [21]. Guidelines help create sustainable and safe neurosurgical practices in LMICs.

There are more opportunities for neurosurgeons in developed countries to provide novel, cost-effective support to those in LMICs. The COVID-19 pandemic has forced the worldwide medical community to treat, connect, teach, and learn while maintaining social distance. International society meetings have continued throughout the pandemic via live-stream platforms such as Zoom Inc. (San Jose, California). Inpatient and outpatient neurosurgical consultations have continued via telemedicine [22, 23]. These pipelines can be employed to educate physicians and treat neurosurgical pathology in LMICs. Neurosurgeons can also support neurosurgical care in LMICs by creating less expensive technology. Great examples include the "Malawi" shunt and "Chhabra" shunt, which are two ventriculoperitoneal shunt systems that can be purchased for a fraction of the cost of the shunt systems commonly used in the United States and Europe [24]. Neurosurgeons need to continue to be creative in developing cost-effective strategies to support the ongoing neurosurgical care in LMICs.

In sum, since the genesis of the neurosurgical subspecialty, neurosurgeons have maintained a global consciousness. Global neurosurgery began as simple traveling societies and international conferences, but it now comprises a worldwide infrastructure to educate the next generation of neurosurgeons and provide neurosurgical care to LMICs. Neurosurgeons will continue to innovate and raise the standard of neurosurgical care across the world, while emphasizing an international awareness.

# References

1. Andrews RJ. What's in a name? "Global neurosurgery" in the 21st century. World Neurosurg. 2020;143:336–8.
2. Harvey Cushing: A Journey Through His Life. Becoming a Neurosurgeon. Yale University Library Online Exhibitions. https://onlineexhibits.library.yale.edu/s/harvey-cushing/page/the-johns-hopkins-years-and-be. Accessed 2 Nov 2020.
3. Parkinson D. Early history of neurosurgery in Manitoba: threads in the tapestry of world neurosurgery. J Neurosurg. 1995;82:900–6.

4. Society of Clinical Surgery – Opening the Door of Science to a New World. https://societyof-clinicalsurgery.com/. Accessed 2 Nov 2020.
5. Hanigan WC. Neurological surgery during the great war: the influence of Colonel cushing. Neurosurgery. 1988;23:283–94.
6. Kulkarni AV, Schiff SJ, Mbabazi-Kabachelor E, et al. Endoscopic treatment versus shunting for infant hydrocephalus in Uganda. N Engl J Med. 2017;377:2456–64.
7. Lepard JR, Dewan MC, Chen SH, Bankole OB, Mugamba J, Ssenyonga P, Kulkarni AV, Warf BC. The CURE protocol: evaluation and external validation of a new public health strategy for treating paediatric hydrocephalus in low-resource settings. BMJ Global Health. 2020;5:1–9.
8. Bagan M. The Foundation for International Education in Neurological Surgery. World Neurosurg. 2010;73:289.
9. Fuller A, Tran T, Muhumuza M, Haglund MM. Building neurosurgical capacity in low and middle income countries. eNeurologicalSci. 2016;3:1–6.
10. Umansky F, Black PL, DiRocco C, Ferrer E, Goel A, Malik GM, Mathiesen T, Mendez I, Palmer JD, Juanotena JR, Fraifeld S, Rosenfeld JV. Statement of Ethics in Neurosurgery of the World Federation of Neurosurgical Societies. World Neurosurg. 2011;76(3–4):239–47.
11. Weiser TG, Regenbogen SE, Thompson KD, Haynes AB, Lipsitz SR, Berry WR, Gawande AA. An estimation of the global volume of surgery: a modelling strategy based on available data. Lancet. 2008;372:139–44.
12. Park KB, Johnson WD, Dempsey RJ. Global neurosurgery: the unmet need. World Neurosurg. 2016;88:32–5.
13. Meara JG, Leather AJM, Hagander L, et al. Global Surgery 2030: evidence and solutions for achieving health, welfare, and economic development. Lancet. 2015;386:569–624.
14. Schmidt FA, Kirnaz S, Wipplinger C, Kuzan-Fischer CM, Härtl R, Hoffman C. Review of the highlights from the first annual global neurosurgery 2019: a practical symposium. World Neurosurg. 2020;137:46–54.
15. THE 17 GOALS | Sustainable Development. https://sdgs.un.org/goals. Accessed 9 Nov 2020.
16. Price R, Makasa E, Hollands M. World health assembly resolution WHA68.15: "strengthening emergency and essential surgical care and anesthesia as a component of universal health coverage" – addressing the public health gaps arising from lack of safe, affordable and accessible surgical a. World J Surg. 2015;39:2115–25.
17. Vaishnavi S, Rao V, Fann JR. Neuropsychiatric problems after traumatic brain injury: unraveling the silent epidemic. Psychosomatics. 2009;50:198–205.
18. Dewan MC, Rattani A, Gupta S, et al. Estimating the global incidence of traumatic brain injury. J Neurosurg. 2019;130:1080–97.
19. Jean WC, Ironside NT, Felbaum DR, Syed HR. The impact of work-related factors on risk of resident burnout: a global neurosurgery pilot study. World Neurosurg. 2020;138:e345–53.
20. Henderson F, Abdifatah K, Qureshi M, Perry A, Graffeo CS, Haglund MM, Olunya DO, Mogere E, Okanga B, Copeland WR. The College of Surgeons of East, Central, and Southern Africa: successes and challenges in standardizing neurosurgical training. World Neurosurg. 2020;136:172–7.
21. Zileli M, Fornari M, Costa F. Lumbar Spinal Stenosis Recommendations of World Federation of Neurosurgical Societies Spine Committee. World Neurosurg X. 2020;7:100080.
22. Bray DP, Stricsek GP, Malcolm J, Gutierrez J, Greven A, Barrow DL, Rodts GE, Gary MF, Refai D. Letter: maintaining neurosurgical resident education and safety during the COVID-19 pandemic. Neurosurgery. 2020; https://doi.org/10.1093/neuros/nyaa164.
23. Greven ACM, Rich CW, Malcolm JG, Bray DP, Rodts GE, Refai D, Gary MF. Letter: neurosurgical management of spinal pathology via telemedicine during the COVID-19 pandemic: early experience and unique challenges. Neurosurgery. 2020; https://doi.org/10.1093/neuros/nyaa165.
24. Ravindra VM, Kraus KL, Riva-Cambrin JK, Kestle JR. The need for cost-effective neurosurgical innovation – a global surgery initiative. World Neurosurg. 2015;84:1458–61.

# Part II
# Neurosurgery Education Around the World

Isabelle M. Germano

Educating the next generation of neurosurgeons is a great privilege and responsibility for our specialty. This evolving educational process will ensure that our patients with neurosurgical disease receive excellent care, no matter where they are in the world. In this Part of the book, authors from five continents highlight differences and similarities in neurosurgical education and training around the world, including new educational tools and paradigms, to reduce inequality and increase access to neurosurgical care.

Africa is arguably the continent that has experienced the steepest change in neurosurgical care over the past couple of decades. At the beginning of the century, the worldwide average ratio of neurosurgeon/inhabitants was 1 /230,000. By contrast, Africa averaged a ratio of 1/1.24 million, with an even lower ratio in Sub-Saharan Africa of 1/6.368 millions [1]. The dedication of African neurosurgeons, in collaboration with world societies, foundations, and neurosurgeons worldwide, allowed increased training of neurosurgeons in Africa, resulting in a phenomenal expansion of the workforce [2]. Chapter 13 provides a summary of all the great educational accomplishments to date and proposes strategies for the way forward.

The vast geographical and population characteristics of the Asian continent contribute to great differences in neurosurgical training. Demographic and economic disparities, along with differences in population size, account for the multifaceted and sometimes divergent opportunities for neurosurgical education in Asia. Chapter 14 reviews highlights of the currently available training provided by 13 Asian countries that account for 87% of the Asian population.

The Australasian neurosurgery workforce faces unique challenges for both training and delivery of healthcare services due to its relatively small population spread across a large land body. Chapter 15 reviews how accomplishments have allowed neurosurgeons there to address present challenges and to pave the way for future expansions.

Standardization of training remains a key point for neurosurgical education in the European continent. Duty hour requirements, increasing expectations of the neurosurgery trainee workforce, and new curricular mandates all had a significant impact over the past few years in shaping the future European neurosurgeon.

Chapter 16 reviews the steps toward cooperation among European countries needed to establish further consolidation of neurosurgical training in Europe.

There is currently little published literature on the current state of neurosurgical education in Latin America and in the Caribbean region. Chapter 17 is a first attempt to collate such data. The evolution of neurosurgery training in this region was influenced by many factors, including political events. Variability in education programs and length of training remain a challenge to address in future years.

In North America, the neurosurgery training in Canada, United States, and Mexico has shown increasing structure over the years. Chapter 18 compares and contrasts the training in these three countries, highlighting both the strengths and weaknesses. Future neurosurgeons need to have the best armamentarium in order to offer the highest quality of care to their patients. In order to provide them optimum care, current neurosurgeons are analyzing opportunities to further improve the training, including incremental use of simulations and subspecialty training.

While no publication can encompass the entire breadth of worldwide neurosurgical education and training, we hope the following chapters give the readers a sense of the accomplishments of and challenges to the education of the next generation of neurosurgeons in different regions of the world.

# References

1. El Khamlichi A. African neurosurgery: current situation, priorities, and needs. Neurosurgery. 2001;48:1344–7.
2. Karekezi C, El Khamlichi A, El Ouahabi A, El Abbadi N, Ahokpossi SA, Ahanogbe KMH, Berete I, Bouya SM, Coulibaly O, Dao I, Djoubairou BO, Doleagbenou AAK, Egu KP, Ekouele Mbaki HB, Kinata-Bambino SB, Habibou LM, Mousse AN, Ngamasata T, Ntalaja J, Onen J, Quenum K, Seylan D, Sogoba Y, Servadei F, Germano IM. Impact of African-trained neurosurgeon on Sub-Sahara Africa. JNS Neurosurg Focus. 2020;48(3):E6. PMID: 3211456021.

# Chapter 13
# Neurosurgery Education Around the World: Africa

**Najia El Abbadi, Rime Al Baroudi, Abdesslam El Khamlichi, Mahmoud Qureshi, Kalango Kalangu, and Jeff Ntalaja**

## Introduction

It is gratifying to note that the issues related to global health have shown a significant progress over the last decades. This resulted in important improvements of human health in many countries. However, a lot of ground to cover still remains, including within the framework of the Sustainable Development Goals (SDGs), a series of global health goals set for 2030, proposed by the General Assembly of the United Nations in 2015 [15]. Some of the major global health issues involve neurosurgery, from noncommunicable diseases like injuries, cancers, hypertension, and its neurological consequences, to communicable diseases when it comes to infectious diseases and congenital malformations. Global surgery as a formal area of universal health-care coverage (UHC) continues gaining international interest since 2015 when the Lancet commission on Global Surgery Report was released and the

N. El Abbadi (✉) · R. Al Baroudi
Department of Neurosurgery, International Cheikh Zaid Hospital, Abulcassis University of Health Sciences, Rabat, Morocco

A. El Khamlichi
Hôpital des Spécialités, ONO Service de Neurochirurgie BP 6444 Rabat-Instituts, Rabat, Morocco
e-mail: elkhamlichi@neurochirurgie.ma

M. Qureshi
Section of Neurosurgery, Department of Surgery, Aga Khan University Hospital, Nairobi, Kenya

K. Kalangu
University of Zimbabwe, College of Health Sciences, Department of Neurosurgery, Harare, Zimbabwe

J. Ntalaja
Hopital Ngaliema, Kinshasa, Democratic Republic of Congo

© The Author(s), under exclusive license to Springer Nature Switzerland AG 2022  179
I. M. Germano (ed.), *Neurosurgery and Global Health*,
https://doi.org/10.1007/978-3-030-86656-3_13

adoption of the World Health Assembly (WHA) resolution WHA68.15 *"Strengthening emergency and essential surgical care and anaesthesia as a component of universal health coverage"* [15, 16].

The philosophers Norman Daniels and Mark Jessen have argued that some basic goods in life are essential, and health is one of them. To secure equal opportunities in life, providing health care and education is an ethical requirement of humanity. The World Health Organization (WHO) defines a health system *as "all the activities whose primary purpose is to promote, restore and/or maintain health. Or it's the people, institutions, and resources arranged together in accordance with established policies, to improve the health of the population they serve."* Hence, one of the main services provided by a health system is a comprehensive emergency care. As described within WHO health system framework (Fig. 13.1), one of the pillars of a well-functioning health system is the health workforce, and one that is in the right place at the right time with the right training, ready to deliver proper care [2].

Global health consists of population-based public health strategies that are implemented in cost-effective ways to serve the most vulnerable members of our population. When this principle is applied to Africa, since the majority of the countries are low-income countries, it is clear that there is a desperate need to implement population-based public health strategies to advance the training of health-care professionals and the availability of material and human resources. While pursuing these goals, it is important to draw from the experience of other countries to ensure that we invest as wisely as possible particularly in the training of the African neurosurgical workforce.

## Historical Background

### The African Legacy

Africa is known as the cradle of humanity and the home of many civilizations. Each participated in the building of human history and cultural capital. Several anthropologists have stated that the greatest evolution in human prehistory has taken place in

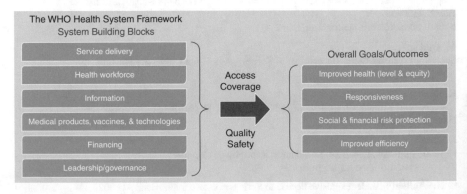

**Fig. 13.1** World Health Organization's (WHO) health system framework [3]

Africa, and that the first civilization in humankind took root around the Nile valley. In the papyrus documents of Pharaonic Egypt, descriptions are made of the way head trauma was treated, endonasal brain aspiration (before mummification), and trephination that pharaohs underwent just before death in order to allow their souls to find their way to paradise. Among the tribes in Africa whose healers have practiced and taught the basic rules of trephination for centuries, we can mention Chaouia and Kabyle tribes (respectively in Morocco and Algeria), the Gouache in the South of Morocco, and the Tuareg in Sub-Saharan Africa and Libya. From Abulqassim Al Zahrawi (Abulcasis) in the tenth century to the current ages, education in African neurosurgery has known many peaks and troughs. Abulcasis is considered to be the pioneer of neurosurgery and wrote a book composed of 30 treatises *"Kitab Al Tasrif Liman Ajaza an Al Talif"* [4] which was later translated into many languages and served as the basis for teaching both medicine and surgery in various schools in Europe during the Renaissance. The Arab-Islamic medicine has greatly contributed to the development of medicine during the Middle Ages as it flourished in North Africa and later allowed for medicine to develop in Europe in the thirteenth century: Hussein Ibn Sina (Avicenna), Abubakr Ar-Razi (Rhazes), Ibn El Haytham, Ibn Tofail, Ibn Zohr (Avenzoar), Ibn Rochd (Averroes), Ibn Maymon (Maimonide), and many others have all marked the Golden Age of Arab-Islamic medicine. The knowledge and practice of those Hakims, meaning "wise man," as doctors were called, have later spread around the Mediterranean, and have been taught in medicine schools (School of Cordoba, Spain; Karaouiyine University in Fez, Morocco; Schola Medica Salernitana in Italy [7]; Ecole de Montpellier in France). Further to this spread of knowledge, the first care facilities were built (also called Maristan, Arabic word meaning "hospital" in that period) [1].

Unfortunately, this historical asset did not necessarily work in favor of the African continent when it came to the scientific advances in the world. From the eleventh to the eighteenth centuries, Africa was marginalized from the important cultural, technological, and economic advances until the beginning of the twentieth century. It woke up to find itself weak and colonized by European powers and to witness a world that had moved forward at high speed without its active participation. Concerning the medical development in Africa in the second half of the twentieth century, the focus was on the setting up of vaccination plans against infectious diseases, such as plague, cholera, tuberculosis, malaria, and HIV/AIDS. The lack of medical professionals and the endless needs in basic health care urged African states to deliver only primary health care to their citizens, therefore marginalizing neurosurgery among all the other surgical specialties, wrongly considered as a "luxury specialty" [1].

## The Dawn of African Neurosurgery

The birth of neurosurgery in Africa, as an independent specialty, just about 60 years ago, was an arduous process. It started in North African countries and South Africa and was introduced in the majority of countries by European neurosurgeons, brought to the continent by citizens of the colonizing countries. When Africa emancipated from the occupational state, there were no native African neurosurgeons, and the number of native physicians did not exceed five [1]. When Africa gained back its independence, it was deemed to fall into a worrying health-care situation. The continent was bound to keep European physicians and even request more assistance to provide much-needed health care for the local population until some pioneers of African neurosurgery took over (Table 13.1).

**Table 13.1** Some of the first neurosurgical departments in Africa by European physicians and native pioneers [1]

|  | First departments by European physicians | Some of the first native neurosurgeons |
|---|---|---|
| **North Africa** | The first units of neurosurgery were set up in Algiers, Algeria, in 1942; and in Casablanca, Morocco, in the 1940's respectively by Doctors P. Goignard and R. Acqua viva [14] | The first local neurosurgeons in north Africa would take over between 1960 and 1975: those are Doctors H. El Kerdoudi, D. Bouchareb. A. El Ouarzari and A. El Khamlichi in Morocco; M. Abada, A. Abdelmoumen, A. Bousalah and Boutmene in Algeria; and M. Betteyeb in Tunisia. The latter set up the first operational department of neurosurgery in Tunisia in 1964. In Egypt, the first neurosurgeons to set up neurosurgery between 1950 and 1960 were Drs. A Abu Zikri, O. Sorour, I. Higazi, A. Benhawy and S. El Guindi in Cairo, and S. Boctor and G. Azab in Alexandria. |
| **West Africa** | The first neurosurgery unit has been set up in Dakar, Senegal, in 1967, by French neurosurgeon B. Courson. | The first Senegalese resident joined up, Dr. M. Gueye, in 1977, and became the first Senegalese Professor and Neurosurgery Department Chairman. The first Ivorian neurosurgeon, Dr. K. Kanga, had already started practicing neurosurgery in 1974. In Ghana, the first Ghanaian neurosurgeon, Dr. J.F. Osman Mustaffah, set up the first neurosurgery department in 1969. In Nigeria, neurosurgery was introduced in the country by local neurosurgeons. The first department was set up in Ibadan in 1962 by Dr. E.L. Odeku. |
| **East Africa** | Neurosurgery was set up by English-speaking neurosurgeons from Europe first in Kenya where it was introduced by Dr. P. Clifford, an ENT surgeon who operated on encephaloceles and hydrocephalus, before an Italian neurosurgeon, Dr. Renato Ruberti pioneered neurosurgery in 1967. | In 1971, Dr. J. Kiryabwire, the first Ugandan neurosurgeon would join come back to Uganda, after training in London |
| **Southern Africa** | In South Africa, things were different, the practice of neurosurgery began with Doctors R.A. Krynauw in Johannesburg in 1940, and H.L. de Villiers Hammann in Cape Town in 1946both born in South Africa and trained respectively in Oxford (United Kingdom) and Munich (Germany). | |

In Morocco, European neurosurgeons started passing on their knowledge to local trainees around in 1962. Local professors gradually replaced them, and over a 20-year span, Moroccan teachers were more than 80% of the teaching workforce within neurosurgery training programs. This encouraged the government to open more Moroccan schools, develop local training, and promote clinical research. Efforts then focused on evenly distributing neurosurgeons all over the country. The aim was to integrate neurosurgery as an important part of the health and academic system. Neurosurgery trainees still went to foreign countries for a limited time for additional training. It rapidly became obvious that a full training in a foreign country was costly and above did not teach the trainees how to adapt their learning to the local conditions. This self-improving system allowed Morocco to go from zero native Moroccan neurosurgeons in 1956, after gaining back its political independence, to 80 neurosurgeons, a number that increased exponentially over the years [1]. In Sub-Saharan Africa (SSA), the training system did not follow the same template over the years, despite neurosurgery being set up as a specialty in most countries by 1960s and the opening of many medical schools after each country's political independence. Instead, most SSA chose to send their trainees to Europe and North America. However, many neurosurgeons who trained abroad continued to practice where they trained. Therefore, the SSA demand of neurosurgeons was not met. In 1998, the neurosurgeon/inhabitant ratio in SSA was 1/7–ten million [1].

## The Neurosurgical Workforce Distribution in Africa: Past and Present

The discrepancy of the regional distribution of neurosurgeons is palpable. In 1998, the neurosurgeon/inhabitant ratio was 1/230,000 in the world, whereas in Africa it averaged at 1/1,238,000. Moreover, most African neurosurgeons (86%) were condensed in the North African countries and in South Africa. This resulted in providing the rest of the African continent, which accounts for 74% of the entire Africa population, with 14% of the neurosurgery workforce and neurosurgeon/inhabitant ratio of 1/6,368,000. Additionally, these countries also suffer a lack of basic neurosurgical equipment and appropriate facilities.

A survey was conducted by A. El Khamlichi in 1998 to establish a comprehensive guide to assessing the status of neurosurgery in Africa. It was published and presented in the different international meetings to inform the neurosurgical community worldwide about the distressing ratio of neurosurgeons in Sub-Saharan Africa. Two years later, a more elaborate version of the survey was conducted to carry out a follow-up in order to have more detailed information regarding already-existing training systems, and the biomedical equipment available, the pathology spectrum but mostly to appraise the kind of help African neurosurgeons needed. The results of the survey in the tables below (Table 13.2) were presented to the WFNS Administrative Council (AC) on February 20, 1999 [5]. The request made by African neurosurgeons was clear: to be supported by the WFNS for the acquisition of basic equipment and to have access to basic training in neurosurgery. Regarding

**Table 13.2** Evolution of African neurosurgery

| | Population (in millions) | Neurosurgeons | Ratio (adjusted) |
|---|---|---|---|
| A. Results of the survey conducted by A. El Khamlichi in 1998 [1] | | | |
| Africa | 800 | 565 | 1/1066666 |
| South Africa | 45 | 86 | 1/ 405,405 |
| North Africa | 140 | 400 | 1/ 380,658 |
| Sub-Saharan Africa | 615 | 79 | 1/ 7,784,810 |
| World | 5.479 | 23.940 | 1/ 230.000 |
| **WHO recommended ratio** | | | **1/100.000** |
| B. Results of the survey conducted by A. El Khamlichi in 2016 [1] | | | |
| Africa | 1.120 (+75) | 1.727 | 1/ 654,000(1/691000) |
| South Africa | 55 | 171 | 1/ 420,000 |
| North Africa | 181 | 1.187 | 1/ 131,000 |
| Sub-Saharan Africa | 884 | 369 | 1/2395663 |
| **WHO recommended ratio** | | | **1/100000** |

the first issue, the WFNS president, Pr. M. Samii, was already able to secure equipment as he already secured two companies to manufacture basic instrument sets for craniotomy and laminectomy at a reduced price.

Regarding the support to training, the WFNS AC members committed to encourage the organization of training courses in Africa and accepted the project presented by A. El Khamlichi to set up a regional training center in Rabat to train African neurosurgeons in their continent. The training in regional centers was an aim for African neurosurgeons and had many advantages. First, it could avoid the "brain drain." The young who trained in Europe or North America rarely went back to their African home countries. Second, the young neurosurgeons could receive their training in an environment more similar to their home countries. Third, the training cost would be a fraction of the cost of training in Europe or North America.

Thanks to the efforts of the new national and regional centers, an exponential growth of the number of neurosurgeons and trainees was witnessed. In the latest inquiry presented in the WFNS Webinar on June 13, 2020, J. Ntalaja showed that in 4 years (2016–2020) the number of neurosurgeons went form 1727 (Table 13.2B) to 2044 in 2020; in addition, there are 1036 residents currently in training. The success witnessed in the development of neurosurgical training supports the original strategy, proposed by Professor A. El Khamlichi, and that supported by the WFNS was a winning proposition.

## Minimizing the Paucity of Neurosurgeons in Africa: From the WFNS Residency Training Center (RTC) to a Widespread African Effort

Born from the cooperation between the WFNS and the Mohammed V University in Rabat in 2002, the WFNS Rabat Training Center (WFNS RTC) aims at ensuring basic training in neurosurgery for postgraduates from Sub-Saharan African countries. The financial support provided by the WFNS RTC aims at two goals. First, it provides the required resources (human and logistics) to achieve the neurosurgery training. Second, it provides financial aid grants to candidates in order to allow them to live decently and focus on their training. The Moroccan authorities shoulder the first part, which accounts for 90% of the total expenses accrued. African doctors benefit from free enrolment at the university, which allows them to complete internships at the hospital. The only cost the trainees need to bear is that of medical insurance, which often does not exceed 1.800 MAD (less than 200 USD) per annum [1].

During these 18 years, 64 young African doctors have enrolled at the WFNS-RTC: 54 to complete the 5-year training and 7 enrolled for a limited complimentary training (6 months to 3 years) since they were already enrolled in a training program in their home countries. All these young neurosurgeons are well-integrated into the national health system in their country and all are able to acquire the required basic equipment that allows them to operate on patients [18]. They also successfully promote and lobby for neurosurgery in their countries and by doing so manage to work with local authorities to launch a local training program. Currently, 64 young African neurosurgeons have been trained or are training in the WFNS-RTC. Neurosurgeons trained at the WFNS RTC upon graduation and reentry in their country of origin are also eligible for receiving a neurosurgical set of instruments by the WFNS Foundation.

Following the footsteps of the first francophone reference training center in Rabat, the Consortium of Collaborative Neurosurgical Sites of Training of the East, Central and Southern African region (C-CNS-ECSAR) was established in 2006 as the second WFNS reference center in Africa, and the first Anglophone. The center incorporates neurosurgical training at major hospitals in the East African region of Sub-Saharan Africa. The initiative was led by Dr. Mahmood Qureshi of Kenya, Prof Paul H. Young of the Foundation for International Education in Neurosurgery (FIENS), and Dr. Benjamin Warf who was working in Mbale, Uganda, at the time [6, 11].

In 2014, Pr. M. Samii's started a program called "Africa 100" aimed at increasing the training of young African neurosurgeons. The program committed to managing the full basic training of 100 young African doctors in neurosurgery by providing them with scholarships and enrolling them in training departments in Africa or elsewhere. In January 2014, the first six trainees of the "Africa 100" program enrolled in the WFNS-RTC, all of whom were sponsored by Pr M. Samii. Since then, four neurosurgery centers are able to train and accept "African 100" trainees. They are located in Dakar (Senegal), Algiers (Algeria), Nairobi (Kenya), and Cairo, Egypt. In 4 years (2014–2018), 15 trainees were enrolled in the "Africa 100" program, all of whom are currently under training. Eight of these have completed their training at the WFNS-RTC. In 2018, the Africa 100 committee accepted the applications of 31 students from the following countries: Somalia, Nigeria, Zimbabwe, Chad, Tanzania, Gambia, Swaziland, Niger, Mauritania, Zanzibar, Cameroon, Guinea Conakry, Benin, Malawi, and the DRC (Fig. 13.2).

**Fig. 13.2** African map representing countries of applicants accepted in the program by Africa 100

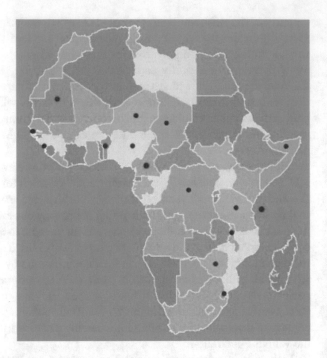

# The Impact of Local Training on the Growth of African Neurosurgery

The two examples to follow are provided to highlight the importance of local neurosurgery training on the growth of our filed in Africa.

*The Nigerian Experience*  Dr. Nasirou was trained in the WFNS RTC from 2002 to 2004. In 2004, after he came back to his home country, and with the help of Pr. Shehou, the Regional Neurosurgical Centre was established in Sokoto. It was commissioned in 2007 and received the WFNS neurosurgical set and a microscope. In the following 10 years, the center trained 14 young neurosurgeons and aimed for 50 more in the years to come. In the same time, the Nigerian Academy of Neurological Surgeons was formed in 2007 with 58 active members. The success of this project was possible because of the commitment and team-building abilities but also local training for human resources and local financial and administrative support.

*The Democratic Republic of Congo (DRC) Experience*  In Congo, where the practice of neurosurgery started in 1976. The DRC has a surface area of 2,345,409 km$^2$, 75,000,000 inhabitants, and only 4 neurosurgeons dispatched in two provinces out of 26 in 2019. Neurotraumatology was the main neurosurgical activity. Before the World Federation of Neurosurgical Societies Rabat Reference Training Center (WFNS RTC) sent its first wave of newly trained neurosurgeons, there was the following equipment in the DRC: one MRI device 0.35 Tesla, four CT scan devices, and one image intensifier. Late Mudjir Balanda M.D. was the first to be trained at the WFNS RTC, who returned to his country, but unfortunately died a year later. Jeff Ntalaja, as soon as he came back home after training at the WFNS RTC in December 2013, witnessed the will to trigger the development of neurosurgery in the country, namely in improving patients' management and equipment purchase. An appeal was written to the political and administrative authorities for the purchase of tools to improve working and patients' management conditions. The permission was given to purchase new equipment: image intensifiers; several CT scan devices, with three including 64 slices; five MRI devices, with two 1.5 Tesla; one digital angiography device; one basic operating microscope; two Medtronic Quadrant systems; etc. Help also came from the neurosurgeons who were practicing outside the country. The diaspora (neurosurgeons outside the country), Professor Kazadi Kalango, Professor Kalala from the University of Gand, Dr Orphee Makiese, a neurosurgeon at Clinique Floreal in France, Dr Hugues Matondo, an interventional radiologist practicing in Belgium, to mention a few, are important partners toward the development of neurosurgery in the DRC, namely by strengthening competence and sharing practical experience in neurosurgery. A Congolese Society of Neurosurgery was established as well as an online information exchange platform with an information website linked to the Congolese Society of Neurosurgery. In March 2018, we set up a National Neurosurgery Excellence Pole whose coordination has been carried out by Jeff Ntalaja M.D. A pole is a unit including neurosurgeons who practice neurosurgery, ranging from minimally invasive surgery to the surgery of malformations, tumors, traumatology, and degenerative surgery. It is a collaboration platform gathering neurosurgeons (three from outside the country), but also specialists from neighboring fields (anesthetists, radiologists, etc.). Currently, the number of neurosurgeons is up to 9 [8].

## The African Neurosurgery Training Curriculum

The WFNS RTC's vision revolves around training African neurosurgeons within their native continent to create a self-sufficient and sustainable system aiming to provide a well-trained neurosurgical workforce. Its main goal is to teach them to work with affordable and low-maintenance technology and expand efforts to improve quality of neurosurgical care throughout the continent. As a result, neurosurgeons' availability increased during the last two decades in Africa due to the joined efforts of senior African senior neurosurgeons and the WFNS [19]. The WFNS RTC welcomes 4–5 Moroccan residents and 1–2 other African residents per hospital per year. One resident stays in Rabat while five others are sent to the hospitals in Casablanca, Fes, Marrakech, and Oujda. Currently, other teaching hospitals are opening their doors to welcome more African residents in Rabat, Casablanca, Agadir, and Tangier, increasing the capacity to welcome more African residents. Other international doctors can become neurosurgical residents by taking the same competitive exam as Moroccan graduates. The neurosurgical curriculum in the WFNS RTC encompasses 5 years of training, including rotations in the five neurosurgical departments of Rabat and 6 months in a neurology department. The residents undergo the exact same curriculum regardless of their nationality. The 5–6-year-long training is predominant in Africa except in Egypt, where it is 6–8 years long, depending on the city, for example.

## The Current Challenges of Neurosurgical Training in Africa

Despite the enormous efforts of the WFNS Foundation, the lack of material resources and equipment remains a major obstacle to the practice and teaching of neurosurgery. The WFNS Foundation has been instrumental in providing basic neurosurgical sets and microscopes. Other international institutions have donated or sold at a reduced rate surgical instruments sets and/or microspores. These programs are to command and propagate. However, to avoid the main drawback, which is that the continuous assistance may result in a lack of incentive by the local health authorities from acquiring the equipment, a regular audit of the facilities seeking help is strongly recommended to establish the needs. Ideally, this should be a joint effort of the WFNS Foundation and CAANS [13, 14].

Cost-effectiveness and a fair and smart distribution of available resources are two sound principles when developing neurosurgery strategies for the African continent. However, ethically speaking, these two concepts might appear to be contradictory. An educated health-care team can help orient the authorities to a more cost-effective management of the health systems.

On-site education after completion of the neurosurgery training program is very important. Prior to the recent COVID-19 pandemic, this required traveling abroad. The registration fee and travel expenses oftentimes were prohibitive to the majority of young neurosurgeons. During the unprecedented global health crisis experienced by the world during 2020 following the COVID-19 outbreak, many questions were raised about the essentials of global health and the management of the health systems all over the planet. At the same time, new opportunities were discovered. Education has shifted to the use of videoconferencing platforms to alleviate the cancelling of all courses formerly requiring attendance. Lectures and conferences as well as case discussions and meetings covering various neurosurgery topics were all held electronically. E-learning appeared to be an attractive, easy, comfortable, cheap solution to replace educational social gatherings, but it has also shown some downsides. Resistance, financial issues, infrastructures, and dedicated IT (Information Technology) personnel in addition to the need for official legalization are a prerequisite. Nevertheless, the rapid increase in the speed of travel and communication, as well as the economic interdependency of all nations, has led to a new level and speed of globalization that can be a driving force.

# Future Opportunities and Unmet Needs

Africa is currently undergoing a demographic transition, at different stages depending on the region, but most of the African population is still young. By 2025, the African population is expected to reach 1.4 billion people with 1.1 billion in Sub-Saharan Africa. Fertility is at its highest but so is mortality. Both these facts have a direct impact on the increase of the already existing need for neurosurgeons. It is also worth mentioning that pediatric neurosurgery here since 45% of the African population will be under 15 years old. Also, more than half of the African population in 2025 will live in cities. This has the potential to increase the number of traffic road accidents and urban violence. The goal is to reach a critical mass of neurosurgeons to speed up the process of increasing the neurosurgical care capacity in Sub-Saharan Africa. Furthermore, the progress and technological advances witnessed recently in neurosurgery have required significant financial, material, and human resources, to grant patients safe and efficient treatment.

As shown in Fig. 13.3, the African population will double between 2015 and 2050 up to 2.4 billion inhabitants. By 2100, the African population will represent more than 25% of the population and Asia will reach almost 50% of the world population. The rest of the world, including Europe, North, Central and South America, will account for less than 25% of the population. In addition, most of the African population itself will be concentrated in East and West Africa accounting for almost 75% of the population.

It is also worth noting that with the epidemiological transition from a majority of communicable diseases, and a fair amount of injuries, to the predominance of non-communicable diseases, but just as many injuries, a change in the neurosurgical pathology spectrum is predicted. Currently, most of the African neurosurgical pathologies are CNS traumas, infections, hydrocephalus, and congenital diseases.

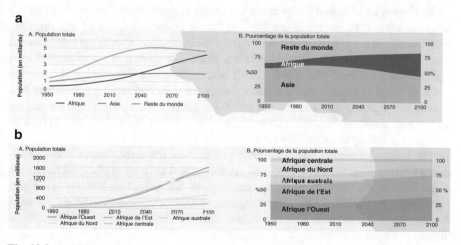

**Fig. 13.3** (**a**, **b**) Estimated evolution of the African population by global neurosurgery during the 2017 conference [10]

The predicted shift in Africa's epidemiological profile includes a lower number of infections and an increase in life expectancy. This in turn could result in a higher incidence in tumors, cerebrovascular diseases, and urban violence. This will itself trigger changes when it comes to choose a subspecialty, which can only be possible if the number of neurosurgeons is sufficient to cover enough ground. In addition, some environmental changes such as climate change and unhealthy eating habits can cause an increased incidence of cancers, which in turn can reveal themselves only when they metastasize to the brain.

There are several important WHA resolutions targeting advancements in surgical care and further providing a mandate to allow LMICs and resource-poor settings to prioritize assessment, development, and restructuring of health-care systems aimed at caring for acutely injured patients at the time of the event and for those whose illness requires urgent care. For example, neurosurgeons continue to be fundamental in international advocacy of patients suffering from traumatic brain injury (TBI) and spinal cord injury (SCI), which represent significant contributors to global morbidity and mortality. TBI and SCI correspond to approximately 55 million (estimated range 53–58 million) and 27 million (estimated range 25–30 million) prevalent cases, respectively [17], and remain a priority in achieving UHC and context-specific priority areas in global neurosurgery, which relies heavily on advocacy by neurosurgeons [15].

Another important consideration are the social and cultural changes around the world, including Africa. With an increase of the levels of literacy, most likely there will be a rise of patients and their families' awareness regarding their medical management. This will likely result in higher societal expectations regarding the quality of care. Another important aspect is that with more trained neurosurgeons in Africa there will be more competition for the best opportunities. Due to limited resources, it is possible that not all neurosurgery trainees will have access to achieve competency in standard neurosurgery, microsurgical, and operative techniques.

The North and South African countries are on the right track to work as a driving force for the rest of the continent through the developing network of training centers. The African neurosurgery is now a fully integrated member in the international neurosurgical community through WFNS and other institutions and has its own regional organizations like the CAANS and the national neurosurgical societies working hand in hand to build a better future for the continent by promoting and developing neurosurgery locally and in Africa. More importantly, when we add up all these parameters, Africa is a young continent, full of potential waiting to be harnessed. It is highly attractive for investment in medical care.

The training program has to be reviewed to meet the future needs of neurosurgeons starting with a reinforcement of education and training in standard neurosurgical techniques, then developing training in subspecialties mainly pediatric neurosurgery (20–30% of neurosurgical activities), neuro-oncology, neuro-endoscopy, spine surgery, and functional neurosurgery. Minimally invasive techniques, as opposed to the classical surgical techniques, should be developed within the availability of appropriate equipment. Simulation centers are highly encouraged, even if costly, to avoid the medical error.

Also, the research gates are yet to be developed in African countries. Research projects are known to be beneficial not only for scientific purposes within themselves, but also for the individual growth of young trainees. Research teaches them to think critically and gain independence. Young trainees are full of energy and driven to change the situation for better, an ambition Africa can only benefit from.

The role of CAANS and national neurosurgical societies is capital as they are the main actors in the advancing and promoting of neurosurgery in the wide variety of socioeconomic and scientific aspects. These include but are not limited to setting up new active neurosurgical societies, institutionalizing inter-African cooperation and exchange (south–south cooperation), exchanging with other continental and international institutions (training, research, organization), and collaborating with an established training program in Africa to exchange faculty and harmonize training standards.

# Conclusion

Sustainability of actions and collaborative partnerships are essential factors to continue improving neurosurgical health care in Africa. Although the neurosurgical workforce in Sub-Saharan countries is increasing, its sustainability is still at risk. The economic reality of an expanding population with limited resources is a complex scenario with challenges and opportunities. Local solutions will be more successful when integrated with the support of the international neurosurgical community. Additional WFNS regional training centers are poised at cost-effectively increasing the neurosurgical capacity with long-term tenable plans. International efforts to organize and secure equipment will continue to be important and needed. However, even if global health is based on the idea of the underserved regions of the world being helped by wealthier countries, a two-way flow is necessary to address the global health challenges that the world faces. A more nuanced and contemporary perception can only allow the striving of global health as a whole [9]. Yet, the neurosurgical community's interfacing with global health governance, policymakers, donors, and other stakeholders lacks a unified, formalized framework for participation in neurosurgical global health advocacy, policy, and research [15].

Additional forces influencing the success of improving neurosurgical care in Africa include providing strategies to address the brain drain, resulting in a dearth of health staff at multiple levels. Additional cultural barriers, such as a high percentage of personnel absenteeism, need to be addressed to improve the shortage of properly trained staff. A culture promoting value-based professional growth of well-trained most likely will result in improved desire to work harder. Such cultural change will also need to rest on the availability of resources to ensure that the neurosurgical workforce can effectively deliver good health care to its own people [2].

# References

1. Emerging neurosurgery in Africa by Pr. Khamlichi A. 2019.
2. Pr. Skolnik Global Health 101, Chapter 5- "Introduction to Health Systems" 2012.
3. WHO "Everybody's Business : Strengthening health systems to improve health outcomes" 2007.
4. Al Zahraoui Abulqassim (Abulkassis) Al tasrif leman ajaza an al taalif. Institute for the History of Arabic Islamic Science at the Johann Wollgang Univrsity. Frankfurt am Main, 198.
5. El Khamlichi A. African neurosurgery: current situation, priorities and needs. Report presented to the WFNS administrative Council, Geneva, Feb 20, 1999.
6. The WFNS Reference Training Center in East Africa . Mahmood QURESHI, MBChB, M.Med (Surgery), FCS-ECSA, FRCSEd (SN), Coordinator, C-CNS-ECSAR.
7. Prof. Franco SERVADEI Milan, Italy in the forewords. Emerging neurosurgery in Africa by Pr. Khamlichi A. 2019.
8. The practice and development of neurosurgery in the Democratic Republic of Congo, Jeff NTALAJA. Emerging neurosurgery in Africa by Pr. Khamlichi A. 2019.
9. Fried LP, Bentley ME, Buekens P, Burke DS, Frenk JJ, Klag MJ, Spencer HC. Global Health is public health. Dis Lancet. 2010;375(9714):P535–7.
10. Estimated evolution of the African population by Global Neurosurgery during the 2017 Conference.
11. World Neurosurgery, 01 Apr 2010, 73(4):261-263 history of Neurosurgery in Kenya, East Africa by MQureshi and D Oluoch Olunya.
12. World Neurosurgery 20 Apr ;136:172–177. doi: The College of Surgeons of East, Central, and Southern Africa: Successes and Challenges in Standardizing Neurosurgical Training.
13. Neurosurgical FOCUS. October 2018. https://doi.org/10.3171/2018.7.FOCUS18287. The challenges and opportunities of global neurosurgery in East Africa: the Neurosurgery Education and Development model.
14. Akhaddar A. Raphael Acquaviva: the forgotten pioneer of modern neurosurgery in Morocco. World Neurosurg. 2020:S1878-8750(20)32074-X. https://doi.org/10.1016/j.wneu.2020.09.066. Epub ahead of print. PMID: 32949804.
15. Rosseau G, Johnson WD, Park KB, Hutchinson PJ, Lippa L, Andrews R, Servadei F, Garcia RM. Global neurosurgery: continued momentum at the 72nd World Health Assembly. J Neurosurg. 2020;17:1–5. https://doi.org/10.3171/2019.11.JNS191823. Epub ahead of print. PMID: 31952031.
16. World Health Organization. WHA68.15: Strengthening Emergency and Essential Surgical Care and Anaesthesia as a Component of Universal Health Coverage. Geneva: WHO; 2015.
17. GBD. Traumatic brain injury and spinal cord injury collaborators: global, regional, and national burden of traumatic brain injury and spinal cord injury, 1990–2016: a systematic analysis for the global burden of disease study 2016. Lancet Neurol. 2016;18(56–87):2019.
18. Karekezi C, El Khamlichi A, El Ouahabi A, El Abbadi N, Ahokpossi SA, Ahanogbe KMH, Berete I, Bouya SM, Coulibaly O, Dao I, Djoubairou BO, Doleagbenou AAK, Egu KP, Ekouele Mbaki HB, Kinata-Bambino SB, Habibou LM, Mousse AN, Ngamasata T, Ntalaja J, Onen J, Quenum K, Seylan D, Sogoba Y, Servadei F, Germano IM. Impact of African-trained neurosurgeon on Sub-Sahara Africa. JNS Neurosurg Focus. 2020;48(3):E6. PMID: 3211456021.
19. Karekezi C, El Khamlichi A, El Ouahabi A, El Abbadi N, Ahokpossi SA, Ahanogbe KMH, Berete I, Bouya SM, Coulibaly O, Dao I, Djoubairou BO, Doleagbenou AAK, Egu KP, Ekouele Mbaki HB, Kinata-Bambino SB, Habibou LM, Mousse AN, Ngamasata T, Ntalaja J, Onen J, Quenum K, Seylan D, Sogoba Y, Servadei F, Germano IM. The impact of African-trained neurosurgeons on sub-Saharan Africa. Neurosurg Focus. 2020;48(3):E4. https://doi.org/10.3171/2019.12.FOCUS19853.

# Chapter 14
# Neurosurgery Education Around the World: Asia

Yoko Kato, Satoshi Kuroda, Rajeev Sharma, Ahmed Ansari,
Dhananjaya I. Bhat, and B. Indira Devi

## Introduction

Asia is characterized by demographic and economic disparities along with differences in population size. The infrastructure at various central and peripheral hospitals is also variable. Though uniformity in medical education and neurosurgery in particular is desirable, it may not always be feasible.

Neurosurgeons are required to be trained for the demands of the region of practice. The education of current and future neurosurgeons in Asia therefore becomes an important consideration because of the size, 4.6 billion people corresponding to 60% of the total world population, and diversity of the population, belonging to 48 different countries.

Y. Kato (✉)
Department of Neurosurgery, Fugita Health University, Bantane Hospital,
Nagoya, Aichi, Japan
e-mail: kyoko@fujita-hu.ac.jp

S. Kuroda
Department of Neurosurgery, University of Toyama, Graduate School of Medicine and
Pharmaceutical Sciences, Toyama, Japan
e-mail: skuroda@med.u-toyama.ac.jp

R. Sharma
Department of Neurosurgery, AIIMS, New Delhi, India

A. Ansari
Department of Neurosurgery, Jawahar Lal Nehru Medical College, Aligarh Muslim
University, Aligarh, Uttar Pradesh, India

D. I. Bhat
Neurosurgery, RV ASTER, Bengaluru, India

B. I. Devi
National Institute of Mental Health and Neurosciences, Bengaluru, India

© The Author(s), under exclusive license to Springer Nature Switzerland AG 2022    193
I. M. Germano (ed.), *Neurosurgery and Global Health*,
https://doi.org/10.1007/978-3-030-86656-3_14

Globally, the discipline of neurosurgery (NS) has evolved during the 1990s (also nicknamed the decade of the brain). During the last few decades, massive developments in science and technology have been directly useful for diagnostics and treatment of NS-related disorders. Unfortunately, this development is not evenly distributed between developed and developing countries. The same is the case with neurosurgical education and training, which developed from only traditional apprentice programs in the past to more structured, competence-based programs with various teaching methods utilized, in recent times.

Currently, there are high disparities in the distribution of 49,000 neurosurgeons worldwide. Data indicate a huge variation in the number of neurosurgeons per million population with Japan (58.9) being highest and rural India being the lowest (1) compared to the world average of 6.5 (Fig. 14.1). Ironically, countries like India with 16% of world population have only 6% of world's share of neurosurgeons. Additionally, within India the disparity between rural and urban parts of the country is staggeringly high.

## Neurosurgical Education

Edward Benzel, in a landmark paper, said that "we retain 90% of what we do or teach while we only retain 50% of what we hear and see." This is especially true with NS: a skills-oriented specialty, which has grown by leaps and bounds to a point where we can proudly gauge on its multiple subspecialties. NS has yet only been defined in terms of the ultimate work, whether it be in terms of quality or quantity. Often for a fresh surgeon it is really tough to strike the right chord and balance the work in terms of free hand, mentorship, and finances. It has become all the more important recently to fine-tune one's skills as per the needs and advancements. Besides having been trained as a competent neurosurgeon, one should also be trained as a good neurosurgery teacher.

Kato Y et al. [1] highlighted the striking difference regarding the neurosurgical training compared to other surgical specialties. The training should not be limited to acquiring textbook knowledge and laboratory work, but also skillful in the surgical

**Fig. 14.1** Number of neurosurgeons per million population

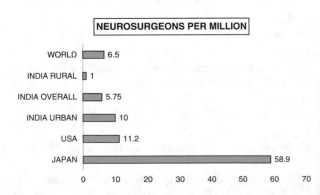

and nonsurgical management of patients with neurological diseases. No surgical training is complete without adequate hands-on exposure and practice.

Training curriculum through regional and international collaboration includes those developed locally and through societies such as the World Federation of Neurosurgical Societies (WFNS) and Asian Congress of Neurological Surgeons (ACNS), which have been formally used to prioritize and teach the young neurosurgeons and faculties from developing countries through its various educational activities. It is the responsibility of the established senior neurosurgeons to teach the next generation of neurosurgeons especially from the developing countries. To fulfill this need, in 2019, over 170 courses have been organized by the WFNS. The organization has also published many guidelines, books, white papers, and newsletters. Another way to decrease the disparity in world neurosurgical services includes the efforts to provide better equipment and resources to the developing countries. There is a need for resourceful countries to help resource-depleted countries in terms of organizing hands-on courses, on-site training, and financial support.

The effort to improve access to journals for publication among neurosurgeons from the low- and middle-income countries to counter the disparity has been implemented. The neurosurgery education should comprise technique of stabilizing their hands during surgery and to review the recordings of their previous surgeries to identify all unnecessary steps. The current generation of neurosurgeons should reduce their dependency on technology and always use anatomy landmarks. A sound knowledge in anatomical landmarks is a good corollary skill to neuronavigation system. A proper risk explained to the patient when required intraoperative neurophysiological monitoring is unavailable should be in common practice.

In the following, we provide a brief description of some of the historical facts and current data about neurosurgical education in 13 Asian countries. These account to 3897.53 million people, equivalent to 87% of the Asian population (data searched on Google and pertinent to 2018).

## Japan

On records, 7933 neurosurgeons in Japan are board certified out of a total of 10,014 neurosurgeons (2019). The average number of neurosurgeons per 100,000 population is 5.5 in each prefecture, and Japan has the highest proportion of neurosurgeons compared with its neighboring East Asian countries. Owing to the historical background of medical practice in Japan, neurosurgeons are not only involved in the surgical work, but a lot also involved in community prevention of diseases, radiation therapy, and rehabilitation.

After passing a national examination, aspiring neurosurgeons in Japan planning to engage in clinical practice are required to undertake general medical training, such as internal medicine, emergency medicine, and community medicine, for no less than 2 years at a university hospital or a Ministry-designated hospital. Only after completing this 2-year training period does training to become a neurosurgeon begins. Residents need to gain experience in disease management with approval from clinical instructors. The minimum requirements are strictly fixed by the Japan Neurosurgical Society (JNS) for each type of disease, such as tumor, cerebrovascular disease, trauma, spinal disease, pediatrics, and functional neurosurgery. The minimum requirements of the surgical cases are also strictly fixed.

The Japan Neurosurgical Society (JNS) is the organization that awards neurosurgical specialty board certification to the graduated trainees. It has approved 94 training programs, and there are a total of 857 training centers. These programs are strictly determined by the JNS according to the total number and variety of surgeries and the recommendation of the Dean of Faculty Neurosciences of the medical staff and equipment, and must be reapproved every 5 years. The objective of the Japan Neurosurgical Society, GIA (General Incorporated Association), is to serve national welfare through neurosurgical practice, to popularize neurosurgical science, to contribute to academic development in Japan by means of presenting neurosurgical theories and research on their application, and to exchange knowledge by cooperating and collaborating with other members and related societies in Japan and foreign countries. As of September 2016, The Japan Neurosurgical Society has 9567 members in total, including 150 honorary/special members (including 43 foreign members), 34 guest members, and 58 supporting members. These members include physicians in training.

The Department of Neurosurgery was established for the first time in June 1, 1951, at the University of Tokyo Hospital as a medical department officially approved by the Ministry of Education. Subsequently, in September 1951, the Third Course of Surgical Medicine, which had been vacant since 1893, became a part of this department. Professor Kentaro Shimizu, head of the First Course of Surgical Medicine, concurrently held the post in the Department of Neurosurgery and the Third Course of Surgical Medicine. The Third Course of Surgical Medicine was established with Julius Scriba who was still in office (never an official professor because of foreign nationality) when the course system was introduced in Japan for the first time in 1893 and had long been vacant since then. In December 1962, Keiji Sano became a professor of the Third Course of Surgical Medicine with a limit on the number of students and was simultaneously appointed the head of the Department of Neurosurgery. On April 1, 1963, the Third Course of Surgical Medicine became the Course of Neurosurgery, and both the course and department were officially approved by the Ministry of Education.

On the other hand, the Second Course of Surgery at Niigata University derived from the First Course of Surgery by Professor Mizuho Nakata in 1953, and Nakata was a professor of the course, which was deemed a neurosurgical course. In reality, however, these two courses used one surgery classroom. In August 1957, Komei Ueki took a post in the Second Course of Surgery. Then, in 1962, the Division of Neurosurgery was established within the Neurosurgical Research Institute, the predecessor to the Brain Research Institute, where Ueki moved from the Second Course of Surgery, and became the Neurosurgical Class both in name and reality. Before long, a neurosurgery course and division were established at Keio University (Professor Tatsuyuki Kudo) in 1963, as well as at Kyoto University (Professor

Hajime Handa) and other universities. Since the inclusion of neurosurgery in the medical departments stipulated in Article 70 of the Medical Service Act, departments of neurosurgery were also established in general hospitals. Now, all university and major hospitals have a department of neurosurgery; and the members of the Japan Neurosurgical Society have rapidly increased.

In 1966 to improve the quality of members, during the 25th meeting of the Japan Neurosurgical Society presided by Prof Tatsuyuki Kudo, it was decided that a board certification system or certification system for physicians specializing should be similar to that of Western societies. The preparatory committee for the first certification system lead by President Keiji Sano was established by 14 dedicated professors from the departments of neurosurgery at that time. These 14 professors were certificated as certified physicians first and drafted regulations on the certification system at the same time. The first review meeting was held on August 31, 1967. After a transient period in 1968, all applicants have been obligated to undergo written and oral examinations starting in 1969.

## India

In India, neurosurgery saw its evolution in leaps and bounds post its independence. Earliest departments were established at CMC Vellore (1949) and Madras Institute of Neurology (1950) by Dr. Jacob Chandy and Dr. B Ramamurthi, respectively. As early as in 1968, India could boast of its first female neurosurgeon Dr. T S Kanaka. Since then, the country has produced about 25 female neurosurgeons till now. Currently in India, neurosurgical training is a well-structured super-specialty program with Master of Chirurgiae (MCh) and Diplomate of National Board (DNB) being the two alternative super-specialty degrees (Fig. 14.2). While MCh is offered mainly by central and state government institutes and some selected private institutions recognized by the Medical Council of India (MCI), DNB is offered mainly by corporate and trust hospitals and only by a few government hospitals. MCh evaluations are done by universities whereas DNBs are conducted by the National Board of Examinations (NBE). The current annual intake in neurosurgery residency across the country is 410, which include 304 MCh and 106 DNB seats. Enrolled trainees

**Fig. 14.2** Neurosurgical training paths in India. DNB Diplomate of National Board, MCh Master of Chirurgiae, NS Neurosurgery, MBBS Medicine Bachelor, Bachelor of Surgery

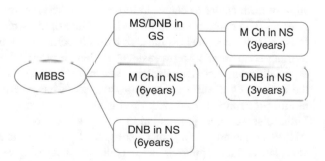

are called Residents. Though around 400 residents are graduating every year, the numbers registered with professional society and/or available in the country do not add up.

This is discussed at the end of the chapter. The different possible neurosurgery training paths are summarized in Fig. 14.2. After the basic medical training (MBBS), one usually joins Master of Surgery (MS)/DNB General Surgery (GS) for 3-year master's degree followed by 3-year MCh/DNB Neurosurgery course, but a direct 6-year integrated MCh/DNB neurosurgery training is an alternative option (less common). The 6-year integrated MCh training is provided only by select central autonomous institutes (AIIMS-D and NIMHANS). Integrated courses have an obligatory 1-year general surgical training during the initial years of the course. The entry introductory neurosurgical training through either ways is uniform and merit-based all over India and is obtained through a single competitive examination [National Eligibility cum Entrance Test Superspeciality (NEET-SS)] organized by the National Board of Examinations at national level with exceptions for institutes of national importance (INIs). INIs are autonomous institutes that conduct their own entrance examinations at national level individually and are only compliant with MCI. The ratio of MCh/DNB-NS to MS/DNB-GS is remarkably low owing to the wider general surgical needs of the country but is on a rise in recent times. This means that there are fewer centers that offer NS training than GS training. Neurosurgical services/training can be seen as largely focused on (1) central institutes such as INIs, (2) state-run prominent government medical colleges, and (3) private, corporate, and trust hospitals in metropolitan and major cities (Table 14.1). The vast majority of these centers are in urban areas and very few in rural/peripheral areas. Central institutes lead the cause of academic excellence by rigorous neurosurgical training and advanced multidisciplinary research. These include AIIMS-D, NIMHANS, PGIMER, JIPMER, SCTIMST, etc. Irrespective of the institute of training, MCh/DNB degree requires the resident to undertake a thesis on a contemporary topic in neurosurgery. Residents work on a rotational basis under various consultants with their own expertise/inclination in subspecialties. They are also rotating in allied neurosciences. During their training, residents are actively engaged in academic seminars, case presentations, and morbidity/mortality meetings. After acceptance of their thesis/dissertation, trainee has to pass the exit examination (theory + practical) at the end of third year in 3-year course and fifth year in 6-year course to be eligible for the award of their respective degree. The academic curriculum though uniform varies slightly from center to center in terms of emphasis on research methodology, basic sciences, and exposure to cutting-edge technologies, which are usually restricted to INIs and top corporate hospitals. To partially compensate this lack of homogeneity in training content, short-term resident exchange programs occur within the country, especially from peripheral centers to the more sophisticated central institutes. Due to the availability of different systems/sources of basic neurosurgery training, a good number of neurosurgeons with varying levels of neurosurgical ability are available in India to serve its huge population. Besides basic NS training, some institutes like AIIMS-D also provide advanced subspecialty training (fellowship) in skull base and vascular, spine, epilepsy, and pediatric neurosurgery. Fellows' selection is

**Table 14.1**  List of institutions with their neurosurgery course

| S no. | Institution (country) | Neurosurgery course, duration (years) | Eligibility criteria | Mode of selection | Thesis/ publication |
|---|---|---|---|---|---|
| 1 | AIIMS, New Delhi, NIMHANS, Bengaluru (India) and other INI (Institute of National importance) | M Ch, 3 years/6 years | MBBS, MS/DNB recognized by Medical Council of India | Online entrance test conducted by institute at national level | Thesis (1) |
| 2 | GTB Hospital, New Delhi (India) | DNB, 3 years | MBBS, MS/DNB recognized by Medical Council of India | National Eligibility cum Entrance Test – Superspeciality | Thesis (1) |
| 3 | BSMMU, Dhaka (Bangladesh) | MS in neurosurgery, 5 years | MBBS recognized by BSMMU plus 2-year (government candidate) and 1-year (nongovernment candidate) service after internship completed | Entrance test at national level | Thesis (1) |
| 4 | Huashan Hospital, Shanghai, China (Neurosurgery Specialist Standardized Training Curriculum) | 7 years | MBBS equivalent | Entrance test at national level | No |
| 5 | Novosibirsk Research Institute of Traumatology and Orthopedics, Novosibirsk (Russia) | License, 2 years | MBBS plus 1-year postgraduate education (surgeon work) | National-level entrance test | Not needed |
| 6 | Universiti Sains Malaysia | Masters of Neurosurgery, 4 years | MBBS equivalent, 12 months house officer, 18 months medical officer in neurosurgery | National-level neurosurgery entrance test | Thesis (1) |

merit-based decided by two-step examination Multiple Choice Questions (MCQs) test followed by clinical exam, organized by the institute at national level.

The Neurological Society of India (NSI), a combined society of all those associated with neurosciences in India, was established in 1951. A total of 1983 neurosurgeons (including trainee surgeons) are registered with NSI. NSI introduced CME system into the academic curriculum and publishes its journal *Neurology India*. Many subspecialty societies have stemmed from NSI such as the Neurosurgery Society of India (NSSI), the Skull Base Surgery Society of India, the Neurospine Society of India, the Indian Society of Stereotactic and Functional Neurosurgery, the Neurotrauma Society of India, the Paediatric Neurosurgery Society of India, and the Indian Society of Cerebrovascular Surgery.

## China

Following Medicine Bachelor, Bachelor of Surgery (MBBS) equivalent bachelor training in medicine lasting 5 or 6 years, neurosurgery training is traditionally done in two stages in China: resident (equivalent to junior resident) for 3 years and attending (equivalent to senior resident) for at least 5 years. These durations are open-ended depending upon the individual performance of the trainee. Prior to 2010, basic neurosurgery training criteria and curriculum were very heterogenous in different regions/institutes of China. Seeing the need of a standardized residency system all over China, the Shanghai Health and Family Planning Commission established a comprehensive program for initial application in Shanghai in 2010. Since 2015, the Neurosurgical Specialist Standardized Training Program (Shanghai model – 7 years training) is introduced in class IIIA hospitals in China and then all over China since 2020. The 7-year training is divided into two steps in this program. Step I (foundation block, 3 years, resident) involves training in general surgery and its allied surgical subspecialties. At completion of step I, resident appears for national examination (written, oral). Only pass candidates are promoted to step II (neurosurgery block, 4 years, attending) to attend various neurosurgery subspecialties and allied branches of neurosciences. Besides internal assessment at the end of each rotation, trainee has to appear for annual examination (written and oral) throughout the course. Step II has been increased to at least 5 years in a recent regulation [2].

## Russia

There are two avenues of neurosurgery training in Russia: teaching and research (3 years – dissertation needed, degree given) or practice (2 years – no dissertation, license to practice given).

### *Novosibirsk Research Institute of Traumatology and Orthopedics, Novosibirsk*

This institute offers 2-year neurosurgery training to MBBS candidates who have undergone 1-year postgraduate education (surgeon work). Annual intake is three residents per year, and selection is done by national-level test. Resident is posted in neurosurgery wards, ICU, emergency, trauma center, neuro-oncology and neuro-orthopedics. He/she is given postings in neurology, neuroradiology, and neuropathology for 1 month each. Besides periodic assessments at the end of every semester, resident undergoes final test examination at the end of 2 years consisting of theory examination (three papers), practical examination including operative case, radiology, and others. Thesis/publication is not an essential prerequisite for appearing in qualifying examination.

## Bangladesh

Bangabandu Sheikh Mujib Medical University (BSMMU), Dhaka, is the premier Postgraduate Medical Institution in Bangladesh. It was established in December 1965 as the Institute of Postgraduate Medical Research (IPGMR). Later, in the year 1998, the government converted IPGMR into a medical university for expanding the facilities for higher medical education and research in the country.

MS course in neurosurgery was started in 1996 (IPGMR) while residency program was started from the year 1998 (BSMMU). The neurosurgery department conducts MS degree course for 5-year duration. The neurosurgery department is located in the C-block of the university. The department has emergency ward and a general ward with its faculty rooms and operation room in the Cabin block.

The candidates for residency program can be either from government, non-government, or from foreign country. Before joining, the candidates have to fulfill criteria as mentioned by the university. Each year, the admission for residency starts in November, while the residency classes start in March 1. The government and nongovernment candidates have to qualify admission test held by the university while foreign students have to appear for an interview to the neurosurgery department after fulfilling all the criteria as mentioned by the university.

The 5-years residency program imparts training in two phases: first 2 years for Phase A (training in neurosurgery allied subjects) and last 3 years for Phase B (exclusive neurosurgery training). Trainee appears for Phase A examination at the end of 2 years and has to pass in all subjects before being promoted to Phase B. After a minimum of 3-year Phase B training and submitting thesis, trainee appears for the final qualifying examination.

## Malaysia

The first center providing neurosurgical services and training in Malaysia began in August 1963, in the capital city of Kuala Lumpur. Initially the general surgeons performed the neurosurgical interventions while general physicians and pediatricians became the archaic neurologists. Dr. Roy Selby, an American neurosurgeon, heralded the beginning of a new era with the establishment of the first Neurosurgical

Centre in Kuala Lumpur Hospital. The first Malaysian trainee was Dr. Nadeson Arumugasamy and started a neurosurgery unit in Kuala Lumpur Hospital in 1969.

The first local training program for neurosurgery was established in 2001 by Professor Jafri Malin Abdullah in the Department of Neurosciences, University Sains Malaysia. This training program consisted of two plus 4 years of focused, comprehensive clinical training in the field of neurosurgery, culminating in a Master of Surgery (Neurosurgery), which was aimed at developing competent neurosurgeons who could provide effective and safe services, fulfilling the needs of a rapidly developing nation.

After medical graduation (MBBS equivalent), aspiring neurosurgeons have to work as house officer for 1 year followed by medical officer in neurosurgery for a minimum of 18 months to be eligible to appear for entrance test for the master's course in neurosurgery (4 years). Neurosurgery training is of minimum 4-year duration. After passing exit examination, he/she has to work for at least 2 years (clinical practice) to be eligible for registration in National Specialist Register.

## Indonesia

The first neurosurgical center in Indonesia was established in Princess Margriet Hospital in 1948, led by Prof. CH Lenshoek from the Netherlands. This was followed by Prof. Handoyo, Prof. Basoeki, Prof. Soewadji, Prof. Padmosantjojo, Prof. Iskarno, and Prof. Satyanegara, who were the pioneers of Indonesian neurosurgeons. The first national neurosurgical training was established in 1977 with twice yearly national board examinations.

The practice of neurosurgery is limited by the licensing system and classification of hospitals – each neurosurgeon is allowed to practice at a maximum of three hospitals. In Indonesia, only government universities are allowed to conduct neurosurgical training program and must have at least one neurosurgical professor and three PhD neurosurgeons with standard facility and minimal number of surgeries per year. The ratio of supervisor to student has been standardized to 1:3. The length of education is 11 semesters. There are currently eight centers for neurosurgery education. The residency education program in Indonesia takes 5.5 years to complete. During the first 3.5 years, residents undergo the first stage in the form of general surgery basic courses, master programs, and basic neurosurgery. Residents may start off assisting in surgery and, as they progress, begin to perform on their own according to the type of case and difficulty index.

## Pakistan

Neurosurgery service in *Pakistan* began in 1951 with a spinal tumor resection surgery. Prof. Bashir Ahmed, Prof. Qazi, and Prof. OV Jooma were the pioneers who started neurosurgery and continued to train young surgeons to provide basic services. Functional and complex surgeries were performed in the 1960s. The Pakistan Society of

Neurosurgeons was established in 1987 with 22 neuro and general surgeons. This was registered with WFNS in 1987, and WFNS interim meeting was held in Lahore in 1989, under the chairmanship of Prof. Iftikhar Raja. Next few decades saw exponential growth of neurosurgery and modernization. Like other postgraduate courses, neurosurgery training in dedicated training centers of Pakistan is called as fellowship (FCPS). After MBBS equivalent medical graduation and 1-year house job, neurosurgery training aspirant is eligible to appear for Neurosurgery Fellowship Entrance Exam (FCPS part I exam) conducted by the College of Physicians and Surgeons, Pakistan (CPSP). FCPS Neurosurgery is of 4–5-year duration and is of two parts: Part I (general specialty training like surgery for initial 2 years) followed by intermediate module exam, and then Part II (exclusive neurosurgery training for later 2–3 years) followed by final FCPS exit exam. Currently, there are 212 neurosurgeons serving 200 million populations with 415 trainees nationwide in Pakistan. The challenge for the Pakistan Society of Neurosurgeons is to retain over 400 trainees by providing them incentives and post-fellowship training.

## The Philippines

Early pioneers in neurosurgery in the *Philippines* were in the 1930s. The Philippine Society of Neurological Surgeons was founded in 1961 by eight fellows, followed by the establishment of the Academy of Filipino Neurosurgeons in 1999.

The neurosurgical residency is a 6-year program. At present, there are 10 accredited training programs. Training is, at minimum, 72 months (6 years) in duration. The first year is spent in general surgery. The next 5 years involve rotations in the neurology, neuropathology, neurodiagnostics, neuroscience, and free electives, and research. A total of 48 months is devoted to neurosurgery, marked by progressively increasing responsibility in clinics. The certifying examinations come in three parts: written, oral, and practical. The written examination covers the subspecialty topics of neurosurgery. Passing this examination is a prerequisite to sitting for the oral examination in the form of an objective structured clinical examination during which the candidates will be expected to show that they have acquired the capability to diagnose and prognosticate neurosurgical disorders, perform major neurosurgical procedures, and manage complications. The practical examination involves demonstrating a neurosurgical procedure to the examiners. This examination is usually waived for graduates of training programs accredited by the Board. Research output is a requisite for graduation. There is a requirement to make one oral or poster presentation at a national or international conference, and to publish at least one clinical paper as the primary author in a peer-reviewed medical journal.

## Other Asian Countries

The *Sri Lankan* neurosurgical services were started back in 1956 with the establishment of 12-bedded neurosurgical wards by Dr. S.A. Cabral at the General Hospital, Colombo. Here, the basic neurosurgery education is three and a half years of general surgical training followed by 2-year local neurosurgery training and 2-year training abroad. The Fellowship of the Royal Colleges of Surgeons Specialty Examination in Neurosurgery (FRCS–SN) program was started in 2018.

The Nepalese Society of Neurosurgeons (NESON) was established in 2008 with 12 members. In *Nepal*, the prerequisite to enroll into the 3-year neurosurgery residency (MCh) program is to have a master's in general surgery (Master of Surgery, MS, or equivalent) qualification. The current deficit is 215 neurosurgeons as per recommended ratio of 1 neurosurgeon to 100,000 population in Nepal.

The services in *Kazakhstan* have been in existence since 1964. In *Uzbekistan*, for those enrolled in master's program, the training period is 3 years, while for those in the residency program, training period is 4 years. The Kazakh National Center for neurosurgery, which was opened in 2008, is one of the 50 neurosurgical specialized centers in Kazakhstan. The ratio of trainer to trainee is 1:3 in the neurosurgery master training program in Uzbekistan. Advance training is compulsory for all practicing neurosurgeons every 5 years.

The Neurosurgical Association of *Thailand* was found in 1982, followed by the establishment of the Royal College of Neurological Surgeons of Thailand in 2013.

Local training program in *Myanmar* started in 2016. At the moment, there are only four well-equipped neurosurgical centers in Myanmar.

## Neurosurgical Training and Care in Asia: Challenges and Opportunities

Analyzing the various curriculums across the countries, a proposal for achieving uniformity in training to attain common standards is warranted with emphasis on minimum number of hours in operating theater/cases operated, optimal exposures to subspecialties and allied branches, and engaging in academic seminars and surgical skill labs. Minimum basic infrastructure needed at the training center includes dedicated neurosurgery ward beds (at least 20) and neuro-ICU beds with ventilator and monitors (at least five), exclusive neurosurgery operation rooms, microscope, C-arm, and surgical drills along with availability of CT and MRI scanners. In high-income countries, neuroendoscopy, stereotaxic equipment, and ultrasonic aspirators along with angiography facilities are desirable. A good teacher to student ratio (e.g., 1:2 per batch), weekly seminars, journal clubs, case conferences, and morbidity/mortality discussion will ensure academic competence irrespective of economic drawbacks. Since the duration of training programs varies across countries, a minimum hands-on exposure of 400 cases during the entire residency program should be set accounting for the difference in patient flow to the hospitals. Exposure to all subspecialties (spinal, skull base, neurovascular, pediatric neurosurgeries, etc.) by rotation even for a brief stint equips the residents with basic knowledge and sets the path for future learning. Maintaining logbooks by each resident keeps themselves documented and tracked during the residency. Short-term posting to another national or international center of excellence via exchange programs in the final year exposes them to a different setup with different protocols and management skills, thus giving them the opportunity to think out of the box.

In countries like India and other low-income or low–middle-income countries, both the demographic diversity and the existence of different kinds of hospitals with respect to infrastructure, curriculum, exposure, etc., affect the training and delivery of care in multiple ways. Lack of insurance impacts the extent people seek neurosurgical treatment. Though an impressive number of graduating neurosurgeons are available per year, one does not see this reflected in the numbers available in hospitals. This is largely due to the unavailability of infrastructure and lack of a neurosurgery department in medical colleges.

Many go abroad for fellowships and never return to country. Thereby lies the crux of the problem. It is estimated that 50–60% neurosurgeons are concentrated in eight major cities of India with 10% population. This is a common problem in most low-income Asian countries. Patients from rural parts often travel long distances to reach tertiary center, which leads to the loss of crucial time window of successful intervention. Even if there are some neurosurgeons in a peripheral center, lack of a dedicated neurosurgery department, funds, and operation rooms limits the delivery of neurosurgical services. Training in private teaching and corporate hospital limits the hands-on training of the residents due to the patients demanding senior surgeons to operate on them and due to limited exposure to complex cases requiring complex procedures. Achieving equity in infrastructure and improving the standards of training by uniform curriculum is essential for good neurosurgical care for any country. To this end, policymakers should consider reforms that ensure increased funds in peripheral hospitals develop dedicated NS departments with basic infrastructure and pay competent incentives to the doctors working in rural/underprivileged communities. Affiliating multiple small peripheral centers to the regional tertiary care hospital can help in streamlining the referral system and training. Interest-free loans should be provided for institutes to develop NS infrastructure. This eventually would reduce the disparity in doctor patient ratio, which is high in urban and low in rural training centers. Proper streamlined segregation of patients by an established national referral system can ensure the optimal usage of all centers with varied sophistication: for example, one can avoid commuting of a patient with disc prolapse to travel 1000 miles to reach an apex center since there is no proper referral system. Technological advances such as telemedicine and tele-neuroradiology could also help a great deal in this regard, which we are already realizing in this COVID-19 era. Brain drain from middle- and low-income countries to the other pastures is a huge concern and has to be tackled with strict policymaking and paying competent salaries and perks.

Another issue is that the number of neurosurgeons trained in these institutes and the neurosurgeons working in the community is not tallying up. This could be because most of them go abroad after getting trained and some of them get into administrative work and stop practicing.

# Conclusion

Most developing countries still lack adequate number of medical workforces in the care of neurosurgical patients, neurosurgical infrastructure, and neurosurgical training. The shortage of neurosurgical facilities includes dedicated neurosurgical beds, intensive care unit beds, and hospitals with adequate neurosurgery capacity. Streamlining the referral system can help in ensuring optimal use of available infrastructure in the resource-depleted countries. To achieve true standards of neurosurgery at the global level, the concept of an international consensus in ensuring sound knowledge and practical competency through a world certifying body is essential. The contributions from all neurosurgical societies across the world to model their training curriculum based on an examination model with high standards and international validity should be the next strategy for neurosurgery around the world. The needs for sub-specialization have been catalyzed by the exponential growth of neurosurgical knowledge.

**Acknowledgments** The authors thank Prof. Kanak kanti Barua, Prof. Akhlaque Hossain Khan, and Dr. Abu Obaida from Bangladesh; Dr. Peleganchuk Aleksey from Russia; and Dr. Regunath Kandasamy, Prof. Zamzuri Idris, and Dr. Mah Jon Kooi from Malaysia.

# References

1. Kato Y, Liew BS, Sufianov AA, Rasulic L, Arnautovic KI, Dong VH, et al. Review of global neurosurgery education: horizon of neurosurgery in the developing countries. Chin Neurosurg J. 2020;6:19. https://doi.org/10.1186/s41016-020-00194-1.
2. Xu T, Evins AI, Lin N, Chang J, Hu G, Lijun Hou L, et al. Neurosurgical postgraduate training in China: moving toward a national training standard. World Neurosurg. 2016;96:410–6. https://doi.org/10.1016/j.wneu.2016.09.034. Epub 2016 Sep 15.

## *Suggested Reading*

Ferraris KP, Matsumura H, Wardhana DPW, Vesagas T, Seng K, Ali MRM, et al. The state of neurosurgical training and education in East Asia: analysis and strategy development for this frontier of the world. Neurosurg Focus. 2020;48(3):E7.
Haglund MM, Fuller AT. Global neurosurgery: innovators, strategies, and the way forward. J Neurosurg. 2019;131(4):993–9. https://doi.org/10.3171/2019.4.JNS181747.
Ganapathy K. Distribution of neurologists and neurosurgeons in India and its relevance to the adoption of telemedicine. Neurol India. 2015;63:142–54.
Banerji AK. Neurosurgical training and evaluation– need for a paradigm shift. Neurol India. 2016;64:1119–24. https://doi.org/10.4103/0028-3886.193841.
Mishra BK, Singh VP. Neurosurgery in India. AANS Neurosurg. 2017;26(1):1–4. Available at URL: https://aansneurosurgeon.org/inside-neurosurgeon/neurosurgery-in-india/.
Raj A, Agrawal A. Neurosurgery in India: success and challenges. Int J Acad Med. 2018;4:89–90. Available from URL: http://www.ijam-web.org/text.asp?2018/4/1/89/230851.

Fuller AT, Barkley A, Du R, Elahi C, Tafreshi AR, Von Isenburg M, Haglund MM. Global neuro-surgery: a scoping review detailing the current state of international neurosurgical outreach. J Neurosurg. 2020;8:1–9. https://doi.org/10.3171/2020.2.JNS192517. Online ahead of print. PMID: 32384268.

Shamim MS, Tahir MZ, Godil SS, Kumar R, Siddiqui AA. A critical analysis of the current state of neurosurgery training in Pakistan. Surg Neurol Int. 2011;2:183. Published online 2011 Dec 26. https://doi.org/10.4103/2152-7806.91138. PMCID: PMC3263003. PMID: 22276237.

Suzuki M, Suehiro E. Questionnaire survey for board-certified neurosurgeons. Jpn J Neurosurg (Tokyo). 2017;26:817–28. (Japanese).

Japan Neurosurgical Society. 16th annual report of general meeting of members. Osaka, Japan: Japan Neurosurgical Society; 2019 (Japanese). https://www.jnss.or.jp/jns_web/html/activity/meeting/pdf/main/78_syainsoukai_1.pdf. Accessed 22 Jan 2020.

Japan Neurosurgical Society. List of training facilities 2019. Tokyo: Japan Neurosurgical Society, 2019 (Japanese). http://jns.umin.ac.jp/jns_wp/wp-content/uploads/2019/11/program-list_2019.xlsx. Accessed 22 Jan 2020.

Gasco J, Braun JD, McCutcheon IE, Black PM. Neurosurgery certification in member societies of the World Federation of Neurosurgical Societies: Asia. World Neurosurg. 2011;75(3–4):325–34.

Gasco J, Barber SM, McCutcheon IE, Black PM. Neurosurgery certification in member societies of the WFNS: global overview. World Neurosurg. 2011;76(3–4):231–8. https://doi.org/10.1016/j.wneu.2010.10.036. PubMed PMID: 21986411.

Zhang Y, Xue C, Mao Y. Present status and development of Chinese neurosurgeons. Literature from The Sixth National Congress of Chinese Congress of Neurological Surgeons. 2011. p. 8–11. (Chinese).

McLaughlin N, Rodstein J, Burke MA, Martin NA. Demystifying process mapping: a key step in neurosurgical quality improvement initiatives. Neurosurgery. 2014;75(2):99–109.

Khan AH, Hossain ATMM, Shalike N, Barua KK. Evolution of neurosurgery in Bangladesh. Bangladesh J Neurosurg. 2019;8(2):57–62.

Wahjoepramono EJ. Editorial neurosurgery in Indonesia. Int Neurosci J. 2015;1:e863.

Takakura K. Asia and the World Federation of Neurosurgical Societies, World Federation of Neurosurgical Societies Chapter 4.3. https://www.wfns.org/WFNSData/Document/Chapter4-3.pdf.

Bakhshi SK, Waqas M, Alam MM, Shamim MS, Qadeer M. Neurosurgery training in Pakistan: follow-up survey and critical analysis of National Training Programmes. J Pak Med Assoc. 2016;66(Suppl 3)(10):S75–77. PubMed PMID: 27895361.

Kolegium Bedah Saraf Indonesia. Standar Nasional Pendidikan Dokter Spesialis Bedah Saraf. KDSI: Jakarta; 2007.

Preparatory survey report on the project for construction of Mongolia–Japan Teaching Hospital in Mongolia, Japan International Cooperation Agency. 2014. https://openjicareport.jica.go.jp/pdf/12185039_01.pdf.

Myint AT, Thu M. Assisted education for specialized medicine: a sustainable development plan for neurosurgery in Myanmar. World Neurosurg. 2019;130:e85461. https://doi.org/10.1016/j.wneu.2019.07.018. Epub 2019 Jul 8. PubMed PMID: 31295600.

Hashimoto N. Asia and Asian neurosurgery. World Neurosurg. 2011;75(3–4):350–1. https://doi.org/10.1016/j.wneu.2010.06.022. PubMed PMID: 21600462.

Roka Y. Neurosurgery in Eastern Nepal: the past, present and future and a near decade of personal experience. Nepal J Neurosci. 2017;14(2):1–2. https://doi.org/10.3126/njn.v14i2.19696.

Country fact sheet: Uzbekistan. 2014 International organization for migration (IOM). https://aus-tria.iom.int/sites/default/files/IOM%202014_%20CFS%20Uzbekistan.pdf.

Benzel EC. Neurosurgery education: the pursuit of excellence. Clin Neurosurg. 2010;57:49–55. PubMed PMID: 21280494.

Ansari A. From the realms of the depths of neurosurgery. Asian J Neurosurg. 2019;14:1057.

https://www.mciindia.org/CMS/information-desk/college-and-course-search.

# Chapter 15
# Neurosurgery Education Around the World: Australasia

Heidi McAlpine, Edward Mee, John Laidlaw, Andrew Kaye, and Katharine Drummond

## Introduction

Neurosurgery is a relatively young specialty, especially in Australasia, which is the geographic region including Australia, New Zealand and Papua New Guinea (PNG). Due to our relatively small population, Australasian neurosurgical education has been closely linked with a single surgical college, the Royal Australasian College of Surgeons (RACS), which unites all surgeons and governs the training of nine surgical specialties, including neurosurgery, in partnership with specialty training boards. We describe the evolution of neurosurgical training in Australasia from a humble offshoot of general surgery to a mature specialty facing the unique challenges of the Australasian region and look to the challenges of the future.

H. McAlpine · J. Laidlaw
Department of Neurosurgery, The Royal Melbourne Hospital, Parkville, VIC, Australia
e-mail: heidi.mcalpine@mh.org.au; john.laidlaw@mh.org.au

E. Mee
Department of Neurosurgery, Auckland City Hospital, Grafton, Auckland, New Zealand

A. Kaye
Department of Neurosurgery, Hadassah University Hospital, Ein Karem, Kyriat Hadassah, Jerusalem, Israel
e-mail: andrewk@hadassah.org.il

K. Drummond (✉)
Department of Neurosurgery, The Royal Melbourne Hospital, Parkville, VIC, Australia

Department of Surgery, University of Melbourne, Parkville, VIC, Australia
e-mail: kate.drummond@mh.org.au

© The Author(s), under exclusive license to Springer Nature Switzerland AG 2022
I. M. Germano (ed.), *Neurosurgery and Global Health*,
https://doi.org/10.1007/978-3-030-86656-3_15

209

## Historical Background

### *The Royal Australasian College of Surgeons*

The first surgeons in the early colonies of Australia and New Zealand came from various backgrounds, including the navy and army, and later free settlers, and were largely trained in Great Britain or Ireland. The first Australian medical school was in Melbourne, with the first cohort of graduates in 1867. In New Zealand, the first medical school was formed in Dunedin, in 1875. All graduates were considered trained in both medicine and surgery; however, those who wished to undertake more dedicated surgical practice commonly travelled, like their teachers before them, to the British Isles, to become fellows of one of the colleges of Great Britain or Ireland [1]. In 1920, Professor Louis Barnett of Dunedin, at a meeting of the New Zealand Branch of the British Medical Association in his home city, proposed that an association should be founded to raise surgical standards and recognise surgical expertise in Australia and New Zealand. This was partly associated with the progressive movement towards independence from the United Kingdom and also inspired by the establishment of the American College of Surgeons. Considerable debate took place, and it wasn't until a group of surgeons from the teaching hospitals in Australasia met in Sydney in 1926 that an Australasian College of Surgeons was proposed. The 19 founders of the college subsequently met in Dunedin in 1927 and took the opportunity to form the College of Surgeons of Australasia [2]. The objectives of the college included "the cultivation and maintenance of the highest principles of surgical practice and ethics, promotion of the practice of surgery under proper conditions, the arrangement of adequate postgraduate surgical training, and the promotion of research in surgery" [1]. Thus, the foundation of the Australasian College was an amalgam of the best of British and American traditions. In 1931, King George V granted use of the prefix "Royal", and thus the Royal Australasian College of Surgeons (RACS) was born at the opening ceremony of the new headquarters in Melbourne in 1935 [1].

The training of all surgeons in Australasia remains the responsibility of the RACS, which defines the minimum training requirements and ensures, by a summative exit examination introduced in 1956 [3], that defined standards are attained on the completion of training. Previous models included a few years of "basic" surgical training rotating through various surgical and critical care specialties, with subsequent admission to "advanced" training in one of nine surgical subspecialties (including neurosurgery) in an accredited hospital post [4, 5]. Specialty surgical training and the curriculum was overseen by specialty training boards. In the final year of training, trainees deemed eligible based on supervisors' reports, logbooks and progressive assessments were able to present for the centralised final examination [4, 6] with written, clinical and oral sections, to receive fellowship of the Royal Australasian College of Surgeons (FRACS). The majority of fellows undertook further training in overseas units, often in the United Kingdom, but now commonly in the United States and other overseas units [1].

In 2008, the basic and advanced surgical training model was replaced by the Surgical Education and Training (SET) program with neurosurgical trainees no longer undergoing a formal period of basic training but accepted directly into neurosurgical training at some period after their internship. The move away from the basic/advanced model of surgical training was influenced by two main factors. The first was that there were insufficient positions for all trainees accepted into basic training to progress to advanced training, creating unrealistic expectations and a cohort of partly trained "perpetual basic trainees". The second was a range of educational, social, regulatory and political factors, informed by the changing demography of medical graduates (older and more likely to have partners and families), as well as commonwealth and state government demands [7]. The SET program incorporates selection directly into the surgical specialty of choice, and a change to competency, rather than time-based training [7]. RACS identified nine competencies of trained surgeons, and the curriculum and assessment of the SET program align to these [8]. They include medical expert, communicator, collaborator, professional, manager-leader, health advocate, technical expert, scholar-teacher and judgement decision-maker [8]. Both generic and specialty-specific eligibility criteria apply, and a single merit-based state, national or bi-national selection takes place in each specialty, depending on the size of the specialty [7]. Neurosurgery selection, training and curriculum are now overseen by the SET Board of the Neurosurgical Society of Australasia (NSA) contracted by RACS who administer and oversee overall governance and the final examination and awarding of FRACS.

## The Neurosurgical Society of Australasia

The first Australasian neurosurgeons, prior to the establishment of the NSA, were general surgeons with an interest in neurosurgery and were largely self-taught. There was neither the population nor the resources to support a dedicated pioneer neurosurgeon, and most surgeons serving this small and far-flung population tried their hand at everything. A small number of these general surgeons had worked in renowned units in the United Kingdom, where the principles of Lister were practiced and the pioneering surgery of Macewan, Horsley and Godlee had been recognised. Probably the first documented posterior fossa procedure for a cyst was carried out in Dunedin, New Zealand, in 1889, and in 1890 a craniotomy was also performed in Dunedin in what was "very probably the first successful operation of its kind to be performed in Australia or New Zealand". In Melbourne, at the St Vincent's Hospital, a convexity meningioma was successfully removed and reported on in 1895 [9]. Dr. (later Sir) Douglas Miller, from St Vincent's Hospital, Sydney, was instrumental in proposing the formation of a neurosurgical society in Australasia, and in 1939 he wrote to seven like-minded surgeons suggesting an organisation. The Neurosurgical Society of Australasia was established by these eight founding members at a meeting in Melbourne on April 19, 1940 (originally named the Society of Australasian Neurological Surgeons) (Fig. 15.1). The first president was Dr. (and

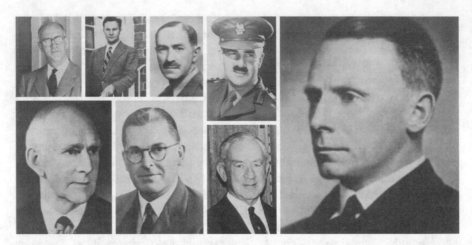

**Fig. 15.1** Founding members of the Neurosurgical Society of Australasia (NSA). Clockwise from top left: D. McKenzie, F. Morgan, G. Phillips, R. Money, A. Coates, D. Miller, L. Lindon, H. Trumble. (With permission from the NSA)

later Sir) Albert Coates, the first neurosurgeon at The Royal Melbourne Hospital [9, 10]. The society was at first conceived as an informal club for scientific meetings and the exchange of views [9]. Over the years, it grew into the governing body for the specialty, an organisation for the training of neurosurgeons in Australia and New Zealand, and in partnership with RACS, responsible for determining the requirements necessary for certification of neurosurgeons [9].

Even after the establishment of the RACS and the NSA, prior to 1960 the majority of Australian neurosurgeons trained overseas (primarily in the United Kingdom), due to the limited opportunities in Australasia. In subsequent years neurosurgery training programs, based in hospitals, were developed in Australia and New Zealand, in concert with the other specialties [11], with the first bi-national neurosurgical training seminar being held in 1970. These seminars continue today, when all trainees from Australia and New Zealand meet for didactic education and networking [11]. In common with comparable programs in other countries, neurosurgical training in Australia and New Zealand is based on the Halstedian apprenticeship model, which implements Osler's principle of learning by practical experience [12, 13].

## Modern Neurosurgical Training

Table 15.1 summarises the components of the neurosurgery selection and training process in Australasia. Australia is a large country with a relatively small population of approximately 25 million people. Neurosurgical units are generally located in the major cities, which lie on the coast, some widely separated and servicing relatively small populations. In Australia, there are 27 training units in 11 cities, none of which are inland, with 49 training positions accredited by the NSA. New Zealand

**Table 15.1** Components of the (**A**) selection process and (**B**) of the neurosurgical training program in Australasia in 2020

| (A) |
| --- |
| Selection to training preceded by 2 or more years of pre-vocational surgical and critical care experience including a minimum of 24 weeks of neurosurgery experience |
| Transparent selection with published assessment standards and criteria |
| Selection based on scores from curriculum vitae, referee reports, neuroanatomy exam and structured interview (Table 15.2) |
| Three referees selected by the SET Board, from recent supervisors proposed by trainee |
| Referees interviewed by two interviewers using structured proforma with marking rubric |
| Interviews are four clinical scenarios with three interviewers scoring against set criteria |
| **(B)** |
| Bi-national (Australia and New Zealand) program administered by SET Board of NSA |
| Competency based not time based |
| Divided into basic (1–2 years), intermediate (3 years) and advanced (1–2 years) training sections |
| Operative competencies and minimum caseload must be achieved for progression |
| Academic, clinical, research and professional standards assessed quarterly and must be achieved for progression |
| Training in a minimum of two, and usually three training units[a], including one paediatric term |
| Compulsory 6 monthly bi-national neurosurgery training seminars at which all trainees gather from Australia and New Zealand for a 2 or 3 day interactive seminar on a selected subspecialty area of neurosurgery with presentations by both trainees and faculty, as well as practice exams |
| Exit examination in the final stage of training administered by RACS |
| Training units accredited every 5 years against multiple criteria (Table 15.4) |
| Performance of training units reviewed annually against trainee logbooks and feedback |

[a]There are currently 32 accredited training units in Australia (27), New Zealand (4) and Singapore (1)

has five neurosurgical units spread over two islands with just under 5 million population. Five training positions are accredited by the NSA in these units with, and four additional positions are filled with senior residents from North American neurosurgical units. The case mix and case load of these various Australasian units led to specific challenges in providing a balanced and broad educational experience in all the accredited units. In the late 1980s the Training Board of the NSA determined that many smaller single neurosurgical units in Australia and New Zealand could not provide the breadth of experience and case load required for adequate training of neurosurgeons. This led to the formulation of a centralised bi-national training program between 1991 and 1994 under the leadership of Professor Peter Reilly, with trainees moving between neurosurgical units every 1 or 2 years, with at least one interstate or international allocation. Most trainees would rotate through three or four training units, with the benefit of training and mentorship by 20 or more individual neurosurgeons, which would not be possible in a single smaller unit. Trainees were selected centrally for the bi-national neurosurgical training program. Central accreditation of training posts by the NSA board had already been instituted under the previous board chair, Professor Leigh Atkinson, and this had informed the need for rotation through a number of training units for a broad and adequate training experience [14]. Neurosurgical training in Australia and New Zealand has subsequently undergone under a number of evolutions. The curriculum has been reviewed regularly, with a major review in 2005 to ensure that "assessment drives learning" [3] and a further update planned for 2022. Training has lengthened from 4 to 5 or more years and has evolved to include competency-based training with the possibility of flexible working hours, and the need for regular in-training assessments, in addition to the long-standing exit exam.

The RACS and the NSA have also been influential in the development of neurosurgery and neurosurgical services in the Pacific region, particularly PNG, but also Fiji, the Cook Islands, Timor-Leste and Samoa. Professor Jeffrey Rosenfeld has been instrumental [10, 15], co-authoring *Neurosurgery in the Tropics: A Practical Approach to Common Problems*, a textbook aimed at neurosurgical knowledge for general surgeons in remote settings [16, 17]. He is an honorary professor at the University of PNG. He and other Australasian neurosurgeons have travelled frequently to PNG as both surgeons and educators of general surgeons in common neurosurgical procedures. Subsequently, neurosurgeons have trained in PNG, including with specialty training at Townsville Hospital under the mentorship of Dr. Eric Guazzo.

## Current Status and Controversies of Neurosurgical Education in Australasia

### Current Status of Neurosurgical Education

Neurosurgical training continues under the basic model described above, with trainees selected across Australia and New Zealand by the SET Board of the NSA, which also oversees the accreditation of training posts and curriculum. The exit examination is conducted by RACS and involves two written papers consisting of five essays and five short answer questions, oral examination in neuroanatomy, neuropathology, neuroradiology and operative surgery, as well as a clinical examination involving actual patients. The chief controversies in Australasian neurosurgical training have been arguably the two most important aspects of producing excellent neurosurgeons, that is, selection of excellent trainees [18, 19] and accreditation of training units or programs for excellence [20–22]. Due to the unique training environment in Australia, these aspects of neurosurgical education have recently been under close scrutiny [14].

Despite general satisfaction with training, there are specific challenges related to a centralised system. The first is the selection of applicants for training. There has never been a rigorous evaluation of neurosurgery (or any other surgical specialty) trainee selection, and no superior method is agreed upon [18, 19, 23]. In the Australasian system, the choice of trainees by a central selection panel, with subsequent allocation of that trainee to an accredited training unit, has led to much discussion, particularly when an underperforming trainee is recognised. While the selection process is arduous and transparent, not all trainees complete training, and disciplinary proceedings due to poor performance, even late in training, are not uncommon. Whether this is due to poor selection processes or a lack of "skin in the game" for the training unit is not clear. For instance, if a particular unit does not take "ownership" of a trainee from the time of appointment to the end of training and early independent practice, then it may be more straightforward to give an excellent reference or pass a trainee in a placement to allow them to move to the next, rather than take the more difficult and sometimes adversarial or litigious path of giving genuine negative feedback, refusing to give a reference or even fail a trainee in a placement. This is in stark contrast to training systems such as in the United States, which are institution based and where ownership of and investment in the trainee is high, possibly leading to a more coordinated oversight of progression. However, limitations of institution-based training may include less transparent selection processes, trainee exploitation and creation of "orphan" graduates if not ultimately employed by their training institution but without broad experience to succeed elsewhere.

Similarly, if trainees, and often their families, are to be moved nationally and internationally between training units, and as trainee experience rightly becomes more appreciated, the quality of training posts is paramount. Thus, the minimum standards for accreditation of a neurosurgical unit as a training post have been strictly defined, and regular feedback is sought from trainees on their experience in each post.

## Selection of Neurosurgical Trainees

In many respects, selection of neurosurgical trainees by the SET Board of the NSA is similar to other international neurosurgical programs. Selection includes analysis of a structured curriculum vitae (CV), including previous research and publications. A major component of the CV is also previous neurosurgical experience, as Australasian medical graduates enter specialty training after internship and a period of pre-vocational training, where they may gain experience in a number of specialties, including neurosurgery. A minimum standard for the CV must be attained, and the applicant must also sit a 70-question neurosurgery anatomy multiple-choice exam. A satisfactory performance in the CV and exam will lead to reference checks from three referees, with the subsequent selection of the 24 total highest-scoring applicants from the first three components for the final semi-structured interviews, all of which are standardised clinical scenario interviews with defined marking rubrics. The weighting of each component of the selection process is shown in Table 15.2. The numbers of applicants in 2019 and their performance in the selection process are shown in Table 15.3.

**Table 15.2** Weighting of the components of the selection process for applicants to neurosurgery training in Australasia

| Component | Weighting | Satisfactory performance |
|---|---|---|
| Structured curriculum vitae | 15% | 50% (5.5 of 11 possible) |
| Neurosurgery anatomy exam[a] | 30% | 70% |
| Referee report | 30% | 50% (36 of 72 possible) |
| Neurosurgery semi-structured interview | 25% | 50% (8 of 16 possible) |

[a]Exam is a 70-question multiple choice exam

**Table 15.3** The numbers of applicants for neurosurgery training in Australasia in 2019 and their performance in the components of the selection process

|  | Curriculum vitae | Anatomy exam | Referee report | Interview |
|---|---|---|---|---|
| Applicants scored | 66 | 66 | 54[a] | 24 (6 female, 25%) |
| Number passed female | 15 (22.7%) | 14 (21.2%) | 11 (20.3%) | NA |
| Number passed male | 48 (72.7%) | 44 (66.7%) | 36 (66.7%) | NA |

Applicants are ranked and allocated according to the number of training positions available, typically 6–11 per year. In 2019, nine places were available with seven male and two female successful applicants

*CV* curriculum vitae, *NA* not applicable

[a]One applicant withdrew following the CV and examination. Of 66 CVs scored, only 63 applicants obtained sufficient points to be further considered. Of 66 applicants who sat the anatomy exam, only 58 obtained a passing mark, leaving 54 applicants proceeding to referee interviews reports. Of the 54 applicants proceeding to referee interview reports, 37 obtained a sufficient score to proceed to interview, and these were ranked based on their total score, and the top 24 applicants were interviewed

Of these components over the previous 10 years, the most contentious has been the referee report. The past experience of the SET Board, and other authors [18, 23], was that standard written references, either using a pro forma or a letter of recommendation, did not discriminate between applicants, with many candidates submitting perfect scores, or overly positive written references, not reflecting their subsequent performance in training.

Thus, the major modification and revolution in the Australasian selection process has been the change to obtaining referee reports using a semi-structured interview process. Referee reports are obtained from three neurosurgeons, often from different neurosurgical units, who have recently worked with the applicant. The applicant does not choose the referees specifically but nominates a selection of recent supervisors who are not SET board members, any of whom may be chosen for interview by the Board. The reference interview is undertaken by two neurosurgeon members of the SET Board, with a member of the executive staff transcribing the discussion and recording scores. The components of each interview are collated into a final score. The reference interview follows a basic script with questions for further probing of answers, and a marking rubric is supplied. While this is an extremely time-consuming process, this method of obtaining referee reports has resulted in a wider spread of scores and is more able to separate high and low scoring applicants than other components of the selection process.

In 2014, using a pro forma written reference, the average score was 33.7/35 (96%, range 24.3–35), and this result was typical of previous years with many applicants obtaining a near perfect score. In 2015, the first year the reference interview was utilised, the average score was 17.1/30 (57%, range 8–25), and this continued in subsequent years with average scores between 58% and 76%. Thus, the references obtained by interview of three referees produce a wider spread of scores and a lower average score than written references, making them more suitable to separate applicants into higher and lower performing groups [14].

The referee report script includes the following components, each with multiple questions, to assess the nine agreed competencies of a RACS surgeon as described above.

*Context* – the relationship of the referee to the applicant, including length, capacity and circumstance of contact.

*Technical skills* – the competence of the applicant for basic neurosurgical procedures, including dexterity, orderly flow, positioning, dealing with complications, evidence of preparatory study, level of supervision required and ability to work under pressure.

*Collaboration and teamwork, medical expertise and judgement* – the quality of the applicant's patient care, including trustworthiness of assessments, recognition of complications, organisation, punctuality, communication skills and interactions with nursing, emergency department and intensive care unit staff.

*Communication and professionalism* – the quality of the applicant's communication with both senior and junior staff and patients, including precision, accuracy and civility. Professional behaviours such as contactability, reliability, workload management and honesty are explored, including a mature response to mistakes and negative feedback, taking personal responsibility and not blaming others.

*Scholarship and teaching, readiness for training* – the applicant's attendance at, level of contribution to and enthusiasm for educational sessions.

Finally, the referee is questioned as whether the applicant is ready for training (or would benefit from further pre-vocational experience before formal training).

## Accreditation of Neurosurgical Training Units

The accreditation of training posts is critical to the success of the training experience. Training units are accredited every 5 years by the SET Board of the NSA in accordance with policies formulated by the RACS (although shorter periods of accreditation may be given if deficiencies need to be rectified). Accreditation involves both site visits, with physical inspection and interview of trainees, neurosurgeons and other staff, and review of application documents for adherence to published criteria (Table 15.4). Accreditation may be of a single site or commonly of two or three collaborating sites with a primary site taking overarching responsibility. For instance, many large tertiary neurosurgical centres have secondary community or private hospitals in close proximity, which act as collaborating training sites.

**Table 15.4** Summary of the NSA SET Board training post accreditation standards

| Standard | Theme | Principles |
|---|---|---|
| 1 | A hospital with a culture of respect for patients and staff | Policies, procedures and staff education to provide a safe training environment free of discrimination, bullying and sexual harassment; actively promoting teamwork and professionalism<br>Policies and guidelines aligned with RACS Code of Conduct<br>Commitment to share complaint and misdemeanour information with the SET Board<br>Robust complaint management and performance review processes |
| 2 | Education facilities and systems | Computer facilities, Internet access and tutorial rooms<br>Private study areas isolated from busy clinical areas |
| 3 | Quality education, training and learning | Coordinated schedule of education without conflicting obligations. Four hours of structured neurosurgeon-led tutorials, one neuropathology session, one Journal Club and 4 h neuroradiology sessions per month<br>Access to simulated learning and basic skills training equipment<br>Educational leave to attend compulsory courses, scientific meetings, biannual trainee seminars and examinations<br>Opportunity to participate in research<br>Supervised management of patients in an emergency department accredited by the Australasian College of Emergency Medicine or equivalent and an intensive care unit accredited by the Australia and New Zealand College of Anaesthetists or equivalent |
| 4 | Neurosurgical training supervisors and staff | A neurosurgical training supervisor who satisfies the requirements of the RACS Surgical Supervisors Policy and NSA Training Program Regulations, with a fellowship in neurosurgery from the RACS, membership of the NSA, compliant with RACS Continuing Professional Development requirements and spending a minimum of 20 h per week at the training site<br>Additional neurosurgical trainers who satisfy all responsibilities and requirements outlined above, but with less time commitment<br>  For a training post with one trainee, a minimum of two additional neurosurgical trainers, spending a combined minimum total of 40 h per week in the site<br>  For a training post with two trainees, a minimum of three additional neurosurgical trainers, spending a combined minimum total of 60 h per week in the site<br>  For a training post with three trainees, a minimum of four additional neurosurgical trainers, spending a combined minimum total of 90 h per week in the site<br>The neurosurgical supervisor and neurosurgical trainers should discuss and agree on goals for the trainee, provide one-to-one clinical supervision, frequent informal feedback, structured constructive feedback and recorded assessment of performance. The trainee must have opportunity to respond to feedback<br>Paid, protected administrative time and secretarial and IT services to undertake neurosurgical supervisor duties and negotiated leave to attend mandated training and meetings |

(continued)

**Table 15.4**  (continued)

| Standard | Theme | Principles |
|---|---|---|
| 5 | Support services for trainees | Work schedules that adhere to local legislation<br>Trainees should:<br>    Be on-call no more than 1 day in 3<br>    Work less than 70 h per week<br>    Be safe and have security provided when necessary<br>    Have access to human resources services, including counselling if required<br>Remuneration should be in accordance with the public sector awards. There should be a commitment to facilitate flexible (part-time or interrupted) employment |
| 6 | Clinical load and operating sessions | A minimum of one outpatient clinic per week to see new and follow-up patients under supervision<br>A defined neurosurgical inpatient unit of sufficient beds (minimum 15) to enable adequate turnover<br>At least three ward rounds or patient care meetings per week with a neurosurgeon<br>The minimum number of major neurosurgical procedures required annually are:<br>*Adult posts*<br>    For one trainee, 400 major cases with a minimum of 200 in the primary site<br>    For two trainees, 600 major cases with a minimum of 300 in the primary site<br>    For three trainees, 900 major cases with a minimum of 450 in the primary site<br>*Paediatric posts*<br>    For 1 trainee, 200 major paediatric neurosurgical cases<br>Significant hands-on involvement in surgical cases, increasing based on skill level to primary surgeon<br>Participation in a minimum of 100 major neurosurgical cases per 6 months in adult posts and 75 in paediatric posts<br>Major involvement in perioperative management of patients<br>Regular weekly involvement in acute/emergency care of neurosurgical patients, with a minimum 1:5 involvement in emergency care required |
| 7 | Equipment and clinical support services | Accreditation of sites by Australian or New Zealand Councils of Healthcare Standards to undertake surgical care<br>Suitable diagnostic and intervention services, including 24 h 7 day access to CT scan, DSA, MRI scan and general pathology<br>Additional specialist neuropathology access<br>Framed and frameless stereotactic equipment, an operating microscope and an ultrasonic aspirator<br>Support and ancillary services including rehabilitation, neuropsychology, neuropsychiatry, neurology and radiology and secretarial support and office space |

(continued)

**Table 15.4** (continued)

| Standard | Theme | Principles |
|----------|-------|-----------|
| 8 | Clinical governance quality and safety | A quality assurance board or equivalent (with a senior external member) reporting to a governance body and documentation published by the hospital on human resources, clinical risk management and other safety policies<br>A designated head of the neurosurgical department with a defined role in governance and leadership and a minimum six-monthly department meeting in each site<br>All medical staff credentialed at least every 5 years in all sites by a hospital credentialing committee<br>Regular (at least quarterly) review meetings of morbidity/ mortality, averaging 1 h per month with all neurosurgical supervisors, neurosurgical trainers and trainees participating and with robust peer review |

*CT* computed tomography, *DSA* digital subtraction angiography, *MRI* magnetic resonance imaging, *NSA* Neurosurgical Society of Australasia, *RACS* Royal Australasian College of Surgeons, *SET* surgical education and training

Trainees are allocated to the primary site but may spend up to 20% of their time in the secondary sites. Each primary site must have a designated neurosurgical supervisor of training for whom there are strict professional and training requirements. Appointment of a neurosurgical supervisor can be reviewed or revoked by the SET Board at any time.

There are currently 32 accredited training units in Australia (27), New Zealand (4) and Singapore (1) with a number accredited for more than one trainee to make a total of 56 training positions. This has increased in the last decade from only 38 posts in 2009. In 2018, two new applications for accreditation for training were denied on the basis of non-compliance to the standards outlined in Table 15.4, largely based on case load. One unit not compliant on reaccreditation has lost accreditation. Five units have been required to rectify deficiencies or been given shorter periods off accreditation to allow for early reassessment.

Analysis of trainee logbook case load data is one mechanism by which the adherence of the training sites to accreditation standards can be analysed and gives valuable information about the breadth and depth of exposure of trainees. A recent analysis of the logbooks of 20 "average" trainees completing their training in the usual 5 or 6 years, in 2016, 2017 and 2018, was examined for case load and case mix, which confirmed that trainees more than fulfil the training requirements in accredited training posts, confirming the robust nature of at least this aspect of unit accreditation and the provision of adequate operative experience for trainees [14, 24].

Additionally, written evaluations of the training experience have been recently reported [14] and can be summarised to reflect:

- An appreciation of the diversity of training due to experience of multiple training units, resulting in a well-rounded trainee with the benefit of a larger professional network

- An appreciation of diversity of skill acquisition, exposure to subspecialties and varying departmental cultures to shape individual future practice
- An appreciation of a relatively uniform standard of training not constrained to a particular hospital's strengths or subspecialty and also fostering relationships between hospitals to facilitate cooperative interests, such as research
- An expression of the logistical challenges of moving away from support networks, critical during early training or the exit exam with resulting isolation, financial burden, relationship challenges (including for the spouse's career, often with periods of separation) and uncertainty regarding future postings
- An expression of the stress of learning new hospital systems, policies and practices

This trainee experience is significantly different to that in systems such as in North America, where training is undertaken largely in a single institution or a few closely allied institutions. Advantages and disadvantages to both systems can be clearly seen from the above evaluation, with the Australasian system notable for breadth of experience and standardisation of the training environment. Despite the challenges, many trainees report positively on rotation between units, citing the clinical exposure and a chance to work with different mentors as advantageous. The experience has improved in recent times, with the establishment of a "home state" whereby the majority of training is performed across hospitals located within that region. Although this reduces interstate or international relocation, this will still occur at least once during training, potentially resulting in significant disruption for the trainee and their immediate family.

## Controversies in Neurosurgical Education

Overall, the bi-national, multi-institutional training scheme seems to have been very successful in improving the diversity, strength and breadth of training for Australasian neurosurgeons. This is evidenced by the case load and case mix [14, 24], which is comparable or superior to programs in Canada [25], the United Kingdom [22] and Europe [26], many of which do not have similar constraints related to vast distances and a small, separated population. However, with the widely agreed benefits has come challenges.

The first consideration, if training is to involve the hardship of moving between multiple institutions, including interstate or internationally, is to ensure excellent training, including an excellent experience for the trainee. There is little in the literature to guide accreditation of neurosurgical units apart from specific considerations for subspecialty training such as endovascular/cerebrovascular surgery [19] or spine neurosurgery [20], and there is little discussion of trainee welfare and satisfaction. The rigorous accreditation process outlined above appears to conform with at least best practice and is monitored by reaccreditation every 5 years and bi-annual trainee feedback, with scores across multiple years aggregated and released to the training unit to highlight deficiencies, while maintaining trainee anonymity. Monitoring of important metrics such as operative experience, professional behaviour and participation in educational activities within the strict framework of a national accreditation oversight may be more rigorous than unmonitored systems that are institution based.

The second consideration is trainee selection, with two chief problems identified in a centralised selection process. The first is the best method for selection, and the second is the lack of ownership and overall oversight of the trainee's career by any single institution.

Trainee selection around the world usually involves a combination of CV, examinations, references, interviews and occasionally psychoanalytic or personality tests. This process is fraught, and there is no agreed standard. In one meta-analysis, Zuckerman et al. [23] studied 21 articles evaluating 1276 resident applicants across five surgical subspecialties (no neurosurgical studies met the inclusion criteria). Of all the common pre-residency selection factors employed, objective standardised test scores correlated well with in-training and board examinations but correlated poorly with subsequent faculty evaluations of the trainee. Subjective factors, such as aggregate rank scores, letters of recommendation and athletic or musical talent, demonstrated only moderate correlation with future faculty evaluations. Similarly, Al Khalil et al. [18] used a questionnaire based on the Electronic Residency Application Service (ERAS) guidelines [27] with 3- or 4-point Likert scales. Of 46 neurosurgery residency program director respondents in August 2011, the most important factors in the selection process (>0.3) were the interview process (mean $\pm$ SD = $3.80 \pm 0.65$), United States Medical Licensing Examination (USMLE I) scores ($3.58 \pm 0.54$) and letters of recommendations ($3.56 \pm 0.54$). However high satisfaction with selected residents was only 60.9%. In multivariate analysis, predictors of long-term satisfaction with resident selection included less emphasis on letters of recommendation ($P = 0.037$) and greater weight on applicant extramural activity ($P = 0.038$). Thus, the NSA efforts to improve the referee process as described above are timely and address a well-recognised deficiency. In particular, the referee reports have a strong emphasis on identifying proficiency in non-technical skills, which are increasingly seen as critical to neurosurgery practice. This is evidenced by initiatives such as "Neurosurgery Boot Camp" which includes training in professionalism and communications skills in addition to traditional skills based teaching [8]. The success of the in-depth referee interviews will, however, only become evident with future analysis of training completion and performance.

The second, as described above, is the lack of "ownership" of centrally selected trainees allocated to a training unit to which they may have no previous or ongoing mentoring or pastoral relationship. This is a recognised deficiency with the Australasian system and may lead to the movement of underperforming trainees along to the next training unit as a path of least resistance, thus avoiding the more difficult and sometimes adversarial or litigious path of giving genuine negative feedback, refusing to give a reference or even failing a trainee in a placement. In addition, there are implications for future employment as an "orphan" graduate with no ties to a specific hospital, with a "home" hospital traditionally the place of first postgraduate employment in the Australia and New Zealand. Solutions to this identified problem are not clear, but creation of smaller training networks or "home" units is suggested and will be vital in the face of an ever-increasing number of applicants to neurosurgery training in Australia and New Zealand who are older and more likely to have a professional partner and children. For this group, constant moves are an increasing hardship, but solutions must be found which do not dilute the excellent breadth and depth of neurosurgical training currently achieved.

## Future Opportunities and Unmet Needs

Upon review, the neurosurgical education in Australasia as it has evolved over the last 80 years produces excellent neurosurgeons, fit for practising in the Australasian system. However, many challenges remain for the future decades.

### *Diversity in the Neurosurgical Workforce*

Gender and racial diversity are ongoing challenges for neurosurgery in Australasia. Although racial diversity with regard to immigrant populations is strong, Indigenous people from Australia and New Zealand continue to be underrepresented. The first RACS surgeon to identify as Indigenous was Dr. Kelvin Kong, who was admitted as a Fellow in Otolaryngology, Head and Neck Surgery in 2007. Currently no neurosurgeons identify as Aboriginal or Torres Strait Islander (ATSI) or Maori. There are current RACS initiatives to address cultural competence and safety, as well as historic and systemic racism in surgical selection and training. These RACS initiatives for people identifying as ATSI or Maori include affirmative action for applicants aspiring to a surgical career and specific programs from undergraduate through to specialist training with scholarships, skills and training courses and mentoring [28].

Since the 1980s, there has been gender parity for medical school graduates in Australasia. However, as is the case internationally, this has not translated to an equal number of women pursuing a neurosurgical career. According to RACS figures, there are 276 active neurosurgeons, of whom 39 are women (14%). For the 2020 training year there are 58 trainees of whom 13 are women (22%). The attitudes of women towards a surgical career was assessed in a recent RACS survey of female medical students and junior doctors [29]. The "Break Barriers" survey demonstrated that surgery was popular amongst women, with 47% of respondents selecting surgery as their career preference [29]. However, the respondents perceived three types of major barriers preventing them pursuing a surgical career. Firstly, they described cultural issues, particularly negative experiences of surgery during medical school from peers, lecturers, clinical tutors and surgeons. Secondly, they described structural issues, including inflexibility and length of the SET program and a need to finish training quickly to offset the cost of medical school. Thirdly, they described personal barriers such as lack of time for dependents, hobbies and leave (travel), lack of protected time for family and friends and partner career constraints [29]. It seems likely that programs similar to those developed for other "minorities" will also need to be instituted for women to enter and complete neurosurgical training if gender parity is to be achieved.

## Flexible Neurosurgical Training

The availability of flexible (part time, less than full time or interrupted) training will address some barriers described by women, but the desire for flexible training is not gender specific. Reasons for undertaking flexible training for all genders include not only parenting and other caring responsibilities but also research and other academic, sporting and cultural pursuits. Both the RACS and NSA training guidelines offer flexible training in principle, but the opportunity has not yet been taken by a neurosurgical trainee, and it is rare in Australasian surgery in general. There is a significant mismatch between surgical trainees in Australasia registering interest in part-time training in one study (31.6%; 54.3% women, 25.9% men) and those actually undertaking part-time training (0.3%) [30]. To pursue flexible training, trainees must find an employer and supervisor willing to offer a suitable position and apply at least 6 months in advance for SET Board accreditation. Therefore, despite policy, institutional and organisational barriers preclude widespread uptake. There are also genuine clinical and supervisory concerns, including that of compromised patient care due to frequent handover and reduced continuity of care and reduced operative experience of part-time trainees compared to their full-time counterparts. Trainees may also be reluctant to prolong years in training with reduced salary potential [30]. However, an important study describing successful implementation of a permanent part-time position for a general surgical trainee in a large tertiary hospital in South Australia directly compared part-time and full-time general surgical trainees and determined that both groups had similar logbooks and operative experience and all passed the RACS fellowship examination [31]. This proof of concept demonstrates that part-time positions may be considered by other surgical specialties. To make the "principle" a reality will, however, require significant institutional and SET Board buy-in and facilitation.

## Research in Neurosurgical Training

The promotion of research in surgery was one of the founding principles of RACS in 1926 and a major focus of the early NSA. Although research remains a requirement of neurosurgery training, this has been significantly diluted in recent decades. Historically, there was a genuine emphasis on research in neurosurgery training, which in the 1990s included a compulsory year of research, often culminating in a research higher degree. There was also a strong emphasis on research for acceptance into neurosurgical training. Due to concerns that research achievement does not necessary correlate with surgical competence, both for acceptance into and completion of training, research in Australasian training has been significantly reduced. The current minimum requirement is a small project undertaken simultaneously with training, rather than during dedicated research years or as part of a research higher degree. Research in neurosurgery has benefits not only for furthering of the profession, but there is an important association between future employment as a neurosurgeon and the attainment of a higher degree [32, 33]. Additionally, there is a positive association between the attainment of a graduate degree and future publication productivity for academic neurosurgeons [34] and attainment of research funding [33]. The Australasian system is an outlier in this regard compared with many international neurosurgery training institutions that mandate at least 1 year of full-time research.

## Innovation in Operative Training

There has been an increasing focus on operative training and skill acquisition in surgery, both in terms of structured intra-operative teaching and the use of simulation and virtual reality. Structured intra-operative teaching methods to improve trainee performance and competency and standardise the operative training experience have been explored in other surgical specialties [35]. One issue with operative training is the greatly varied experiences between centres and surgeons, leading to varied trainee experience and skill acquisition. An operative surgery training intervention was undertaken in Australia within an obstetrics and gynaecology unit, using a surgical encounter template, with briefing, goal setting and intra-operative teaching aims, as well as debriefing [36]. This structured intra-operative teaching model was found to be feasible and lead to learning objectives being met in 85% of cases following the intervention and trainees reporting clarity of feedback and more surgical opportunities using this method [36].

Operative skills can also be augmented by the provision of quality simulation and virtual reality models [19, 25, 26, 37, 38]. With the obvious benefits of practising surgical technique without patient risk, this adjunct to operative skill acquisition may also provide benefits for trainees with regard to skills practise at convenient times and places and individualised focus on an area requiring improvement. In cardiothoracic surgery, simulation is being widely used for training worldwide, with some provision of simulation workshops and skills laboratories for SET trainees in Australia [39]. As technology advances and opportunities for quality simulations become available, simulation should be considered as an adjunct to future neurosurgery training.

## Conclusion

Neurosurgical education in Australasia has evolved from a loose association of surgeons trained largely in the United Kingdom and based in single institutions to a rigorous bi-national training program overseen by the SET Board of the NSA (selection, curriculum, in-training assessment, accreditation of training posts) and the RACS (exit examination, principles and standards). Recent areas of focus have been methods to select excellent trainees, a planned curriculum update and the trainee experience, particularly as it relates to the practice of rotating trainees through two or three national or international training posts. Future challenges will include further improvement of the trainee experience, with reduction of the number of interstate or international moves, gender and racial diversity of trainees, fostering research and academic neurosurgical practice within training and beyond and innovative operative training methods.

## References

1. Clunie GJA. Surgery in Australia. Arch Surg. 1994;129(1):13.
2. Beasley AW. The mantle of surgery: the first seventy-five years of the Royal Australasian College of Surgeons/A. W. Beasley. Royal Australasian College of Surgeons, editor. Melbourne: Royal Australasian College of Surgeons; 2002.
3. Morgan MK, Clarke RM, Lyon PMA, Weidmann M, Law A, Laidlaw J, et al. The neurosurgical training curriculum in Australia and New Zealand is changing. Why? J Clin Neurosci. 2005;12(2):115–8.
4. Ham JM. Advanced surgical training in Australia and New Zealand and the part II FRACS examination. ANZ J Surg. 1988;58(12):937–40.
5. Heslop JH. The history of basic surgical science examinations in the Royal Australasian College of Surgeons. ANZ J Surg. 1988;58(7):529–36.
6. Ham J. Recent changes in the Part II FRACS Examination. ANZ J Surg. 1991;61(12):878–80.
7. Collins JP, Civil ID, Sugrue M, Balogh Z, Chehade MJ. Surgical education and training in Australia and New Zealand. World J Surg. 2008;32(10):2138–44.
8. Collins JP, Gough IR, Civil ID, Stitz RW. A new surgical education and training programme. ANZ J Surg. 2007;77(7):497–501.
9. Simpson DA, Jamieson KG, Morson SM. The foundations of neurosurgery in Australia and New Zealand. Aust N Z J Surg. 1974;44(3):215–27.
10. Rosenfeld JV, Kaye AH. Neurosurgery at the Royal Melbourne Hospital. Neurosurgery. 2000;46(4):978–85.
11. Curtis JB, Miller D, Simpson D. The Neurosurgical Society of Australasia: the first forty years. Aust N Z J Surg. 1980;50(4):434–7.
12. Long DM. Competency-based training in neurosurgery: the next revolution in medical education. Surg Neurol. 2004;61(1):5–14; discussion −25.
13. Cameron JL. William Stewart Halsted, our surgical heritage. Ann Surg. 1997;225(5):445–58.
14. Drummond KJ, Hunn BHM, McAlpine HE, Jones JJ, Davies MA, Gull S. Challenges in the Australasian neurosurgery training program: who should be trained and where should they train? Neurosurg Focus. 2020;48(3):E10.

15. Kaptigau WM, Rosenfeld JV, Kevau I, Watters DA. The establishment and development of neurosurgery Services in Papua New Guinea. World J Surg. 2016;40(2):251–7.
16. Rosenfeld JV, Watters DAK. Neurosurgery in the tropics: a practical approach to common problems. London: Macmillan; 2000.
17. Rosenfeld JV, Watters DAK. Neurosurgery in the tropics: a practical approach to common problems for the isolated practitioner. XLIBRIS AU; 2019.
18. Al Khalili K, Chalouhi N, Tjoumakaris S, Gonzalez LF, Starke RM, Rosenwasser R, et al. Programs selection criteria for neurological surgery applicants in the United States: a national survey for neurological surgery program directors. World Neurosurg. 2014;81(3–4):473–7.e2.
19. Alamri A, Chari A, McKenna G, Kamaly-Asl I, Whitfield PC. The evolution of British neurosurgical selection and training over the past decade. Med Teach. 2018;40(6):610–4.
20. Boszczyk BM, Mooij JJ, Schmitt N, Di Rocco C, Fakouri BB, Lindsay KW. Spine surgery training and competence of European Neurosurgical Trainees. Acta Neurochir. 2009;151(6):619–28.
21. Day AL, Siddiqui AH, Meyers PM, Jovin TG, Derdeyn CP, Hoh BL, et al. Training standards in neuroendovascular surgery: program accreditation and practitioner certification. Stroke. 2017;48(8):2318–25.
22. Lindsay KW. Neurosurgical training in the United Kingdom and Ireland: assessing progress and attainment. Neurosurgery. 2002;50(5):1103–13.
23. Zuckerman SL, Kelly PD, Dewan MC, Morone PJ, Yengo-Kahn AM, Magarik JA, et al. Predicting resident performance from preresidency factors: a systematic review and applicability to neurosurgical training. World Neurosurg. 2018;110:475–84.e10.
24. Starke RM, Asthagiri AR, Jane JA, Jane JA. Neurological surgery training abroad as a progression to the final year of training and transition to independent practice. J Grad Med Educ. 2014;6(4):715–20.
25. Tso MK, Dakson A, Ahmed SU, Bigder M, Elliott C, Guha D, et al. Operative landscape at Canadian neurosurgery residency programs. Can J Neurol Sci. 2017;44(4):415–9.
26. Reulen HJ, Marz U. 5 years' experience with a structured operative training programme for neurosurgical residents. Acta Neurochir. 1998;140(11):1197–203.
27. Applying to Residencies with ERAS 2020. Available from: https://students-residents.aamc.org/applying-residency/applying-residencies-eras/.
28. RACS Indigenous Health. Indigenous scholarships, awards, prizes and indigenous pathways into specialisation. 2020. Available from: https://www.surgeons.org/about-racs/indigenous-health/aboriginal-and-torres-strait-islander-health/scholarships-and-awards.
29. Survey report: breaking barriers; developing drivers for female surgeons. https://www.surgeons.org/-/media/Project/RACS/surgeons-org/files/operating-with-respectcomplaints/Break-barriers-report_2020.pdf. Royal Australasian College of Surgeons; June 2020.
30. McDonald RE, Jeeves AE, Vasey CE, Wright DM, O'Grady G. Supply and demand mismatch for flexible (part-time) surgical training in Australasia. Med J Aust. 2013;198(8):423–5.
31. Neuhaus S, Igras E, Fosh B, Benson S. Part-time general surgical training in South Australia: its success and future implications (or: pinnacles, pitfalls and lessons for the future). ANZ J Surg. 2012;82(12):890–4.
32. Tso MK, Max Findlay J, Lownie SP, Chris Wallace M, Toyota BD, Fleetwood IG. Recent trends in neurosurgery career outcomes in Canada. Can J Neurol Sci. 2019;46(04):436–42.
33. Choi BD, Delong MR, Delong DM, Friedman AH, Sampson JH. Impact of PhD training on scholarship in a neurosurgical career. J Neurosurg. 2014;120(3):730–5.
34. Keough MB, Newell C, Rheaume AR, Sankar T. Association between graduate degrees and publication productivity in academic neurosurgery. Can J Neurol Sci. 2020;47(5):666–74.
35. Timberlake MD, Mayo HG, Scott L, Weis J, Gardner AK. What do we know about intraoperative teaching? Ann Surg. 2017;266:251–9.
36. Leung Y, Salfinger S, Mercer A. The positive impact of structured teaching in the operating room. Aust N Z J Obstet Gynaecol. 2015;55(6):601–5.

37. Bernardo A. Virtual reality and simulation in neurosurgical training. World Neurosurg. 2017;106:1015–29.
38. Davidson B, Alotaibi NM, Guha D, Amaral S, Kulkarni AV, Lozano AM. Studying behaviors among neurosurgery residents using Web 2.0 analytic tools. J Surg Educ. 2017;74(6):1088–93.
39. Villanueva C, Xiong J, Rajput S. Simulation-based surgical education in cardiothoracic training. ANZ J Surg. 2020;90(6):978–83.

# Chapter 16
# Neurosurgery Education Around the World: Europe

André Grotenhuis, Katarzyna Świątkowska-Wróblewska, Francesco Sala, and Marianne Juhler

## Historical Background

Education and training of neurosurgeons in Europe started more than hundred years ago and developed, based upon Halsted's triad of educational principles, namely, knowledge of the basic sciences, research, and graduated patient responsibility for the resident [10, 15]. Although these principles have been the essential requirements of residency training programs for decades, training programs in Europe were organized rather individually and were often unstructured. From the centers where neurosurgery prospered in the first half of the twentieth century, e.g., Stockholm, London, Berlin, Wrocław, Paris, Vienna, Budapest, Bucharest, and Lisbon, it spread out over the individual European countries but without much of an international cooperation. This changed in the second half of the twentieth century. From the ruins of Europe after the Second World War, a profound change started in the way of thinking and in attitude toward interrelations between European nations, both in political terms and also in the medical field.

The Treaty of Rome, or officially the Treaty establishing the European Economic Community, brought about the creation of the European Economic Community

A. Grotenhuis (✉)
Radboud University Center Nijmegen Medical Center, Nijmegen, The Netherlands

K. Świątkowska-Wróblewska
Szpital Świętego Wojciecha, Poznań, Poland

F. Sala
Department of Neuroscience, Biomedicine and Movement Sciences, Section of Neurosurgery, University of Verona, Verona, Italy
e-mail: francesco.sala@univr.it

M. Juhler
Department of Clinical Medicine, Rigshospitalet – Neurocentret, Copenhagen, Denmark
e-mail: marianne.juhler@regionh.dk

© The Author(s), under exclusive license to Springer Nature Switzerland AG 2022
I. M. Germano (ed.), *Neurosurgery and Global Health*,
https://doi.org/10.1007/978-3-030-86656-3_16

(EEC). The treaty was signed on March 25, 1957, by Belgium, France, Italy, Luxembourg, The Netherlands, and West Germany. Under the name "Treaty on the Functioning of the European Union," it remains one of the most important treaties in what is now the European Union (EU).

On July 20, 1958 – 1 year after the treaty of Rome was signed – the representatives delegated by the professional organizations of medical specialists from the six member countries of the European Community met in Brussels and founded the European Union of Medical Specialists (UEMS). On the European level, the UEMS is responsible for the harmonization of the training of medical specialists in the member states of the EU, and its statutory purpose is the formulation of a common policy in the field of training [17].

The UEMS has formulated guidelines and criteria (published in the European Training Charter for Medical Specialist). The UEMS has sections for each specialty. They have developed specific recommendations to set and maintain standards of training, training quality, and accreditation of training institutions for the respective specialty. This aids harmonization of the training level in the EU [17].

With a current membership of 37 national associations and operating through 43 Specialist Sections and European Boards, the UEMS is committed to promote the free movement of medical specialists across Europe while ensuring the highest level of training which will pave the way to the improvement of quality of care for the benefit of all European citizens. The UEMS areas of expertise notably encompass continuing medical education, postgraduate training, and quality assurance [17].

The idea of a European Union of Neurosurgeons had been discussed already in Brussels 1957, where the First International Congress of Neurological Surgery was held. The concept of a European Association of Neurosurgical Societies was discussed after the Rome meeting 1963 and in Madrid 1967, and a committee was established with the task of preparing the definitive constitution. The European Association of Neurosurgical Societies (EANS) was founded in 1971 in Prague, by delegates from 18 national societies present at the Fourth European Congress of Neurosurgery. Right from the start, neurosurgical education and its harmonization within Europe were one of the main objectives, and during the inaugural session of the foundation of the EANS a training committee was established [9].

EANS national membership has expanded significantly in recent years and currently includes 39 countries. It represents around 8500 certified neurosurgeons, who serve a population of about 750 million. The EANS is now involved in all aspects of neurosurgical training both at preboard certification level and at special interest training level. For nearly 50 years it has arranged congresses, scientific meetings, symposia, and workshops, including the now annual European Congress of Neurosurgery and the European Neurosurgical Training Courses.

Neurosurgery training could be defined as the period during which a trainee will be exposed to all technical and cognitive aspects of neurosurgical disease, focusing in the most prevalent and relevant aspects of the brain, spine, and peripheral nerve pathology and becoming competent in the unsupervised practice of such techniques. The primary goal of a training program in neurosurgery is to provide the trainee with a broad theoretical knowledge base, the necessary operative and procedural skills and experience, as well as professional judgment for independent neurosurgical practice. A further goal is to teach him/her self-criticism, critical assessment of his/her results, and the ability to self-directed learning which will eventually lead to continued progression, expert practice, and professionalism.

In the Directive 93/16 EEC of April 5, 1993, the European Commission laid down the general guidelines for improvement of the quality of medical specialist practice in the EU, EFTA (European Free Trade Association, which is the intergovernmental organization of Iceland, Liechtenstein, Norway, and Switzerland), and associated member states.

In 1994, the UEMS adopted its Charter on Post Graduate Training aiming at providing the recommendations at the European level for good medical training. Made up of six chapters, this Charter set the basis for the European approach in the field of postgraduate training. With five chapters being common to all specialties, this Charter provided a sixth chapter, known as "Chapter 6", where each Specialist Section was to complete according to the specific needs of their discipline [11, 17].

More than 20 years after the introduction of this Charter, the UEMS Specialist Sections and European Boards have continued working on developing these European standards in medical training that reflects modern medical practice and current scientific findings. It did not aim to supersede the national authorities' competence in defining the content of postgraduate training in their own state but rather to complement these and ensure that high-quality training is provided across Europe. At the European level, the legal mechanism ensuring the free movement of doctors through the recognition of their qualifications was established back in the 1970s by the European Union. Sectorial directives were adopted, and one directive addressed specifically the issue of medical training at the European level [6, 17].

However, in 2005, the European Commission proposed to the European Parliament and Council to have a unique legal framework for the recognition of the professional qualifications to facilitate and improve the mobility of all workers throughout Europe. This Directive 2005/36/EC established the mechanism of automatic mutual recognition of qualifications for medical doctors according to training requirements within all member states; this is based on the length of training in the specialty and the title of qualification [17].

## Current Status: What Was Accomplished Until Present

At a general training level, the EANS' main activity is the European Neurosurgical Training Courses. These consist of four annual courses of 5 days each, covering the key topics of vascular neurosurgery, tumor, head injury/functional, and spine/peripheral nerves. Initially, there was one course every year; nowadays, there are three courses starting every year, with around 240 participants in each of the courses from all EANS member countries and a small percentage also from outside Europe. The trainees are selected by their national representative to the training committee. They start with the course preferably in their second, third, or fourth year of residency. The number of attendees per country differs and depends, among other things, on the total number of neurosurgeons per country.

The whole course cycle takes 4 years to complete, followed by European examinations in neurosurgery. The European examination is mandatory for all trainees who have completed the 5-year cycle of training courses, at least part one (written examination), but the vast majority also take part two (oral examination). A candidate who receives a passing grade for this examination is granted the European Diploma in Neurosurgery and become a Fellow of the European Board of Neurological Surgery.

However, board certification is still regulated by every individual country according to their local laws and board examinations organized on a national level. Some countries, e.g., Switzerland, have decided to make the European examinations mandatory for their own board certification process. So, the European examination, although a good attempt for certification of young neurosurgeons in Europe, is not binding nor significantly adopted in many countries yet.

The Joint Residency Advisory and Accreditation Committee (JRAAC), a joint committee of the EANS and the Section of Neurosurgery of the UEMS, was founded by both organizations with the task of developing standards and guidelines for the European Training Program in Neurosurgery, to establish matching training curriculum and to try to standardize training in the different European countries [5, 16]. However, only 17 neurosurgical departments, from 10 countries, have currently the European accreditation of their training program.

Although progress has been made in the past few years, the current situation in terms of the unification of training of neurosurgical residents in Europe has much work remaining. The diversity of European countries, historical facts, different nationalities, and languages has caused the diversity and specificity of neurosurgical schools.

There are currently 50 states in (or partially in) Europe, of which 44 states have their capital within Europe. All the states, except Belarus, Kazakhstan, and Vatican City, are members of the Council of Europe. Since 2007, 27 of these countries are also member states of the European Union (EU). There is no unified model of neurosurgical training program in the EU, and it is also quite different in non-EU countries [3, 7]. Despite some similarities, the duration of the program, the selection of new trainees, the number of new recruits, and the manner of their training are specific for almost every country [7]. Some of the factors currently interfering with harmonization of neurosurgical training are summarized in Table 16.1.

But there is increasing interest for a more structured training, identifying a minimum level of competence for a neurosurgeon. At the moment, the EANS is developing a three-stage curriculum, describing the requirements for the training program director as for the program itself, and the educational setting that should offer a supportive, academic environment, together with continuous, competency-based assessment and feedback on performance (Table 16.2). In the first stage, with an indicative duration of 1–2 years, the program should provide breadth of experience allowing to develop core clinical and professional skills and early operative skills. In the second stage, with an indicative duration of 3–5 years, emergency, and

**Table 16.1** Factors possibly interfering with harmonization of neurosurgical training in Europe

| |
|---|
| Differences in NS training duration [2–10 years] |
| Yearly acceptance rate to neurosurgery training is widely variable among EU countries |
| Differences in adhering to the 48 h/week work restriction |
| Differences in availability of sophisticated equipment (neuronavigation, IONM) |
| Differences in access to CME |

**Table 16.2** The three-stage neurosurgical curriculum under development by EANS

| Neurosurgery training stage | Duration | Goals |
|---|---|---|
| Stage 1 | 1–2 years | Development of diagnostic and ward-based clinical skills<br>Learning of basic operative skills and principles |
| Stage 2 | 3–5 years | Acquisition of emergency and elective operative skills<br>Further inpatient and outpatient skills<br>Team working skills |
| Stage 3 | 1–2 years | Full competence in inpatient/outpatient care, multidisciplinary team working, and elective and emergency surgical care<br>Development of transferable microsurgical and special interest skills (subspecialty) skills |

elective operative skills, next to further inpatient and outpatient skills as well as team working skills should be developed. In the third and last stage, with an indicative duration of 1–2 years, there is room for development of specialty interest skills, and the trainee should achieve full competence in inpatient care, outpatient care, multidisciplinary team working, and elective and emergency surgical care, finally at the level of a Day 1 specialist.

National neurosurgical societies should align their programs with those recommendations. In this way, it will be possible to better train neurosurgeons with uniform basic programs, even if they are from different European countries. These would benefit the society, and the licensing of neurosurgeons at the European level would be simplified [16].

Consistency across national training programs in Neurosurgery, however, may remain a chimera. There are various reasons for this incompleteness. First, and most important, the duration of residency programs varies substantially across Europe with obvious implications in terms of surgical training. In addition, criteria to establish the demand for neurosurgeons in each country are also largely undetermined and variable. This is likely due to the fact that different institutional bodies are responsible for planning the number of new neurosurgeons required in a given time. In some countries, this is addressed at a governmental level with no clear involvement or consultation of the national, academic, and neurosurgical community, and this represents an obvious limitation to a rational recruitment plan.

**Work Weeks, Department Staffing, and Neurosurgical Training**
With the rapid progress in diagnostic and therapeutic possibilities, e.g., introduction of CT, microsurgery, MRI, neuronavigation, deep brain stimulation, etc.,

continuous professional education to stay informed about the actual "state of the art" became mandatory for every neurosurgeon, but it also changed the education and training of the next generation of neurosurgeons.

In Europe, the introduction of the European Working Time Directive 2003/88/ EC has led to a significant reduction of working hours to first 58 h/week and from 2009 onwards a 48 h/week with distinct and inevitable impact on the exposure of residents in training to the operative environment [3].

In a survey on neurosurgery resident training in Europe from 2015, Stienen et al. [12, 13] concluded that the theoretical and practical aspects of neurosurgical training are highly variable throughout European countries and also that less than 40% of the >500 responders participate in training programs that adhere to the European Working Time directive with a maximum weekly working time of 48 h.

Besides these duty hour requirements, increasing expectations about attending involvement during surgery and new curricular mandates have put programs under stress to ensure adequate training, in less time, in an environment of limited resident independence. Unfortunately, the most important element of the Halsted triad, graduated responsibility for patient care leading to the role of the resident as the surgeon, can no longer be offered to residents as it was in the past due to social and economic changes in medical care. Thus, the heart and soul of the system of graduate surgical education has been lost, and a drastic change of education and training of neurosurgeon became inevitable.

As conceivable consequence neurosurgical trainees finish their residency with less practical experience or unable or less likely to achieve competency in all areas of neurosurgery [1, 16]. The number of cases performed by residents has gradually come below a critical number, and graduating residents feel inadequately prepared [14] (Fig. 16.1).

This paradigm shift comes in a time of increasing expectations from patients, who are well informed about modern high-tech developments. Ultimately, increasing societal demands for a safer operating environment and optimized outcomes must be fulfilled by less-trained future physicians, which stresses the importance of earlier and more goal-oriented surgical training.

A need for increasing the number of trainees to fulfill daily and on-call staffing requirements is another consequence of shorter working hours. This adds to the decrease in number of surgical cases per trainee. In addition, there is an inherent risk of producing too many certified neurosurgeons compared to European job availability, and future neurosurgeons trained in Europe may have to rethink their job options into other areas of the world.

## Future Opportunities/Unmet Needs

We must take into consideration that the field of neurosurgery is now expanding at an exponential rate. The advances made in specialties that, e.g., consider minimal access (endoscopy, endovascular neurosurgery, minimally invasive spine, and

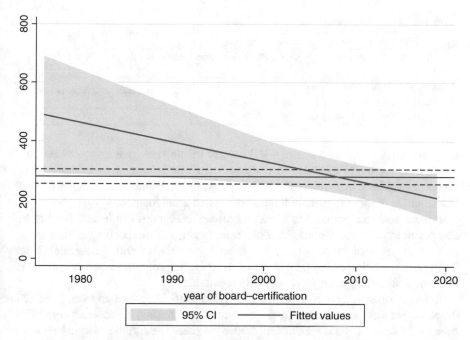

**Fig. 16.1** Linear prediction plot with 95% confidence intervals (CI), illustrating time trends (x-axis, year of residency graduation) in annual caseload (y-axis, number of procedures/year) for European neurosurgical residents. The fitted line indicates a decrease in caseload over time. The red reference lines indicate the proposed threshold for adequate surgical training, ranging around 275 (250–300) per year and resident. From Stienen et al. [14]

functional neurosurgery) make it virtually impossible to make someone competent in all of them [2].

There are (at least) three challenges:

The *first challenge* is to have all subspecialties covered within the specific time that a society deems necessary to train competent specialists.
The *second challenge* is to determine the "break point" between required general knowledge in each field for all neurosurgeons and advanced knowledge and competencies acquired by neurosurgeons subspecialized in particular areas.
The *third challenge* is how to verify that competency indeed has occurred at either the general or the advanced level.

Table 16.3 summarizes some of the key points that might influence the neurosurgery training of the future.

### Subspecialization

The basis for subspecialization rests on concentration of certain rare cases into fewer hospitals which creates the necessary "critical volume" for physicians and regional centers. The principle of "centralization" has already become a reality in some EU countries and obviously has relevant implications for training programs. For example,

**Table 16.3** Training the neurosurgeon of the future

| |
|---|
| Subspecialty training integrated in the training curriculum |
| Certification or licensing through demonstration of competence rather than just by time in training |
| Integration of virtual simulation into training |
| Application of telemanipulated neurosurgery (robotics) |
| Application of artificial intelligence into practice |

the primary institution of a neurological surgery training program may not have sufficient case volume to meet the current case minimum requirements in some areas. Residents will have to travel to other departments for exposure to cases that are either less common or more regionally focused (so-called away rotations) [3, 4].

It is not realistic anymore to think that all neurosurgeons can be and have to be competent in all areas of our field. Therefore, the idea of establishing a three-stage training program as has now been developed by the EANS with a dedicated 1- to 2-year specialization in the final stage of the training program in one or two areas becomes not only appealing but probably inevitable!

In an editorial in *Acta Neurochirurgica* from 2016, Brennum and van Loon [2] describe this also as a change in the organizational future of neurosurgery: "The time of the neurosurgical "jack of all trades" is past. The future must be based on increased sub-specialization and teamwork. Neurosurgery has long surpassed a degree of complexity where a single neurosurgeon can master the theoretical knowledge and practical skills of all subspecialties at a sufficiently high level. Accordingly, most neurosurgical units have already implemented sub-specialization, where the individual neurosurgeons work together as a team to deliver high-quality services. Furthermore, collaboration between units is called for when dealing with rare conditions. In order to support this sub-specialization a neurosurgical training program needs to deliver basic neurosurgical training that allows the further development into subspecialties."

Credentialed postgraduate subspecialty training therefore becomes more important than ever, since we will be publicly claiming that those graduates can practice that subspecialty in a competent and unsupervised fashion [16].

The last 1–2 years of the three-stage curriculum reminds, to some extent, of the North American fellowship programs where graduated residents have the opportunity to become subspecialized in a specific area of neurosurgery, through a fully dedicated clinical and surgical training. Usually, no more than one or two fellows per year are trained at every accredited institution, and they have operative privileges which warrant them appropriate surgical exposure to increasingly complex cases. However, this may potentially interfere with the residency training program, and a careful fine-tuning is needed to adjust the needs of a residency program with those of postgraduate subspecialization. The European perspective to integrate these needs into a unique, extended, residency program is therefore promising.

Surgical training and education will evolve substantially over the next decade in response to new technologies, regulations, practices, and the changing demographics and needs of resident education. A variety of different educational strategies and teaching and assessment methods, each implemented with the aim of updating operative skills assessment and instruction to maximize teaching opportunities in the OR, have recently been described in the literature [8] and will lead to modifications in the current neurosurgery training landscape. Each of these methods varies in terms of focus and mode of implementation, but they all share a common goal of maximizing the development of the neurosurgical resident by encouraging proficiency in neurosurgery.

Effective use of these novel educational tools, e.g., training models, simulators, and virtual reality by surgical educators, may serve to improve the quality and efficiency of intraoperative resident education [2]. Educators and institutions that embrace these new methods of teaching place themselves in an optimal position to train the next generation of neurosurgeons. Cooperation on a European level in the use of such modern teaching techniques will be needed, and it will help to establish further harmonization of neurosurgical training in Europe.

# References

1. Brennum J. European neurosurgical education—the next generation. Acta Neurochir. 2000;142:1081–7.
2. Brennum J, van Loon J. Neurosurgical education in Europe. Acta Neurochir. 2016;158:1–2.
3. Burkhardt JK, Zinn PO, Bozinov O, Colen RR, Bertalanffy H, Kasper EM. Neurosurgical education in Europe and the United States of America. Neurosurg Rev. 2010;33(4):409–17.
4. Gephart MH, Derstine P, Oyesiku NM, Grady MS, Burchiel K, Batjer HH, Popp AJ, Barbaro NM. Resident away rotations allow adaptive neurosurgical training. Neurosurgery. 2015;76(4):421–5; discussion 425–6.
5. Lindsay K. Accreditation of neurosurgical training programmes in Europe: report of JRAAC. Acta Neurochir. 2010;152(11):2013–4.
6. Long DM. European Union of Medical Specialists. The ideal neurosurgical training curriculum. Acta Neurochir (Wien). 2004;90 Suppl:21–31.
7. Omerhodzic I, Tonge M, Matos B, Musabeliu E, Raspanti C, Ferdinandov D, Galimova R, Muroi C, Balik V, Kursumovic A. Neurosurgical training programme in selected European countries: from the young neurosurgeons' point of view. Turk Neurosurg. 2012;22(3):286–93.
8. Perin A, Galbiati TF, Gambatesa E, Ayadi R, Orena EF, Cuomo V, Riker NI, Falsitta LV, Schembari S, Rizzo S, European Neurosurgery Simulation Study Group (ENSSG), Luciano C, Cappabianca P, Meling TR, Schaller K, DiMeco F. Filling the gap between the OR and virtual simulation: a European study on a basic neurosurgical procedure. Acta Neurochir. 2018;160(11):2087–97.
9. Pia HW. Chronicle of the European Association of Neurosurgical Societies Wien: Springer; 1983.
10. Reulen HJ, editor. Training in neurosurgery in the countries of the EU. A guide to organize a training programme. Wien: Springer; 2004.
11. Reulen HJ, Lindsay KW. UEMS charter on training of medical specialists in the EU—the neurosurgical training charter (as of February 2007). Acta Neurochir. 2007;149:843–55.

12. Stienen MN, Netuka D, Demetriades AK, Ringel F, Gautschi OP, Gempt J, Kuhlen D, Schaller K. Neurosurgical resident education in Europe--results of a multinational survey. Acta Neurochir. 2016;158(1):3–15.
13. Stienen MN, Netuka D, Demetriades AK, Ringel F, Gautschi OP, Gempt J, Kuhlen D, Schaller K. Working time of neurosurgical residents in Europe--results of a multinational survey. Acta Neurochir. 2016;158(1):17–25.
14. Stienen MN, Freyschlag CF, Schaller K, Meling T, EANS Young Neurosurgeons and EANS Training Committee. Procedures performed during neurosurgery residency in Europe. Acta Neurochir (Wien). 2020;162(10):2303–11.
15. Sure U, Miller D, Bozinov O. Neurosurgical training in Europe, problems and possible solutions. Surg Neurol. 2007;67(6):626–8; discussion 628–633.
16. Trojanowski T. Certification of competence in neurosurgery – the European perspective. World Neurosurg. 2011;74(4–5):432–3.
17. UEMS 2015/34 European Training Requirements for the Specialty of Neurosurgery. European standards of postgraduate medical specialist training in neurosurgery. https://www.uems.eu/__data/assets/pdf_file/0011/27839/UEMS-2015_34-Training-Requirements-for-the-Specialty-of-Neurosurgery-2015-corr.pdf. Accessed 15 Aug 2020.

# Chapter 17
# Neurosurgery Education Around the World: Central and South America

**Andrés M. Rubiano, Diana Marcela Sánchez Parra,
Luis Ernesto Ricaurte Arcos, and Rodrigo Ramos Zúñiga**

## Introduction

The foundation and development of neurosurgery as a specialty and as a training program in the Latin American and Caribbean region have been influenced by several factors, including local and regional trends in public health and educational policies. In the 1950s most programs started after the return of surgical pioneers who traveled overseas for additional training in well-stablished services of USA and Europe. The first policy influence for these pioneers was the so-called Flexner Report of 1910, which generated a road map for most of the public institutions of higher education that further develops postgraduate programs in the region. After this trend, the II Edinburgh Declaration of 1993 also marked a new context for

A. M. Rubiano (✉)
Neuroscience Institute, INUB-MEDITECH Research Group, Universidad El Bosque, Bogotá, Colombia

Neurological Surgery Service, Vallesalud Clinic, Cali, Colombia

NIHR Global Health Research Group on Neurotrauma, Universidad de Cambridge, Cambridge, UK

D. M. S. Parra
NIHR Global Health Research Group on Neurotrauma, Universidad de Cambridge, Cambridge, UK

Neurotrauma and Global Neurosurgery Fellowship Program, Meditech Foundation, Cali, Colombia

L. E. R. Arcos
University of Medical Sciences, Habana, Cuba

R. R. Zúñiga
Department of Neurosciences, Translational Institute of Neuroscience, University Center of Health Sciences, University of Guadalajara, Guadalajara, Mexico

© The Author(s), under exclusive license to Springer Nature Switzerland AG 2022     239
I. M. Germano (ed.), *Neurosurgery and Global Health*,
https://doi.org/10.1007/978-3-030-86656-3_17

curriculum changes not only at these types of institutions but also for private ones, including clinics and hospitals that develop their own training programs in countries like Argentina, Brazil, Cuba, Uruguay, and Mexico. These two postulates were generated with a common goal, which was and is to be able to generate the necessary conditions and guidelines to optimally educate medical students and future health professionals in a country [1]. Since the introduction of the medical specialties format in the early twentieth century, these standards have been maintained for graduate education in most areas of the region. The local development of academic programs to train fully competent neurosurgeons was established to share a common goal while having different mechanisms to achieve it. In the last decade, an important influence of virtual education and globalization of the curriculums has allowed the specialty training to evolve into a more complex educational model with less access to hours of practice and more access to observational programs. This involves bi-learning models of support for additional competences like research and subspecialty trainings [2]. With this being the specialty of neurosurgery, one of the most competitive specialties, and with very few available placements in the region, our aim is to present a brief historical perspective that will allow for a better understanding of the context of the current state of the neurosurgical medical education in the region. This historical foundation is essential to understand the unmet needs and future opportunities for the specialty training in the Latin American and Caribbean region.

## Brief Historical Background

Modern neurosurgery as a medical specialty is currently considered in full development [3]. It is agreed that its formal birth only occurred during first half of the twentieth century due to the academic and healthcare contributions of the well-known pioneers from North America and Europe. Similarly, as the other specialties, the pathway traveled for the consolidation of neurosurgery as a specialty has evolved from magical and empirical thinking to formal scientific knowledge. According to the four evolving periods of the neurosurgery as specialty proposed and presented by Dr. Jesús LaFuente in the open lecture of the Real Academy of Doctors in Spain in 2018 [4], the early period was called "diagnosis and prevention." Between 1885 and 1915 in the Latin American and Caribbean region, there are many anecdotal events from different medical practitioners developing occasional surgeries of head and spine with most of them related to trauma and infectious diseases. In Argentina, for example, Andrés Llobet, in 1885, published one of the early books on surgical treatment of disorders of the brain with trephination [5], and in 1901, an article related to cranioplasty procedures [6]. In Colombia, among others, Juan Nicolás Osorio, in 1866, published local articles related to the management of syphilitic tumors of the brain and management of brain inflammation after a cranial injury [7]. In Brazil, Luis Gomez Ferreyra described the management of a cranial fracture with multiple fragment restoration in 1710 and published the case in an early medical book in 1735 [8]. Some of these pioneers traveled overseas to achieve more knowledge related to this novel, growing specialty in the USA and Europe. When they returned, younger physicians came under the new practices as local assistants and learned these techniques. With increased motivation, these physicians worked to advance in the field and presented in early medical conferences in different regions of the world (Fig. 17.1).

The second period has been called by LaFuente, "microsurgery and training," and lasted from 1930 to 1970. During this period, the development of microsurgical techniques evolved with the development of the microscope, the improvement of anesthetic techniques, the refinement of coagulation techniques, the evolution of antibiotic therapy, and the development of neuroradiology. This period was the golden period of development of neurological surgery programs in Latin America and the Caribbean, being developed by several apprentices of the pioneers, who also traveled overseas to receive additional training. This training was both theoretical and practical and exposed the physicians to neurosurgical procedures performed on a grander scale at academic, university hospitals, and some private centers. During this period, the teacher-apprentice-patient figure was based on the close and hierarchical observation and imitation of the disciple to his teacher with the idea that the apprentice would take progressive autonomy and assume the teacher's new role. A good example of this type of neurosurgeon includes Dr. Fernando Cabieses. He was born in Mexico but assumed his role as physician in Perú. He did his neurosurgical residency in the USA in the 1940s and then traveled back to found the Cayetano

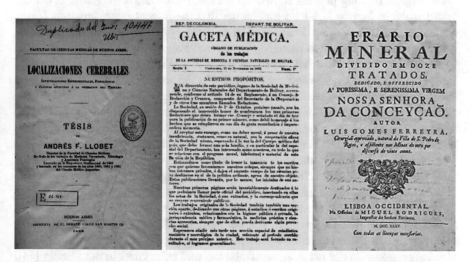

**Fig. 17.1** Brief sample of informational sources from the early period of the neurosurgical education in Latin American and the Caribbean region. From left to right: Dr. Llobet's Thesis at University of Buenos Aires Library from year 1885, Early Medical Journal in Colombia, with surgical descriptions called Gaceta Médica from the year 1890s and textbook of Dr. Luis Ferreyra from Brazil in 1735, describing neurotrauma surgical cases in Brazilian slaves. (Images obtained by authors from original manuscripts in PDF files from Buenos Aires University Library, Colombian National Library, and Mukharajj Institute Library)

Heredia University in Lima, in addition to founding neurological surgery services in at least six of the main hospitals in the Peruvian capital [9]. In 1939, Dr. Alfonso Asenjo from Chile, after being trained in North America at Johns Hopkins University under the guidance of Walter Dandy, and in Berlin with Dr. Wilhelm Tönnis, formed the neurosurgery and neuropathology service in Santiago de Chile. In 1943, he achieved the creation of the famous Central Institute of Neurosurgery and Neuropathology, being one of the first private reference centers for training neurosurgeons in a large number in Latin America. Later, he linked the Institute with the Medicine Training Program at the University of Chile, endowing the educational process with academic rigor [10]. In Uruguay, in 1926, Dr. Alejandro H. Schroeder, who was trained as a neurosurgeon in Breslau (Poland), began the educational process for neurosurgeons training under the Halsted model vision in Montevideo. He developed a new vision for a neurologic institute with the centralization of patients and developed an educational training program which demonstrated the relevance and importance of a reference center [11]. In Brazil, Dr. Alfredo Alberto Pereira Monteiro, among others, was the first professor to promote neurosurgical training and published two neurosurgical technical documents in 1937. He and some of the other Brazilian pioneers began neurosurgical training with the creation of neurology and neurosurgery services in well-established university hospitals like Hospital Das Casas and Hospital Das Clinicas. Posteriorly, more neurosurgical training programs were organized at the Faculty of Medicine in Minas Gerais, the University of Brazil, and the Institute of Neurology of the University of Rio de Janeiro [12]. In 1934, the neurosurgical training process started in Cuba with Dr. Carlos M. Ramirez Corría, who trained in France and who trained the first three local neurosurgeons (Jesús Melendez, Jorge Picaza, and Francisco García) in Hospital Calixto García in Havana city [13]. In Colombia, two pioneers, Dr. Alvaro Fajardo, who trained in 1939 at Columbia University and at Mt Sinai Hospital in New York, and Dr. Mario Camacho Pinto, who traveled as a "volunteer assistant" in the services of Walter Dandy and Freeman Watts, traveled back to Bogotá in the 1940s and subsequently created the academic services in most of the university hospitals in Bogota. Dr. Camacho Pinto returned to the USA and was formally trained as a resident in the Bellevue Hospital under the training of Dr. Foster Kennedy in addition to the Presbyterian Medical Center. After them, many other pioneers were trained in different services. Some of these include Dr. Alejandro Jimenez (trained with Asenjo in Chile and in Montreal) (Fig. 17.2), Dr. Salomon Hakim (trained initially in Colombia and then in the Brigham's and Women's Hospital in Boston), Dr. José Mora Rubio (trained initially in Colombia and then in Sweden), and Dr. Fernando Rosas (trained at the Illinois Neurological Institute in the USA). Most of these physicians developed different training programs in the 1960s at the capital city and other cities in the country [14]. In Panama, Dr. Antonio González Revilla trained with Walter Dandy at John Hopkins, returned to Panama City, and in 1948 created the Institute of Neurology and Neurosurgery at Hospital Santo Tomas, being one of the initial services to train neurosurgeons in the country. His first local resident was Mario Bemporad [15]. In Bolivia, Dr. Mario Michele Zamora, in 1940, graduated with a thesis titled, "Surgical Treatment of Brain Hemorrhage," and founded the first neurological surgery service

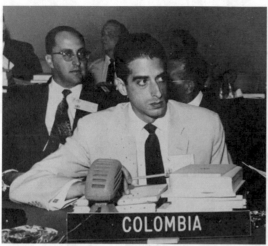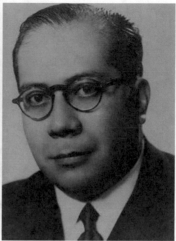

**Fig. 17.2** Several Latin American neurosurgery pioneers were appointed as ministers of health in the second period of the development of neurosurgery education in the Latin American and Caribbean region including countries like Brazil, Argentina, and Colombia. Professor Alejandro Jimenez Arango (right), Colombian Minister of Health between 1952 and 1953, was a neurosurgical trainee in Chile, under the mentorship of Dr. Alfonso Asenjo. In the 1940s, after finishing his training, he returned to Colombia and created the first neurosurgical training programs at National University and the Military Hospital in Bogota. He was also the developer of the first National Medical Professional Council, office in charge of validation of medical titles in the country. In Argentina, Dr. Ramón Carrillo (left) was the first ever Minister of Health, appointed by Juan D. Perón in 1946. Dr. Carrillo was trained as neurological surgeon in Europe in the early 1930s and then returned to Buenos Aires as a cornerstone for the development of the modern healthcare system in Argentina. He promoted the construction of more than 234 hospitals between 1946 and 1954, including the development of specialized training institutes and neurosurgical training programs. (Images courtesy of Dr. Enrique Jimenez Hakim in Colombia and the Health Studies Institute in Argentina)

in the old hospital in La Paz. Then, Dr. Hugo Rodriguez, trained in Brazil, Chile, and the USA, returned in 1953 to develop the first neurological surgery service at the National Hospital in La Paz. Additionally, Dr. Nestor Enriquez, who trained with Asenjo, was the first professor of neurosurgery at Universidad Mayor de san Francisco in La Paz [16] (Fig. 17.3).

The third period according to Dr. LaFuente is called "diagnostic imaging" and occurred between 1970 and 1990. It represented the improvement of equipment and the development of obtaining brain images. The structural detail level allowed the recognition of surgical indications in a more significant number. This increased the number of operations and, therefore, the specialty's learning curve. During this period most of the training programs became consolidated in the region, generating more academic interaction by visiting professors. More educational events were held at the regional level, and a majority were supported by the local neurosurgical societies and the regional societies like the Latin American Federation of Neurosurgical Societies (FLANC) (Fig. 17.4), established in 1981, and the

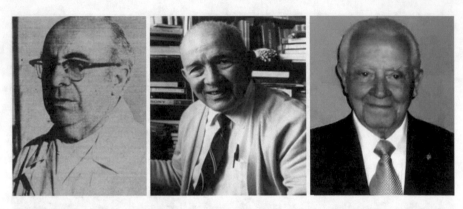

**Fig. 17.3** Example of pioneers of neurosurgery training programs during the second period of evolution of neurosurgery in Latin American and the Caribbean region: Alfonso Asenjo, Chile (1906–1980); Fernando Cabieses, Perú (1920–2009); Ernesto Bustamante, Colombia (1922–2021). (Images courtesy of Chilean National Library in Chile, Fernando Cabieses Peruvian Association from Peru, and the Colombian Association of Neurosurgery in Colombia)

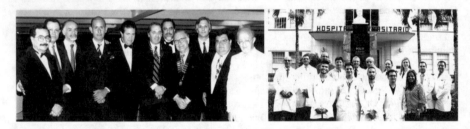

**Fig. 17.4** The Latin American Federation of Neurosurgical Societies (FLANC) has played a leading role in the neurosurgical education in the Latin American region. In 1994, (right picture), FLANC officers meet in Cartagena, Colombia, during the XXVI Latin American Neurosurgical Congress. All of them representatives of the third period of neurosurgical educators generation: (From right to left: Dr. German Peña (Colombia), Dr. Marco Molina (Honduras), Dr. Fernando Rueda (Mexico), Dr. Hector Giocoli (Argentina), Dr. Tito Perilla (Colombia), Dr. Jorge Mendez (Chile), Dr. Juan Mendoza (Colombia), Dr. Armando Basso (Argentina), Dr. Fredy Holzer (Chile), Dr. Cesar Castellanos (Honduras), and Dr. Manuel Dujovny (USA)). During this period, several neurosurgical training programs moved in a transformative process where the trainees of the pioneers became leaders of the educational activities, mentoring young generations of future neurosurgeons. The neurosurgery program at Universidad del Valle in Cali, Colombia, was an example of this transition process (left picture). From right to left: (Back row with instructors and visiting neurosurgeons: Dr. Antonio Montoya, Dr. Gustavo Vásquez, Dr. Carlos Jiménez, Dr. Jorge Aristizabal, Dr. Alfredo Pedroza, Dr. Miguel Velázquez, Dr. Carlos Llanos, Dr. Iris Montes, Dr. Javier Orozco, and Dr. Alejandro Herrera. Front row, neurosurgery residents: Dr. Juan Mier, Dr. Juan Rivera, Dr. Juan Salcedo, Dr. Fernando Peralta, and Ms. María Becerra, administrative assistant of neurosurgery). (Images courtesy of Latin American Federation of Neurosurgical Societies and the Neurological Surgery Service from Universidad del Valle and University Hospital in Cali, Colombia)

Caribbean Association of Neurological Surgeons (CANS) created in 1973. During this same period, and associated with multiple changes in political views of regional countries, there was a move from a public-based educational model toward new private training programs. As an example, in Uruguay between 1973 and 1985, there was a progressive deterioration in the care capacity of the university hospital, which generated delays in the medical progression of the specialty in the period 1973–1985. Due to this, neurosurgery began in private institutions, which was a different way of working for departments. With this came the creation of subspecialties. At the end of the 1990s neurosurgery postgraduate training improved. Due to the crisis in public health, a mandatory neurosurgical residency was introduced [17]. In Chile, after the military dictatorship in 1973, the country reformed their health and education systems under the neoliberal philosophy. The change brought with it administrative adjustments in public health institutions and the development of private institutions with a public missionary component. This began the limitation of education and training programs access to less resourced populations [18]. In Brazil, there was an explosion of private training programs based on the same political issues of the region. This allowed for the evolution of traditional models to new models, with a greater emphasis on research-track training. In 1980, the São Paulo School of Medicine began the programs for training neurosurgeons at the masters and doctoral levels in Sao Paulo, under the direction of Professor Mattos Pimienta [19]. In Argentina, the public model remained reinforced until the policies of military dictatorships ended in 1983. Then, a mixed model allowed the development of more private programs. However, with this, the associations wanted more participation in the national leadership for defining educational procedures. In the 1990s, Dr. Martín Giraldo ensured the local society was recognized by the Argentine Medical Association, the Secretariat of Public Health of the Nation, and the Province of Buenos Aires as the primary reference to establish the norms for the accreditation and control of the practice of the specialty [20]. In Colombia, the same trend was present, debilitating the public training system. It was impacted by several strikes by educational unions and the deep social conflict generated by the internal armed rebel fights and the golden age of the drug traffic business. Social violence was associated with shortages of funds in education and healthcare at public sector level. This situation generated a growing opportunity for new private programs mostly centered in Bogota, as the public programs remain during this period as the only possibility for training in other cities like Cartagena, Cali, and Medellin [21–23] (Fig. 17.4). During this time, the only country that did not suffer this transformation was Cuba, where after the regime change for the actual model, most of the original programs of the 1970s were reinforced as training programs. The neurotransplant center (CIREN) was founded in the 1980s, and new services were opened in other regions different from La Havana. In the 1990s, most of these schools were reinforced as training programs for the region, generating an option for students with economical capabilities. These students came mostly from the Caribbean and the Andean region and also in specific programs for Venezuelan physicians since the starting of the actual regime in 1999. These programs have been receiving trainees from African countries and Middle East [24]. The same trend, but mostly based on private universities, has been an option for medical students of the region pursuing a career in neurological surgery in programs of Brazil, Argentina, and Chile, where more positions are available.

## Current Status: What Was Accomplished Until the Present

The current, fourth period, described by LaFuente as the period of "preservation of function and improvement of the quality of life," occupying the end of the twentieth century and the beginning of the twenty-first century, represents the exponential growth of diagnostic technologies and innovative management strategies to preserve the patient's functional state. The best clinical evidence that research resources can provide is devoted to this. Therefore, the previously inaccessible brain areas now have fewer limitations. As mentioned in the previous section, the neurosurgery education process in Latin America and the Caribbean has had significant influence from the European and North American schools from what is considered the starting point. To date, it has been possible to modify the structure of medical education aimed at training neurosurgeons, through the formal creation of medical residency programs linked to universities. Furthermore, the application of the competency training model, with initial practice scenarios through simulation laboratories, inanimate skills training stations, and animated models, has provided opportunities to become familiar with instruments, improve agility, and provide the student with the opportunity to gain knowledge of surgical management, techniques, and potential complications. The student is then permitted to move on to direct patient practice, with clarity in the principles, focus, and previous experience [25, 26].

The traditional Halsted model, based on three principles of surgical training that the resident should have, i.e., (a) intense and repetitive opportunities to care for surgical patients under a trained surgical master's supervision, (b) the understanding of the scientific basis for surgical disease, and (c) the management of patients and technical operations of increasing complexity with greater responsibility and progressive independence, has been transformed into the competency model. This requires the teacher to guide and support the young person's learning in the dimensions of being, doing, and knowing, considering that he or she puts into practice what is acquired in the teaching and learning process. The six essential competencies that the resident must achieve and master are medical knowledge, patient care, interpersonal and communication skills, professionalism, practice-based learning and improvement, and finally a systems-based practice.

This training model aims to have a comprehensive approach that seeks to link the educational sector with the productive sector. This raises the potential of individuals with the ability to face the transformations of contemporary society, which is considered a strength since it seeks to end the existing gap between the world of academia and the labor market. The strengths of the actual model is the capacity for internationalization and the possibility of allowing the flow of students and professionals from one country to another and the validation of degrees and degrees according to international criteria. However, this model tends to generate certified students in an accumulation of competencies so that they have efficient and effective job performances, without reinforcing the humanistic and professionalism competences required to lead and take difficult decisions in complex surgical cases in areas were resources are scarce [27, 28].

To describe the current status of neurosurgery medical residency, we developed two tables, presenting the sociodemographic characteristics of the countries in the region according to the income level proposed by the World Bank (Table 17.1) and also some characteristics of the neurological surgery training programs in the region (Table 17.2).

Of the 24 countries in the region, some general data was found. Physician density had a variation from 2.3 to 81.9 doctors per 10,000 habitants, with the lowest concentration in low-income countries. Health expenditure as a percentage of gross domestic product (GDP) ranged from 3.22% to 12.19%. The rural population rate rank from 5% to 73%, as is shown in Table 17.1. It was found that there are more than 1063 residents of neurosurgery and more than 6637 neurosurgeons in Latin America and the Caribbean [29–31]. Seventy-six neurosurgery programs were described in 13 countries in Latin America and the Caribbean, mostly distributed in

**Table 17.1** Sociodemographic characteristics of Latin American and Caribbean countries

| Income level | Country | Rural population (% of the total population) | Physicians (per 10,000 population) | Density of neurosurgeons per 100,000 population | Health expenditure % GDP |
|---|---|---|---|---|---|
| Low income | Haiti | 45 | 2.3 | 0.378 | 5.39 |
| Lower middle income | Bolivia | 31 | 16.1 | 3.313 | 6.86 |
| | El Salvador | 28 | 15.6 | 0.409 | 6.96 |
| | Honduras | 43 | 3.1 | 0.540 | 8.40 |
| | Nicaragua | 41 | 10 | 0.665 | 8.75 |
| Upper middle income | Argentina | 8 | 39.6 | 0.843 | 7.55 |
| | Brazil | 13 | 21.4 | 1.59 | 11.77 |
| | Belize | 54 | 11.2 | 0.852 | 6.12 |
| | Colombia | 19 | 20.8 | 0.414 | 5.91 |
| | Costa Rica | 21 | 11.4 | 0.840 | 7.56 |
| | Cuba | 23 | 81.9 | 0.940 | 12.19 |
| | Dominican Republic | 19 | 15.6 | 0.720 | 6.16 |
| | Ecuador | 36 | 20.5 | 0.622 | 8.39 |
| | Guatemala | 49 | 3.5 | 0.187 | 5.82 |
| | Guyana | 73 | 7.9 | 0.130 | 4.24 |
| | Jamaica | 44 | 13.1 | 0.441 | 6.07 |
| | Mexico | 20 | 22.4 | 0.373 | 5.47 |
| | Paraguay | 38 | 13.6 | 0.396 | 8.02 |
| | Peru | 22 | 12.7 | 0.862 | 5.14 |
| | Suriname | 34 | 12.2 | 0.000 | 6.06 |
| | Venezuela | 12 | 19.2 | 0.208 | 3.22 |
| High income | Chile | 12 | 10.8 | 1.373 | 8.53 |
| | Panama | 32 | 15.6 | 0.129 | 7.26 |
| | Uruguay | 5 | 50.4 | 0.965 | 9.06 |

**Table 17.2** Characteristics of postgraduate programs in neurosurgery in Latin America and the Caribbean

| Country | Number of programs | Duration (years) | Total number of residents | Salary | Weekly hours | Number of neurosurgeons | Research requirement | Examination strategy |
|---|---|---|---|---|---|---|---|---|
| Haiti | 0 | NA | 0 | NA | NA | 4 | NA | NA |
| Bolivia | 3 | 5 | ND | ND | ND | 350 | ND | ND |
| El Salvador | 3 | 3 | 5 | ND | ND | 39 | ND | ND |
| Honduras | 1 | 5 | 6 | ND | ND | 45 | ND | ND |
| Nicaragua | 1 | 5 | 18 | ND | ND | 40 | ND | ND |
| Argentina | ND | 5 | ND | ND | <60 | 208 | ND | ND |
| Brazil | 24 | 5 | 650 | $816 monthly | >100 | 3298 | Thesis | ND |
| Belize | 0 | NA | 0 | NA | NA | 3 | NA | NA |
| Colombia | 11 | 5 | 110 | $0, and residents must pay for their training | >100 | 320 | Thesis | ND |
| Costa Rica | 1 | 6 | 9 | $5900 | 66 | 31 | No | ND |
| Cuba | ND | 4 | ND | $50 Foreign residents must pay for their training | >100 | 107 | Thesis | Annual general oral exam |
| Dominican Republic | ND | 4 | ND | ND | ND | 75 | ND | ND |
| Ecuador | 1 | 5 | 18 | ND | ND | 99 | ND | ND |
| Guatemala | 2 | 5 | 16 | ND | ND | 35 | ND | ND |
| Guyana | ND | 5 | ND | ND | ND | 1 | ND | ND |
| Jamaica | ND | 5 | ND | ND | ND | 12 | ND | ND |
| Mexico | 16 | 5 | ND | ND | >100 | 1146 | ND | ND |
| Paraguay | ND | 3 | ND | ND | ND | 23 | ND | ND |

| | | | | | | | | |
|---|---|---|---|---|---|---|---|---|
| Peru | ND | 5 | ND | ND | ND | 269 | ND | ND |
| Suriname | ND | ND | ND | ND | ND | 0 | ND | ND |
| Venezuela | 13 | 5 | ND | $4 | >100 | 250 | Thesis | Weekly oral evaluation, every 4 months a general oral/written exam |
| Chile | ND | 4 | 247 | ND | ND | 244 | ND | ND |
| Panama | ND | 5 | ND | ND | ND | 5 | ND | ND |
| Uruguay | ND | 6 | ND | ND | ND | 33 | ND | ND |
| Total | 7€ | NA | 1063 | NA | NA | 6637 | NA | NA |

*NA* Not available, *ND* no data

large cities, with little or no coverage of rural areas. Approximately 31% were in Brazil, 21% in Mexico, and 18% in Central America and the Caribbean. Additionally, we found no training programs in Haiti and Belize, as shown in Table 17.2. The approximate duration of neurosurgery programs in Latin America is 3–6 years, 5 years in most countries. The places with shorter period require prior training in general surgery and a year of work in a rural environment. In Uruguay and Costa Rica alone, the training is 6 years, while in Paraguay and El Salvador, it lasts 3 years. Also, the workload varies in a significantly way; in some countries such as Venezuela, Brazil, or Colombia, residents work more than 100 hours a week, while in countries like Argentina and Costa Rica, they work less than 70 hours a week, while in the USA or Europe, where there are specific rules on the workload of residents [32, 33].

For each country there are guidelines for postgraduate programs not specific to neurosurgery. There are recommendations from the neurosurgical scientific societies, and they are not fully integrated with government guidelines. The main elements in the structure of the training programs were identified in three main aspects, medical care, educational activities, and research, where significant gaps are evident in these areas in general, mainly in research, where the language is a significant barrier, since most of the available biomedical literature is in English. The countries of Latin America and the Caribbean speak Spanish, Portuguese, and, to a lesser extent, English or French [32, 33]. Class presentations and readings were optional; besides this, there are significant differences in each country's qualification methodology.

Periodic and theoretical evaluations are carried out in most programs, but there is no overall evaluation system established in most countries. Neither is the training time. It was found that most residents received payment, supported mainly by the government and some alliances with the private sector. Salaries ranged start from USD 5 in Venezuela up to USD 5900 in Costa Rica. The only country where neurosurgery residents do not receive salary was Colombia; however, in 2018, a law was created, regulating residents' payment. To date, this payment has not yet materialized in all of them. On the other hand, graduate students in neurosurgery in the Dominican Republic, Chile, Cuba, and Colombia must pay for their training; tuition payment was reported in Cuba only for foreign residents [32–35]. Currently, most fellows are trained in the skull base, spine, and vascular-endovascular surgery. Less offered are subspecialties like pediatric neurosurgery, peripheral nerve surgery, trauma, intensive care, and global neurosurgery. As in other low- and middle-income countries of the world, there are few subspecialists in these regions. With large, concentrated urban centers, many patients must travel to other countries to compensate for the lack of services. Of the programs already mentioned, only four of them include salary support for the student, including one for skull base surgery in Brazil, one for pediatric neurosurgery in Chile, and the global neurosurgery and trauma fellow from Colombia [34, 35].

## Future Opportunities and Unmet Needs

The evolution of neurosurgical education in the Latin American and Caribbean region has entered into the new era of the global neurosurgery trends. As more programs become part of international collaborations and as more universities and hospitals become integrated with global knowledge and research networks, a clear pathway for integration of curriculums is required [36–38]. Regional and local neurosurgical societies have been supporting these types of activities as the expansion of new programs fills specific local requirements. Standardized curriculums for subspecialty educational tracks and better balance between humanitarian and technical skills have been identified as key aspects, in order to move to a future that has been forced by the recent reality of a new world during pandemics [39]. The COVID-19 reality has pushed healthcare systems at the edge, especially in regions like Latin America and the Caribbean region where workforce and resources are scarce (Fig. 17.5) [40]. The challenges of moving surgical training into a new paradigm of virtual education are now a status quo for most of the world training centers (Fig. 17.5). Basic and advanced surgical skills training requirements has increased the number of virtual and augmented reality tools into this process, where engineering and computer sciences skills meet the traditional surgical ones [41, 42]. A recent forum of the larger universities in Latin America discussed how the "new normal" will include a modular training system approach where residents can select virtual credits so long as it fits into a specific curricular design. Several international

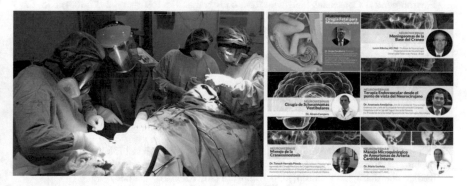

**Fig. 17.5** The new reality of neurosurgical training during the COVID-19 era has accelerated the trend of virtual education in surgical careers. New residents and fellows will be exposed to a new reality of performing surgical procedures with additional occupational risk factors, generating a larger burden of burnout during training, especially in regions like Latin America and the Caribbean where human resources and advanced care technology are scarce (right picture). New models of virtual education supported by educational institutions and specialized societies have arrived to stay. The new webinars program for neurosurgical education of the Latin American Federation of Neurosurgical Societies is a good example of this new trend (left picture). (Images courtesy of the Neurotrauma and Global Surgery Fellowship Program (Meditech Foundation, Cali) and the Latin American Federation of Neurosurgical Societies)

universities and hospitals are now offering credits through short virtual programs fulfilling high academic standards and are available all over the world [43]. The unmet needs remain. Neurosurgery training opportunities are still a luxury or an almost impossible pathway for some physicians in the region. Differences between public education and private ones will be shortened because of the new normal as virtual education is available for all. North-south collaborations between more-developed areas and less-developed areas will remain as an important process of balancing educational needs and offers. New collaborations inside the same region will create a strong academic process minimizing traveling costs for the students and preparing them for a more context-based scenario. Educational technology will decrease the gap for students and teachers in order to be connected to a global neurosurgery environment where we all continue empowering the training of future neurosurgeons worldwide.

# References

1. Pinzón CE. Los grandes paradigmas de la educación médica en Latinoamérica. Acta Med Colombiana. 2008;33(1):33–41.
2. Nicolescu R. The Influences of Globalization on Educational Environment and Adjustment of National Systems. Procedia Soc Behav Sci. 2015;180:72–9.
3. Kim DH, Dacey RG, Zipfel GJ, Berger MS, McDermott M, Barbaro NM, Shapiro SA, Solomon RA, Harbaugh R, Day AL. Neurosurgical Education in a Changing Healthcare and Regulatory Environment: A Consensus Statement from 6 Programs. Neurosurgery. 2017;80(4):S75–82.
4. LaFuente J. De la neurocirugía mística de la antiguedad a los retos que afronta en el siglo XXI: Los cambios de paradigma según la evolución de la Neurocirugía en el tiempo. 1ª ed. Barcelona: Real Academia Europea de Doctores; 2018. p. 33–55.
5. Llobet AF. Localizaciones cerebrales. Investigaciones experimentales, neurológicas y clínicas aplicadas a la operación del trépano. Tesis. Facultad de Medicina, Universidad de Buenos Aires; 1885.
6. Llobet AF. La prótesis en la cirugía moderna. Obturación craneana con placas de celuloide. Anal Sanidad Militar. 1901;3:9–16.
7. Peña G. Apuntes para la historia de la neurocirugía en Colombia. 1ª ed. Bogotá: Ed. Kimpres; 1999. p. 12–15.
8. Ferreyra LG. Erário mineral. Lisboa: Na officina de M. Rodrigues; 1735.
9. Espinoza Concha PM, Lagos Labbé PS. Entrevista al doctor Fernando Cabieses (76 años), médico neurocirujano y antropólogo. Chungará (Arica). 2010;42(2):357–36.
10. Sfeir F, Villanueva PR, Tagle P. History of the Neurosurgery Department of Pontificia Universidad Católica, Santiago de Chile. World Neurosurg. 2017;97:645–51.
11. Turnes AL. Creadores de la Neurocirugía Uruguaya: Alejandro H Schroeder and Roman Arana Iñiguez. In: Wilson E, editor. Historia de la Neurocirugía en Uruguay. 1ª ed; 2007.
12. Silva Guzmao S, De Souza JG. Historia Da Neurocirurgia No Brasil. 2ª ed. Editorial SBN, Sociedad Brasileira de Neurocirurgia; 2008. p. 41–100.
13. Goyenechea FF, Pereira R: Neurocirugía: lesiones del Sistema Nervioso. 1ª ed. La Habana: Editorial Ciencias Médicas; 2014.
14. Burgos de la Espriella R, Ahumada Y. La Neurocirugía en Colombia 50 años de Asociación: 1962–2012. 1ª ed. Bogotá: Asociación Colombiana de Neurocirugía; 2012.
15. Gonzalez Revilla A. Historia de la Neurocirugía en Panama. Neuroeje. 1990;8(2):49–57.

16. Dabdoub CF, Dabdoub CB. The history of neurosurgery in Bolivia and pediatric neurosurgery in Santa Cruz de la Sierra. Surg Neurol Int. 2013;4:123.
17. Sociedad de Neurología de Uruguay. Historia de la Sociedad de Neurología de Uruguay. [Online]; 2019. Available at: https://neurologiauruguay.org/web/index.php/inicio/institucional/historia.
18. Noriega M, Castillo M, Santolaya M. Formación de especialistas en Latinoamérica. Rol de las universidades chilenas. Educ Méd. 2018;19(S1):25–30.
19. Scheffer MC, Dal Poz MR. The privatization of medical education in Brazil: trends and challenges. Hum Resour Health. 2015;13:96.
20. Tujanski L. Historia de la Neurocirugía Argentina. Rev Argent Neurocir. 2004;18(Supl 1):s1–7.
21. Castillo M, Montoya J, Castillo L. La educación, una mirada desde el conflicto social en Colombia. Rev Educ Hum. 2018;20(34):216–32.
22. Arias-Castillo L. Reflexión sobre la educación médica en Colombia. FEM: Rev Fund Educ Méd. 2019;22(3):97–102.
23. Restrepo-Espinosa MH, Lara-Orduz JM, Diaz-Serrano E. Educación médica colombiana en la segunda mitad del siglo XX: entre el modelo Flexneriano y la Medicina Social Latinoamericana. Nova et Vetera. 2017;3(26). Available at: https://www.urosario.edu.co/Revista-Nova-Et-Vetera/Vol-3-Ed-26/Omnia/Educacion-medica-colombiana-en-la-segunda-mitad-de/.
24. Goyenechea F. Historia de la Neurocirugia en Cuba. Neurocuba. 2008;1:49–62.
25. Polavarapu HV, Kulaylat N, Sun S, Hamed O. 100 years of surgical education: The past, present, and future. Bull Am Coll Surg. 2013;1(1):22–7.
26. Kadmon M, Cate OT, Sigrid H, Berberat PO. Postgraduate Medical Education: an increasingly important focus of study and innovation. GMS: J Med Educ. 2017;34(5):Doc70.
27. Reussi R. Pre and post-graduate education in Latin America. Educ Méd. 2018;19(S1):1–3.
28. Sánchez W. Tendencias y modelos en la educación superior en Cirugía. "Reingeniería en Educación Quirúrgica". Rev Med. 2010;18(2):266–69.
29. Punchak M, Mukhopadhyay S, Sachdev S, Hung YC, Peeters S, Rattani A, et al. Neurosurgical care: availability and access in low-income and middle-income countries. World Neurosurg. 2018;112:e240–54.
30. Liang KE, Bernstein I, Kato Y, Kawase T, Hodaie M. Enhancing neurosurgical education in low- and middle-income countries: current methods and new advances. Neurol Med Chir (Tokyo). 2016;56(11):709–15.
31. Loyo M. Neurosurgery in Mexico and Latin-America. Int Neurosci J. 2015;1(1):45–6.
32. Rickard J. Systematic review of postgraduate surgical education in low- and middle-income countries. World J Surg. 2016;40:1324–35.
33. Murguia-Fuentes R, Husein N, Vega A, Rangel-Castilla L, Rotta JM, Quinones-Hinojosa A, Guinto G, Esquenazi Y. Neurosurgical residency training in Latin America: current status, challenges, and future opportunities. World Neurosurg. 2018;120:e1079–97.
34. Miller EI, la Riva D, Ortega JE, Sansivirini Valle F, Lungo Esquivel R, Salgado Pérez M, et al. Current situation of neurosurgery in Central America: an analysis and suggestions for improvement. World Neurosurg. 2013;80(5):E53–7.
35. Vera D, Clavijo A, Rubiano AM. Survey for Latin American residents in neurological surgery. Internal working document. INUB Meditech Research Group; 2019.
36. Gasco J. Present and future of neurosurgery training and education. Malays J Med Sci. 2013;21(1):1–3.
37. Kato Y, Liew BS, Sufianov AA, et al. Review of global neurosurgery education: horizon of neurosurgery in the developing countries. Chin Neurosurg J. 2020;6:19. https://doi.org/10.1186/s41016-020-00194-1.
38. Ashfaq A, Lazareff J. Language and style: a barrier to neurosurgical research and advancement in Latin America. Surg Neurol Int. 2020;8:308.
39. Calero-Martinez SA, Matula C, Peraud A, Biroli F, Fernández-Alén J, Bierschneider M, Cunningham M, Hawryluk GWJ, Babu M, Bullock MR, Rubiano AM. Development and

assessment of competency-based neurotrauma course curriculum for international neurosurgery residents and neurosurgeons. Neurosurg Focus. 2020;48(3):E13.

40. Fontanella MM, Saraceno G, Lei T, Bederson JB, You N, Rubiano AM, Hutchinson P, Wiemeijer-Timmer F, Servadei F. Neurosurgical activity during COVID-19 pandemic: an experts' opinion from China, South Korea, Italy, the USA, Colombia, and the UK. J Neurosurg Sci. 2020;64(4):383–8.

41. Tagaytayan R, Kelemen A, Sik-Lanyi C. Augmented reality in neurosurgery. Arch Med Sci. 2018;14(3):572–8.

42. Fiani B, De Stefano F, Kondilis A, Covarrubias C, Reier L, Sarhadi K. Virtual reality in neurosurgery: "can you see it?"-a review of the current applications and future potential. World Neurosurg. 2020;141:291–8.

43. Orr D, Weller M, Farrow R. Models for online, open, flexible and technology enhanced higher education across the globe – a comparative analysis. International Council for Open and Distance Education, Oslo, Norway. Technical Report. Accessed online on Dec 1st of 2020. Available at: https://static1.squarespace.com/static/5b99664675f9eea7a3ecee82/t/5bb8e52e24a6941855f8d039/1538843963467/Models-report-April-2018_final.pdf.

# Chapter 18
# Neurosurgery Education Around the World: North America

**Bárbara Nettel-Rueda, Stephan A. Munich, Mojgan Hodaie, Sergio Moreno-Jiménez, and Richard W. Byrne**

## Introduction

Neurosurgery education in North America has evolved through the years. The United States and Canada are among the most influencing countries not only in the field of surgical techniques and evolution of technology applied to the operating room but also in clinical and basic research. Although Mexico belongs to North America, it is one of the most influencing countries in Central and South America in terms of education. In this chapter, we present a scope about the historical background of neurosurgery education in each country, which is the current status of neurosurgical training and which are the future opportunities and what needs to be improved in order for future neurosurgeons to have the best armamentarium to offer the highest quality of attention to their patients. Every topic is analyzed in each country since education in either one has particular characteristics.

B. Nettel-Rueda (✉)
Department of Neurosurgery, Hospital de Especialidades, Centro Médico Nacional Siglo XXI, IMSS, Mexico City, Mexico

S. A. Munich · R. W. Byrne
Department of Neurosurgery, Rush Medical College, Rush University Department of Neurosurgery, Chicago, IL, USA

M. Hodaie
Division of Neurosurgery, Toronto Western Hospital, University of Toronto, Toronto, ON, Canada

S. Moreno-Jiménez
Instituto Nacional de Neurología y Neurocirugía, Mexico City, Mexico

I. M. Germano (ed.), *Neurosurgery and Global Health*,
https://doi.org/10.1007/978-3-030-86656-3_18

## Brief Historical Background

### Canada

Canada is geographically a very large country, where the vast majority of the population is located in the southernmost fringe of land within relative proximity to the United States border and along the Atlantic and Pacific rims. The northern part of Canada is much less inhabited, and there is a significant part of the land where road access is not available. This effectively renders the great Canadian North with significant limitations to access to healthcare. Canada is also a new country in historical terms, having just recently completed its 150th anniversary since its birth. A third important note about the country of Canada is its bilingual nature. Canada is thus divided into French-speaking, primarily Québec, and English-speaking Canada. All of these three factors have significantly influenced the development of our neurosurgical programs.

By all accounts at the first Canadian neurosurgeon was Dr. Kenneth McKenzie, who left Canada to train with Harvey Cushing in Boston in the 1920s [1, 2]. Upon his return from Boston, he became the first staff neurosurgeon in Toronto [1]. His portrait, as painted by the famous Canadian Group of Seven artist Frederick Varley, still hangs on the walls at the Toronto Western Hospital. Wilder Penfield, the preeminent neurosurgeon, set up his practice in Montreal at the fame; however he was not at the first Canadian neurosurgeon [2]. Penfield was American by birth and established himself in Montreal Neurological Institute, where he rose to scientific fame with his studies of the cerebral cortex and epilepsy [1]. Kenneth McKenzie returned to Toronto in 1923 and dedicated his work to operating on neurosurgical cases after 1929. A large number of key figures of the Canadian neurosurgical scene trained under the hands of Kenneth McKenzie Including Harry Botterell and Charles Drake [2]. Drake established himself in London on where he masterfully developed the subspecialty of vascular neurosurgery, operating on very difficult vascular lesions and in turn training a large number of neurosurgeons who arrived from around the globe to learn his unique skills [1]. Within a short span of time, neurosurgical centers flourished across the country, with key hubs remaining as Toronto, Montreal, and London. To the West, Calgary and Vancouver have remained as the major sites of clinical care and academic activity.

### The United States

American neurosurgery and, therefore, the education of American neurosurgeons are most commonly thought to have begun with its father, Harvey Cushing. Yet, the way in which Dr. Cushing educated is quite different from the way formalized neurosurgical education has evolved. Rather than enroll trainees in a regimented, prescribed residency program, Cushing provided a training comparable to a trade apprenticeship. Trainees spent variable amounts of time with him and then "gained additional exposure to other inspirational educators" [3].

Despite this training paradigm employed by the father of American neurosurgery, neurosurgical training and education developed similarly to that of other surgical specialties – according to the Halsted approach – the familiar, well-structured, gradually progressive march through a training program. In this way, trainees progressed through general education in neurology, neuropathology, and neuroradiology, with, historically, "at least 24 months as a neurosurgeon" [3]. This was followed, at the conclusion of residency training, by "practice for 2 years" prior to board certification by the American Board of Neurosurgery. Formalization of this method of training occurred in 1953 with the foundation of the Residency Review Committee [4].

Opposition to this "Halstedian" method of neurosurgical education prompted Bergland to catastrophize in 1973 in the *New England Journal of Medicine* (at time when the United States had 95 approved residency programs and 662 available resident positions) that "Neurosurgery May Die." His treatise begins simply with "Neurosurgery has stopped evolving." He further argued that while "most trainees are…capable of generalized practice at a standardized level; few are directed into neurosurgical subspecialities or neurosurgical research which will lead to neurosurgical progress." Whether it was due this article, or the public discourse that followed, neurosurgical training since the 1970s (and particularly in the last two decades) has emphasized both the pursuit of subspecialty and research interests. The success of these developments in neurosurgical education may be best illustrated through contemplation of one of the replies to Dr. Bergland's article:

> I can visualize that in the not too distant future neurosurgeons will be able to implant visual receptors into the occipital cortex…or auditory receptors into the temporal cortex…as a result of the cooperative research in artificial sensory organs. A new subspeciality of neurosurgical fetology may be able to diagnose myelomeningocclcs in early intrauterine life so that the embryo or fetus can be removed from the uterus, the deformity corrected, and fetus returned to the mother before neurological deficit has occurred… [5]

## Mexico

In Mexico, from the late nineteenth and early twentieth centuries, neurosurgical procedures were already performed by general surgeons, although it is not accurately known where some type of neurological surgery was first performed [6]. Neurosurgical procedures have been documented since 1842, with the publication by Doctors José María Terán and Luis Hidalgo y Carpio on the theme "a case of skull-brain trauma" in the Newspaper of the Academy of Medicine (sic) and in 1864 the work published by Dr. Luis Hidalgo and Carpio on "Attention of Skull Wounds" published in the *Gaceta Médica* [7]. It was the Juarez Hospital of Mexico, founded in 1847, one of the first centers, where neurosurgery was practiced in a systematized way [8].

In the early and mid-twentieth century, specifically in the 1930s, before a formal residency program began, there were doctors who were already engaged in learning the practice of neurosurgery. They did so through training in general surgery and with studies carried out in the area of neurology; this informal training in neurological surgery was guided by Dr. Mariano Vázquez and Dr. Clemente Robles at the General Hospital of Mexico. They were the ones who after having traveled through all the surgical disciplines decided to focus especially on the study and knowledge of the "delicate and difficult techniques of neurosurgery" [9, 10].

From the end of the nineteenth century and the early years of the twentieth century, neurosurgery in Mexico was predominantly influenced by European neurosurgery, mainly the French, English, and German schools; however, after the first third of the twentieth century, it began to receive influence from the North American school, which was increased until it became to be considered the one that has the most influence in the modern practice of neurosurgery in Mexico [7].

The first neurosurgery department in Mexico was founded at the General Hospital of Mexico in 1937 by Dr. Clemente Robles Castillo and Dr. Mariano Vázquez Rodríguez as a neurology and neurosurgery unit [11].

Dr. Clemente Robles Castillo was one of the most recognized physicians, who is considered the main driver of neurosurgery in Mexico. He began his career as a general surgeon, where he also made great contributions. Later in his career, in the area of cardiology he was the one who started cardiovascular surgery. Dr. Clemente Robles studied neurosurgery in both American and European schools [9, 11].

Medical training through a medical residence was created by the Austrian surgeon Theodore Billroth, starting in the second half of the nineteenth century. In Mexico, the first medical residency program was inaugurated in 1942 at the General Hospital of Mexico with 20 residents of various specialties [6].

Before 1955, the year in which Mexico began with the first neurosurgery residency program, neurosurgeon specialists, who had gone abroad for formal specialization courses, were already available in the country. That was the time when the influence of North American neurosurgery increased as most young Mexican doctors went to large medical centers such as the Massachusetts General Hospital, Johns Hopkins University Hospital, and Mayo Clinic, just to name a few. There were also those who emigrated South, to carry out their specialization studies, such as Dr. María Cristina García Sancho, who trained at the Institute of Neurosurgery and Brain Research of Santiago de Chile and, on her return to Mexico in 1951, became the first woman neurosurgeon in our country.

The first formal program of neurosurgery residency in Mexico was instituted at Hospital "La Raza" of the Mexican Institute of Social Security (IMSS) in 1955, and it was followed in 1960 by the General Hospital of Mexico and Hospital Juárez of Mexico. Over the years, new neurosurgery schools have been added in the different health institutions of the country, all incorporated into the National Health Public Service, summarized in Table 18.1 [12].

In April 1965, the Mexican Council of Neurological Surgery A.C. (MCNS) was founded, being the second oldest in Mexico. Its founders were Horacio Martínez Romero, Daniel Gonzálezy González, Jesús López Lira Castro, José Humberto

**Table 18.1** Neurosurgery in Mexico: historical landmarks

| Year of creation | Hospital · |
|---|---|
| 1955 | Hospital La Raza, IMSS |
| 1960 | Hospital General de México, SSA |
| 1960 | Hospital Juárez de México, SSA |
| 1961 | Centro Médico Nacional "20 de Noviembre," ISSSTE |
| 1963 | Centro Médico Nacional SXXI, IMSS |
| 1964 | Instituto Nacional de Neurología y Neurocirugía, SSA |
| 1964 | Hospital Civil de Guadalajara "Fray Antonio Alcalde," SSA |
| 1970 | Hospital regional "Lic Adolfo López Mateos," ISSSTE |
| 1970 | Hospital Universitario "José Eleuterio González," UANL |
| 1980 | Centro Médico Nacional de Occidente, IMSS |
| 1985 | Hospital "Ángel Leaño," SSJ (closed in 2000) |
| 1989 | UMAE Hospital No. 25, IMSS |
| 1990 | Hospital regional "Ignacio Zaragoza," ISSSTE (closed in 2003) |
| 1991 | Hospita Central Sur de Alta Especialidad, PEMEX |
| 1994 | Hospital Regional "Valentín Gómez Farías," ISSSTE |
| 2011 | Hospital Central Militar, Colegio Militar |
| 2012 | Nuevo Hospital Civil de Guadalajara "Juan I. Menchaca," SSA |
| 2012 | Centro Médico Adolfo López Mateos, ISEM |
| 2013 | Hospital Regional 1° de Octubre, ISSSTE |
| 2015 | Hospital General 450, SSA |
| 2016 | UMAE 71 Centro Médico Nacional Torreón, IMSS |
| 2017 | Instituto de Seguridad Social del Estado de México y Municipios, GDEM |

*IMSS* Instituto Mexicano del Seguro Social, *SSA* Secretaria de Salubridad y Asistencia, *ISSSTE* Instituto de Seguridad y Servicios Sociales para los Trabajadores del Estado, *PEMEX* Petróleos Mexicanos, *ISEM* Instituto de Salud del Estado de México

Mateos Gómez, Ignacio Olivé, Clemente Robles, Manuel Velasco Suárez, Ramón del Cueto, Humberto Guzmán West, Juan Cárdenas y Cárdenas, José María Sánchez Cabrera, and Francisco Gómez Méndez, all of them well recognized neurosurgeons at that time. In 1995, the National Regulatory Committee of Medical Specialty Councils A.C. (CONACEM for its acronym in Spanish) was conformed. This is a tripartite instance that is made up of the Medicine National Academy of Mexico, the Mexican Academy of Surgery, and the Group of Medical Specialty Councils. The CONACEM is responsible for issuing both certification and recertification diplomas that need renovation every 5 years [13, 14].

Each of the neurosurgery specialization programs are endorsed and recognized by a public university and the Mexican Secretariat of Public Education (Table 18.2). In 1992, the National Autonomous University of Mexico designed the Single Plan of Medical Specialties (PUEM for its acronym in Spanish) which came into force in 1994 and currently serves as a pedagogical model for the training of specialists throughout the country. Both the MCNS and PUEM ensure the systematization of academic programs, verify that they are met, and monitor that headquarters have the

**Table 18.2** Subspecialty training programs in Mexico with university endorsement

| Course/duration | Headquarters | University |
|---|---|---|
| Skull base surgery Endoneurosurgery/1 yr | Centro Médico Nacional "20 de Noviembre" | UNAM |
| | Instituto Nacional de Neurología y Neurocirugía | UNAM |
| Spine surgery/2 yr | Centro Médico ABC | UNAM |
| | Centro Médico Nacional "20 de Noviembre" | UNAM |
| | Hospital Central Sur de Alta Especialidad | UNAM |
| | Hospital de Traumatología y Ortopedia "Lomas Verdes" | UNAM |
| | Hospital General Villa | UNAM |
| | Hospital Juárez de México | UNAM |
| | Hospital Regional "1° de Octubre" | UNAM |
| | Hospital Regional de Alta Especialidad de Ixtapaluca | UNAM |
| | Instituto Nacional de Neurología y Neurocirugía | UNAM |
| | Instituto Nacional de Rehabilitación | UNAM |
| | Hospital de Traumatología "Victorio de la Fuente Navarro" | UNAM |
| | Hospital Civil "Fray Antonio Alcalde" [a] | UDG |
| | Hospital General de México | UNAM |
| | ISSSEMYM Centro Médico de Ecatepec | UNAM |
| Epilepsy surgery/1 yr | Instituto Nacional de Neurología y Neurocirugía | UNAM |
| Neuro-oncological surgery/1 yr | Instituto Nacional de Neurología y Neurocirugía | UNAM |
| | Instituto Nacional de Cancerología | UNAM |
| Functional and stereotactic neurosurgery/1 yr | Centro Médico ABC/Instituto Nacional de Neurología y Neurocirugía | UNAM |
| | Centro Médico Nacional "20 de Noviembre" | UNAM |
| | Hospital General de México | UNAM |
| Vascular neurosurgery/1 yr | Centro Médico Nacional "20 de Noviembre" | UNAM |
| | Instituto Nacional de Neurología y Neurocirugía | UNAM |
| | UMAE Hospital de Especialidades CMN SXXI | UNAM |
| Radiosurgery/1 yr | Instituto Nacional de Neurología y Neurocirugía | UNAM |

*UDG* Universidad de Guadalajara, *UNAM* Universidad Autónoma de México, *UMAE* Unidad Médica de Alta Especialidad, *ISSEMYM* Instituto de Seguridad Social del Estado de México y Municipios, *CMN SXXI* Centro Médico Nacional Siglo XXI
[a] Will start in 2021

**Table 18.3** Neurosurgery pediatrics and endovascular training programs in Mexico

| Course | Duration (years) | Headquarters | University |
|---|---|---|---|
| Neurologic endovascular therapy | 2 | Hospital Universitario de Nuevo León Instituto Nacional del Neurología y Neurocirugía Hospital Juárez de México | UANL UNAM UNAM |
| Pediatrics neurosurgery | 2 | Hospital Infantil de México Instituto Nacional de Pediatría Hospital de Pediatría CMNSXXI | UNAM UNAM UNAM |

*UANL* Universidad Autónoma de Nuevo León, *UNAM* Universidad Nacional Autónoma de México

minimum necessary infrastructure to comply with the curriculum of the specialization course. This guarantees that neurosurgeons who train in Mexico, regardless of the institution where they carry out their residency program, have the same academic opportunities.

From 1991 the National Graduate Quality Program (PNPC for its acronym in Spanish) was instituted by the National Council of Science and Technology (CONACYT for its acronym in Spanish) and a branch of the Secretariat of Public Education. The PNPC, in addition to recognizing the quality of the specialization courses, grants scholarships to resident physicians [15].

In 1999, the courses of pediatric neurosurgery (PedNc) and neurological endovascular therapy (NET) were recognized as subspecialties of neurosurgery (Table 18.3). They have their own PUEM and graduates process. At present there are three locations to study PedNc's residence and also three locations to carry out NET's residence.

## Current Status: What Was Accomplished Till Present

### Canada

As of September 2020, there are 14 neurosurgery training programs throughout Canada with less than 20 residents accepted every year. Most programs accept 1 or 2 residents per year except for Toronto, the largest program which on average has greater than 30 residents and accepts approximately 4 residents every year. Neurosurgery residents do not need to complete a year of general internship and apply instead directly into a program from medical school. Training is of 6 years duration, of which 1 year at least is dedicated to research. Frequently this year is extended toward the pursuit of a graduate degree – either a master's or PhD. A requirement for the completion of residency includes the Royal College of Physicians and Surgeons of Canada examination. The Royal College of Physicians and Surgeons of Canada is the body overseeing Canadian subspecialties (http://www.royalcollege.ca/rcsite/home-e). It was established in 1929, and eventually in 1945 it included a subspecialty committee of neurosurgery. One of the key features of Canadian neurosurgery is that training is highly centralized. This means there are many university hospitals where neurosurgery is not available and certainly there is a dearth of community hospitals with neurosurgery services. This directly relates to the population of Canada access to care and a socialized health structure that prevents or mix prohibitive the availability of new research a neurosurgery service in small community hospitals. The implication of this is that patients at times need to travel to seek a neurosurgeon, and this results in a significant new surgery workload issue with the sizable backlogs and waiting lists.

Despite its size, Canadian neurosurgery has been an important force in academic neurosurgery. The University of Toronto has routinely ranked in the top of research papers per year, competing only with UCSF in this category [16]. Neurosurgery residents in Toronto take the opportunity of participating in the surgeon-scientist program which allows integrated and protected research time for the completion of a graduate degree during residency. The vast majority of Toronto residents therefore remain within academic neurosurgery with careers that span clinical work and include basic science research. Key figures in this area include Charles Tator (spinal cord injury), Charles Drake (vascular neurosurgery), RR Tasker (functional neurosurgery) [17], James Rutka (pediatric neurosurgery), and Michael Fehlings (complex spinal neurosurgery), all of which have trained in Toronto and hold up important international notoriety in their subspecialty fields, both in research and international organizations.

Academic neurosurgery requires subspecialty training at which is directly linked to fellowship training. Subspecialty fellowship training is therefore a key component in the large academic sites such as Toronto, Montreal, London, Calgary, and Vancouver. Neurosurgery in French-speaking Canada is primarily concentrated in Québec with sites such as *Université de Montreal, Université de Sherbrooke*, and *Université Laval*. For those in French Canada, Royal College examinations are taken in French.

A key feature of neurosurgery training in Canada is successful completion of the Royal College Fellowship examinations. These exams, consisting of 2 days of written examination followed by an oral exam, are necessary for all Canadian neurosurgeons prior to independent practice.

Fellowship training in subspecialty neurosurgery is widely available in Canada and is primarily offered based on the subspecialty strength and caseload of the hospitals. The Toronto Western Hospital, for instance, hosts approximately 12 fellows each year, in a variety of subspecialty fields such as functional, vascular, neuro-oncology, skull base, and spine subspecialties. The components of a strong residency program, high volume of cases, and a rich fellowship program with broad international representation result in a dynamic environment focused on excellent patient care and clinical and research advances in the field.

## The United States

From 2000 to 2018 the number of neurosurgery residency training programs in the United States increased from 100 to 115. This resulted in an increase in the number of trainees from 1112 to 1462. This increase in resident complement was paralleled by an increase in the mean number for neurosurgery faculty per program from 5.6 to 17.5.

The last decade of neurosurgical training in the United States has seen many changes designed to both improve standardization while also permitting opportunities to pursue individual interests. In 2009, the PGY1 year was incorporated fully into all American neurosurgical residency (whereas it previously had been considered a preliminary training year under the purview of general surgery). In 2010, the Society of Neurological Surgeons introduced boot camp courses for incoming PGY1 residents, with the stated goal of teaching "a systematic core of skills" (Table 18.4) [18]. This boot camp course has been expanded since to include another course for residents in the beginning of their PGY2 year.

Beginning in 2019, PGY2 residents are administered a written exam of surgical anatomy. They are permitted to take the exam three times and ultimately must attain a 100% score. The intention of this is increase the focus toward practical and relevant neurosurgical knowledge. This sentiment is also reflected on the written board exam (that must be passed prior to the chief year of residency) – recently, exams echo a move toward practical neurosurgical knowledge and away from esoteric, pedagogic questioning.

Another change designed to standardize the training within American neurosurgical programs was the introduction of the Milestone program in 2012. The Milestone program was an ACGME initiative designed to "create a logical trajectory of professional development in essential elements of competency and meet criteria for effective assessment..." [19]. The categories of Milestones include patient care, medical knowledge, systems-based practice, practice-based learning

**Table 18.4** Content of didactic and procedural sessions at PGY1 neurosurgical boot camp

| Didactic session topics | Procedural session topics |
| --- | --- |
| Unstable neurosurgical patient | Ventriculoperitoneal shunt tap |
| Intracranial pressure management | Lumbar puncture, lumbar drain insertion |
| Emergency cranial radiological assessment | Intracranial pressure monitor placement |
| Emergency evaluation/management of hydrocephalus patient | External ventricular drain placement simulator |
| Neurological and neurotrauma assessment | Cervical spine traction and reduction |
| Emergency spinal radiological assessment | Cranial fixation and positioning basics |
| Professionalism, supervision, pearls | Spinal positioning basics |
| Making the incision | Basic neurosurgical instrumentation |
| Patient safety and communication | Lines: Central venous, arterial |

and improvement, professionalism, and interpersonal and communication skills [20, 21]. Milestones progress through Levels 1 to 5, with Level 4 being the goal for graduation from residency and Level 5 being subspecialty fellowship-level goals. Implementation of the Milestone program resulted in identification (and design of individual improvement plan) of struggling residents, revision of residency curricula based on identified training gaps, and an increase in the number of logged cases among residents [22, 23].

In 2014, the American Board of Neurological Surgeons mandated implementation of 84 months (7 years) of postgraduate training. Prior to this mandate, 80% of neurosurgery training programs were already 7 years, while 20% were 6 years in duration. While the length of training was standardized, this mandate also served to foster the pursuit of individualized interests since this training period invariably included at least 1 year of protected research time. During this time, US residents have pursued basic science research, clinical research, subspecialty fellowship training, and advanced degrees (e.g., masters of business administration, masters in public health).

In an effort to combat physician burnout, over the last two decades there has been increased attention given to resident wellness [24]. The first major change with this in mind was the establishment of the 80-h workweek for trainees across all medical and surgical specialties, including neurosurgery, by the ACGME. In addition to a strict mandate of less than 80 h work per week, trainees were no longer permitted to work more than 24 h per shift and were mandated to have 1 day without patient care responsibilities per week [25]. Since that time, more attention has been given not just to work hour restrictions but also to the concept of "wellness," which is meant to "emphasize that psychological, emotional, and physical well-being are critical in the development of the competent, caring, and resilient physician" [26]. While the benefits (or detriments) of work hour restrictions remain a subject of debate [27–29], the implementation of resident wellness programs is becoming more prevalent as the success of these programs on trainee well-being is realized [30, 31].

In addition to training at the resident level, changes have been made to the process of board certification. Recently, the American Board of Neurological Surgeons changed oral board certification to include review of the candidates own surgical cases. In this way candidates are evaluated according to their own practice and not exclusively according to hypothetical cases.

## Mexico

All neurosurgery residency programs in Mexico consist of 6 years of preparation: 1 year of general surgery plus 5 years of neurosurgery. The process for a surgeon physician, national or foreign, to enter the specialty of neurosurgery will take several mandatory and systematized steps; it is a single process that is followed, regardless of the educational institution to which the candidate will apply. This process has changed over the years, but at present time the steps to be followed are summarized in Fig. 18.1. The approval of the National Examination of Medical Residence Applicants (ENARM for its acronym in Spanish) will allow the applicant to enter first the specialty of general surgery from which he may be referred to neurosurgery by a selection exam and an interview.

Once neurosurgery training is finalized, the new neurosurgeon may choose to continue with a subspecialty in pediatric neurosurgery or neurologic endovascular

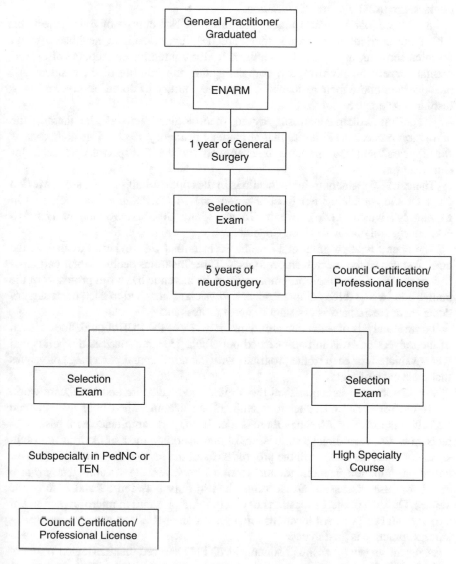

**Fig. 18.1** Neurosurgical training process in Mexico flowchart. *ENARM Examen Nacional de Aspirantes a Residencias Médicas* (National Examination of Medical Residence Applicants), *PedNC* pediatric neurosurgery, *TEN* neurologic endovascular therapy

therapy for two more years; at the end a subspecialty license is granted (Table 18.2). Neurosurgeons who do not choose to continue in a residency program for subspecialty but aspire to expand their preparation in a specific area have the option to take a high specialty course; most of these courses have a minimum duration of 1 year, except the high specialty course in spine surgery, which lasts for 2 years without being given a specialist license as a spine surgeon (Table 18.3). There is also the option to hold diplomas on different disciplines, which, unlike high specialty courses, are usually shorter in duration.

In all headquarters neurosurgery programs, PUEM consist of four subjects on which the curriculum is based; these are healthcare seminar, healthcare work, research seminar, and education seminar. It also contemplates a course of experimental surgery or microsurgery, complementing the training of the resident. All headquarters allow their residents to leave the country to do an observer training lasting on average 3 months [32].

Regarding pediatric neurosurgery and neurological endovascular therapy, the admission process is similar to that of medical residency. Each of the courses lasts for 2 years, and the graduate is examined by the Subspecialty Council for Certification.

There are 20 resident training locations in the country, half of them are in Mexico City. Of the remaining ten locations, four are in Guadalajara (Jalisco), two in Monterrey (Nuevo León), two in Toluca (State of Mexico), one in Durango (Durango), and one in Torreón (Coahuila).

The operational program of 17 of the 20 locations was reviewed to analyze the current status of the specialization courses. Three locations declined their participation or did not submit their program on time. Each venue has a full professor of the course and two or three adjunct teachers. Physicians attached to each neurosurgery department participate as assistant or guest professors.

For the analysis of academic programs, a review of the PUEM guidelines of each of the universities was initially carried out. Table 18.5 summarizes the points that were evaluated for each of the programs with the number and percentage of venues that meet each of them.

All 17 locations accomplished the seminar on healthcare and healthcare work, while the research and education seminars are accomplished only by 94% and 52.90%, respectively. Although there is a deficiency in compliance with basic subjects, however, regarding specific issues of neurosurgery, most of the trunk and subspecialty areas are met by all the programs. In all the revised venues residents have active participation in monographic sessions; however, the sessions that are provided for case discussion are accomplished in only between 52 and 84% of the venues. Only 13 of the 17 locations have a training program in microsurgery and/or experimental surgery. All locations are high-volume patient care centers, so neurosurgical practice is guaranteed.

A recent survey by Yoshua Esquenazi MD PhD showed that in Mexico 76 out of 130 (58.4%) neurosurgeons who responded to the survey have performed an overseas rotation, mainly to the United States or Germany, and all of them underwent a local rotation. The working hours were 60–80 in 20 neurosurgeons (15.4%),

**Table 18.5** Neurosurgery training in Mexico: academic subjects and rotations compliance

| Subject | Hospitals | % |
|---|---|---|
| *Basic seminars (PUEM)* | | |
| Healthcare seminar | 17/17 | 100% |
| Healthcare work | 17/17 | 100% |
| Research seminar | 16/17 | 94% |
| Education seminar | 9/17 | 52.90% |
| *Rotations* | | |
| Lessons according year of residency | 17/17 | 100% |
| National rotations | 16/17 | 94% |
| International rotations | 17/17 | 100% |
| *Basic subjects* | | |
| Anatomy/physiology/ embryology | 17/17 | 100% |
| Neurology/neurological exploration | 17/17 | 100% |
| Neuropathology | 17/17 | 100% |
| Pharmacology | 8/17 | 47.05% |
| Intensive care | 9/17 | 52.90% |
| Neuroradiology | 15/17 | 88.23% |
| *Specific areas training* | | |
| Pediatric neurosurgery | 17/17 | 100% |
| Neuro-oncology/skull base | 17/17 | 100% |
| Vascular neurosurgery | 17/17 | 100% |
| Spine neurosurgery | 17/17 | 100% |
| Trauma neurosurgery | 17/17 | 100% |
| Functional neurosurgery | 16/17 | 94% |
| Stereotactic radiosurgery | 12/17 | 70.58% |
| *Discussion sessions* | | |
| Monographic sessions | 17/17 | 100% |
| Clinical and surgical sessions | 14/17 | 82.35% |
| Bibliographic sessions | 15/17 | 88.23% |
| Morbi-mortality sessions | 9/17 | 52.94% |
| Experimental surgery/ microsurgery | 13/17 | 76.47% |
| High volume hospital | 17/17 | 100% |

*PUEM Plan Único de Especialidades Médicas* (Single Plan of Medical Specialties)

80–100 in 59 (45.4%), and more than 100 in 51 (39.2%) during residency. The teaching hours reported per week were less than 1 by 3 neurosurgeons (2.3%), 1–3 by 21 (16.2%), 3–5 by 55 (42.3%), 5–10 by 48 (36.9%), and more than 10 by 3 (2.3%). Only 17 (13%) neurosurgeons experienced a research exclusive time during the residency (information provided by Yoshua Esquenazi).

## Future Opportunities and Unmet Needs

### *Canada*

The future of neurosurgery includes continued excellence in training, as well as greater incorporation of tools such as surgical simulation, cadaveric labs, and virtual training methods. These will be of particular value in the setting of preparation and teaching of complex, rare procedures, and fellowship level training.

### *The United States*

Neurosurgery is one of the most rapidly evolving fields in medicine. Within a generation of neurosurgeons, endovascular techniques have emerged (and expanded) as a means to effectively treat cerebrovascular pathology. Minimally invasive spine surgery is often replacing more extensive surgical procedures, and deep brain stimulation has offered hope to those with previously inevitably progressive neurodegenerative (and, even *more* recently, psychiatric disorders). As such, it is imperative that the training of American neurosurgeons similarly evolve.

However, this begs the question – will "new" trainees adequately develop the "old" skills? As more aneurysms are coiled rather than clipped, will trainees finish their residency with the skills to safely and effectively clip an aneurysm? As more spine surgery is performed through minimally invasive techniques, will residents have the same understanding of spinal anatomy that is gained through the visualization afforded by open techniques?

One potential way to address these future training gaps is through surgical simulation [33–35]. Surgical simulators are becoming more prevalent, sophisticated, and affordable, making them reasonable ways to confront this issue. It will be critical for neurosurgical training programs to ensure that these skills do not become "a lost art."

### *Mexico*

In neurosurgery residency programs in Mexico, there are still many opportunity areas that can be opened to improve the quality of education that Mexican residents receive. While it is true that all the headquarters hospitals where Mexican residents are trained guarantee a high volume of patients to be able to train them, the truth is that not all the facilities develop all areas of neurosurgery despite the fact that they have highly trained neurosurgeons among their staff. Most of the time this is due to the lack of infrastructure and technology; however, this weakness has been dealt with by allowing residents to visit other facilities either in the same country or abroad where they can complete their training.

In the review of the academic programs that we carried out, it was observed that there is quite a homogeneity in them, all covering the basic areas for training residents. Notwithstanding, it is striking that the microsurgery training program is not covered in all the venues. A microsurgery course is a fundamental subject for the training of a specialist in which more than 80% of the surgeries performed are under the use of a microscope, so this is an unmet need that should be improved not for the future but in the short term.

Even though all the venues comply with a research seminar in their academic programs, the actual practice does not designate a specific time for clinical o basic research, so residents do not get involved in research trails in a regular way, being this an unmet need that is important to fulfill.

None of the PUEM in neurosurgery contemplates within the training program the practice of surgical approaches and dissections in anatomical specimens (cadaveric lab) nor are there programs for practice in surgical simulators, which have been shown to be useful in other countries where the training hours for residents have been reduced and consequently so do are the hours spent in the operating room. In Mexico these situations have not yet occurred (reduction of working hours per week); nonetheless, what is certain is that the resident will not arrive at the operating room to practice microsurgical techniques or surgical approaches, or both, in the patient itself. We found here another unmet need that should be solved in a short-term period, opening the opportunities for neurosurgery residents to have a safe way to improve surgical skills avoiding an increased risk for the patient and legal issues [36, 37].

**Acknowledgments**  The author wants to express special gratitude to Dr. Gerardo Guinto Balanzar, Dr. Ángel Martínez Ponce de León, Dr. Yoshua Esquenazi Levy, Dr. Antonio Zárate Méndez, Dr. Rafael Mendizabal Guerra, Dr. Erika Dalila Ascencio Gil, Dr. José Damián Carrillo Ruíz, Dr. Gustavo Melo Guzmán, Dr. Francisco López González, and Dr. Sophie d'Herbemont for their invaluable support during the preparation of this manuscript.

# References

1. Ramnath S. Cerebrovascular neurosurgery in Canada: an historical review. Can J Neurol Sci. 2018;45:227–34.
2. Weir B. A history of neurosurgery in Canada. Can J Neurol Sci. 2011;38:203–19.
3. Friedman WA. Resident duty hours in American neurosurgery. Neurosurgery. 2004;54:925–33.
4. Neurological Surgery Milestones. 2018. https://www.acgme.org/Search-ACGME?searchterm=neurological%20surgery%20milestones%202018&sort=score%7CDESC&page=1&pagesize=10. Accessed 10 Sep 2020.
5. Clark K. Accreditation and approval of residency positions in neurological surgery in the United States: an overview. Neurosurgery. 1981;9:601–3.
6. Quijano-Pitman F. Origen y desarrollo de las residencias hospitalarias. Gac Med Mex. 1999;1351:73–6.
7. Calvo-Fonseca JR. Dr. Manuel Velasco Suárez. EL hijo predilecto de Chiapas. Científico, Político, Humanista (1914–2001). 2017. ISBN: 978–607-8413-57-9.
8. Mendizábal-Guerra R, Hernández-Moreno JL. La neurocirugía en el hospital Juárez de México. In: Rodrigo Ramos-Zúñiga, editor. Tractos históricos de la neurocirugía en México. 2012. p. 131–40.

9. Carrillo-Ruíz JD. Historia de la neurocirugía funcional, estereotaxia y radiocirugía en el Hospital General de México. Rodrigo Ramos-Zúñiga, editor. Tractos históricos de la neurocirugía en México. 2012. p. 165–40.

10. Rivero-Serrano O. Homenaje al académico doctor Clemente Robles con motivo del cincuentenario de su ingreso a la Academia Nacional de Medicina. Gac Med Mex. 1991;127:521–34.

11. Robles-Castillo C. Nuevo Académico Dr. Clemente Robles Castillo. Gac Med Mex. 1940;70:541–2.

12. Loyo-Varela M. La neurocirugía en el Instituto Mexicano del Seguro Social. Rodrigo Ramos-Zúñiga, editor. Tractos históricos de la neurocirugía en México. 2012. p. 141–6.

13. Consejo Mexicano de Cirugía Neurológica AC. 2020. http://www.cmcn.org.mx/historia.php . Accessed 20 August 2020.

14. Ramos-Zúñiga R. Educación y formación de recursos en neurocirugía. Rodrigo Ramos-Zuñiga, editor. Tractos históricos de la neurocirugía en México. 2012. p. 49–72.

15. PNPC CONACYT. 2020. https://www.conacyt.gob.mx/index.php/becas-y-posgrados/programa-nacional-de-posgrados-de-calidad. Accessed 20 August 2020.

16. Lozano CS, Tam J, Kulkarni AV, et al. The academic productivity and impact of the University of Toronto Neurosurgery Program as assessed by manuscripts published and their number of citations. J Neurosurg. 2015;123:561–70.

17. Tasker RR. One man's recollection of 50 years of functional and stereotactic neurosurgery. Neurosurgery. 2004;554:968–76.

18. Babu R, Thomas S, Hazzard MA, et al. Morbidity, mortality, and health care costs for patients undergoing spine surgery following the ACGME resident duty-hour reform: clinical article. J Neurosurg Spine. 2014;21:502–15.

19. Nasca TJ, Philibert I, Brigham T, et al. The next GME accreditation system — rationale and benefits. N Engl J Med. 2012;366:1051–6.

20. Bergland R. Neurosurgery may die. N Engl J Med. 1973;288:1043–6.

21. Dacey RG Jr. Resident duty hour regulations: time for reassessment and revision. J Neurosurg. 2016;124:840–1.

22. Shakir HJ, Cappuzzo JM, Shallwani H, et al. Relationship of grit and resilience to burnout among U.S. neurosurgery residents. World Neurosurg. 2020;134:e224–36.

23. Sachs E. Graduate training in neurosurgery. J Neurosurg. 1974;40:554–5.

24. Pelargos PE, Nagasawa DT, Lagman C, et al. Utilizing virtual and augmented reality for educational and clinical enhancements in neurosurgery. J Clin Neurosci. 2017;35:1–4.

25. Selden NR, Abosch A, Byrne RW, et al. Neurological surgery milestones. J Grand Med Educ. 2013;5(Suppl 1):24–35.

26. ACGME. Common Program Requirements. 2020. https://www.acgme.org/What-We-Do/Accreditation/Common-Program-Requirements . Accessed 10 Sept 2020.

27. Yaeger KA, Munich SA, Byrne RW, et al. Trends in United States neurosurgery residency education and training over the last decade (2009-2019). Neurosurg Focus. 2020;48(3):E6.

28. Bodani VP, Breimer GE, Haji FA, et al. Development and evaluation of a patient-specific surgical simulator for endoscopic colloid cyst resection. J Neurosurg. 2020;133:521–9.

29. Conforti LN, Yaghmour NA, Hamstra SJ, et al. The effect and use of milestones in the assessment of neurological surgery residents and residency programs. J Surg Educ. 2018;75:147–55.

30. Babu R, Thomas S, Hazzard MA, et al. Worse outcomes for patients undergoing brain tumor and cerebrovascular procedures following the ACGME resident duty-hour restrictions. J Neurosurg. 2014;121:262–76.

31. Selden NR, Origitano TC, Burchiel KJ, et al. A National Fundamentals Curriculum for neurosurgery PGY1 residents: the 2010 society of neurological surgeons boot camp courses. Neurosurgery. 2012;70:971–81.

32. Plan Único de Especializaciones Médicas, UNAM. 2020. http://www.sidep.fmposgrado.unam.mx:8080/fmposgrado/Cursos.jsp?medicallevel=ESPECIALIDADES. Accessed 20 July 2020.

33. Bina RW, Lemole GM, Dumont TM. On resident duty hour restrictions and neurosurgical training: review of the literature. J Neurosurg. 2016;124:842–8.

34. Spiotta AM, Fargen KM, Patel S, Larrew T, et al. Impact of a residency-integrated wellness program on resident mental health, sleepiness, and quality of life. Neurosurgery. 2019;84:341–6.
35. Gasco J, Holbrook T, Patel A, et al. Neurosurgery simulation in residency training: feasibility, cost, and educational benefit. Neurosurgery. 2013;73(Suppl 1):S39–45.
36. Rehder R, Abd-El-Barr M, et al. The role of simulation in neurosurgery. Childs Nerv Syst. 2016;32:43–54.
37. Ganju A, Aoun SG, Daou MR, et al. The role of simulation in neurosurgical education: a survey of 99 United States neurosurgery program directors. World Neurosurg. 2013;80:e1–8.

# Part III
# The Economics of Neurosurgery

Isabelle M. Germano

This Part of the book is focused on analyzing a few aspects of economics that influence neurosurgery globally. Economics is the study of how humans make decisions in the face of scarcity. These can be individual, family, business, or societal decisions. Scarcity is a fact of life and has no geographical boundaries. Scarcity means that human needs for goods, services, and resources exceed is the resources available. Resources such as labor, tools, land, and raw materials are necessary to produce the goods and services we want, but they are all, to some extent, limited in supply. Therefore, every society, at every level, must make choices about how to use its resources and how to prioritize its choices.

It is important to underscore the difference between economics and business. Based on an understanding of economics, a business can decide what products to produce and how best to make the enterprise prosper. Medicine and neurosurgery are both an art and a science. The *art* is the *know how to care for our patients*. The *science* is the *know how to treat specific conditions based on evidence*. However, especially in recent years, we also need to take into account a third sphere: business. *Business* is the *know how to pay/get paid for the services provided*. All three of spheres- the art, the science and the business- need to coexist and balance for our field to stay level and prosper.

This Part of the book will introduce and review fundamental aspects of the economic forces shaping neurosurgery globally. The study of economics helps us understanding the major forces influencing our economy. It provides theories, models, and tools helpful to use when seeking a solution to an economic problem. Economics does not provide the answer to the problem rather it provides the tools to find an answer, or, ideally, multiple possible solutions.

In Chap. 19, we will define the neurosurgery enterprise and review its stakeholders. This will allow a deeper understanding of the economic forces that can influence decisions important to our field. It is key for a neurosurgeon to be aware of such forces to understand how best to leverage them when caring for their patients, in order to enhance the art, the science, and the business of their practice.

Part of the science of being a neurosurgeon is not only the ability to treat our patients according to scientific evidence but also to advance the field with discovery.

Since our field is heavily dependent on technology, neurosurgeons are best positioned to understand the unmet technological needs and create the scientific solutions to meet such needs. It is important to note that, by and large, technological advances result in safer/better care and possibly in lower care costs. Chapter 20 reviews some of the steps required to navigate this path and presents successful examples of neurosurgeons on different continents who were able to develop technology that has had a global impact.

In the last decade, through unprecedented technological advancement, digital technology has become a crucial component of many industries, including medicine and neurosurgery. Some of the digital solutions are more cost-effective than ever. Due to the widespread use of computer technology worldwide, digital solutions are readily available to most. Chapter 21 reviews some of the concepts of digital technology, how these are pertinent to neurosurgery, and how they can enhance education.

Nonprofit institutions and foundations constitute a fundamental force influencing medicine. These private entities often serve as a link between healthcare providers/patients and government/industry by providing bridging funds and/or education necessary to initiate important programs. Partnerships between private foundations and government/industry allow us to better align available resources to address some of the unmet needs and to provide progress in delivery of care. Chapter 22 reviews the history, current work, and future direction of nonprofit and academic institutions in global neurosurgery. Collaboration is the central theme for the development of impactful and sustainable global neurosurgery with academic and nonprofit partnerships.

The government represents a central force in any economy around the world. To address topics common across the globe, representatives from 193 countries, members of the United Nations (UN), meet to find shared solutions. The World Health Organization (WHO) is the health technical arm of the UN. The WHO is involved in many health-related projects including surgical care and anesthesia requirements. In neurosurgery, the ability to readily and safely treat traumatic brain and spine injuries are at the top of the list for global unmet needs. Chapter 23 reviews several other aspects of neurosurgical care included within the scope of the WHO.

More than ever before, the uncertainty due to the Covid-19 pandemic has impacted all global market sectors. As first remarked by Kenneth Arrow, recipient of Nobel Prize in Economics in 1972 and one of the founders of healthcare economics, uncertainties affect health care more than other industries. The COVID-19 pandemic started ot disrupt the globe in 2020. Its full impact on global neurosurgery still remains unknown. Neurosurgery globally has been affected in many ways, including case prioritization, workforce redistribution, pre- and intraoperative safety, and the development of new technology. Research training and publications were also significantly affected. Chapter 24 reviews these changes and assesses how these will impact the future of our field.

# Chapter 19
# The Neurosurgery Enterprise and Its Stakeholders

**Kurt Yaeger and Isabelle M. Germano**

## Introduction

With the heavy clinical responsibility as a practicing neurosurgeon, neurosurgery resident, or other healthcare provider, it can be easy to overlook the many complex, interlocking parts that allow a neurosurgical organization to function smoothly in the delivery of surgical services, both locally and worldwide. Standards for surgical technique, quality of care, and patient safety apply to all neurosurgeons regardless of environment, cultural content, and socioeconomic status. From the rural primary care hospital to the technologically advanced, urban subspecialized practices, and anywhere in between, practicing neurosurgeons have to conform to such standards and are thus influenced by economic forces that shape our field. Key stakeholders in the current healthcare delivery model worldwide include, but are not limited to, hospitals, state and local governments, pharmaceutical and technological industries, insurance companies, and other externalities. On the direct care delivery level, providing safe and efficacious care in neurosurgery depends on many healthcare providers beside the neurosurgeon, including anesthesiologists, nurses, therapists, and more.

Practicing neurosurgeons, trainees, and other providers within any institutional structure around the world can take for granted the complexity of the neurosurgical

K. Yaeger (✉)
Department of Neurosurgery, Icahn School of Medicine at Mount Sinai,
New York City, NY, USA
e-mail: kurt.yaeger@mountsinai.org

I. M. Germano
Department of Neurosurgery, Icahn School of Medicine at Mount Sinai,
New York City, NY, USA

Department of Neurosurgery, Icahn School medicine at Mount Sinai and Department of
Economics, NYU Stern School of Business, NYU, New York City, NY, USA

© The Author(s), under exclusive license to Springer Nature Switzerland AG 2022
I. M. Germano (ed.), *Neurosurgery and Global Health*,
https://doi.org/10.1007/978-3-030-86656-3_19

care delivery dynamics. While performing brain and spine surgery and other neuro-surgical procedures is key to directly improving patient health on the individual level, it is the end product of what a complex neurosurgery enterprise has been built to deliver. It is important to understand not only the different stakeholders in this model but also the organization of the neurosurgery enterprise in order for the healthcare providers to best offer neurosurgery services in any setting, including those with limited resources.

## Defining the Neurosurgery Enterprise and Its Complexity

The neurosurgery enterprise can be defined as an organization whose specialized purpose is the delivery of surgical care for patients with neurological disorders. Table 19.1 outlines several complexities of neurosurgical care that can complicate delivery.

Due to the range of complexity of pathologies and procedures, the neurosurgery enterprise is oftentimes part of a larger medical institution rather than a stand-alone independent facility. Neurosurgical procedures vary from minimally invasive such biopsy, cyst/abscess drainage, embolization, or ablation to complex procedures such as brain tumor resections and spine instrumentation. Overall, the neurosurgery enterprise has many defined personnel specialized for the different components of the delivery of such care, with some outside the surgical management. These include but are not limited to anesthesia, pathology, neurology, radiology, and radiation oncology. While surgeons and other neurosurgical providers enact direct patient care, they are employed by the larger healthcare institution that may have a financial directive. This institutional incentive may impede the provider to care for each

**Table 19.1** The neurosurgery enterprise and its complexity

| Element | Complexities |
| --- | --- |
| Neurosurgeon | Works are part of multidisciplinary team to directly affect patient outcomes. Part of an institution with nonclinical administration and a business objective |
| Healthcare institution | Must maintain financial solvency in order to continue providing care to patient populations. Profits allow for expansion to help different communities |
| Government | Regulatory oversight for drugs, devices, and procedures. Provides healthcare coverage for disenfranchised patients. Often negotiates with healthcare institutions over costs and quality standards |
| Equipment | Technology for neurosurgical interventions range from basic (ventilator, microscope) to more sophisticated (intraoperative image guidance, augmented reality). Different institutions have ranges of technological capacity. Often dependent on supply chain dynamics |
| Care delivery | Pre- and postoperative care is as important as the surgical intervention itself to ensure successful outcome. Reliant on ancillary staff and other healthcare providers |
| Patients | The impact of the neurosurgical care delivered depends on the patient's overall health determined by socioeconomic factors |

patient, limited by regulation, cost, availability, and other obstacles. These institutions themselves may be run primarily by nonclinical administration, with a focus on investment and return on capital. Thus, incentives between hospital and provider are not always aligned. One role of government in this enterprise is to better align the priorities of patient, physician, and hospital administration, by setting regulations for cost and standardization of quality.

The complexity of neurosurgery care delivery at the time of the surgical intervention is only one piece of the enterprise. Pre-, intra-, and postoperative care for most neurosurgical interventions are as important as the surgery itself and contribute to its ultimate success of the surgery. Preoperative care depends heavily on an ancillary team of nurses, technologists, and other providers to ensure the patient is healthy enough to undergo a neurosurgical operation. Intraoperative care goes beyond the surgical technique itself. For any given surgery, the medical supply chain will have delivered the necessary equipment, the operating room will have been prepared by environmental services, and the instruments will have been adequately sterilized according to national and local standards, with the necessary technology installed in the room by a team of experts. Since the beginning of our discipline, neurosurgeons have relied on various technological innovations such as ventilators, operating microscopes, and newer resources such as augmented reality and intraoperative and image-guided navigation to enhance the surgical technique. All in all, this results in a more complex relationship than just the patient and the doctor.

As introduced by Michael Grossman in 1972 [1], one of the founders of healthcare economics, health is seen as stock with a production process and an output, the latter concept typically being measured as "healthy days." Healthcare delivery is only one of the items necessary for the production process. These include diet, exercise, environment, income, and time. Of note, in recent years, it has become evident that within the environment category, the family support is a cardinal factor influencing healthcare outcome. Additionally, since his model was first introduced, we have further defined a fundamental concept of biomolecular signature and genetics. Thus, as a neurosurgeon part of a neurosurgery enterprise, when delivering our care, we need not to forget that our role is only one tassel in the complex mosaic of each patient's health stock (Fig. 19.1).

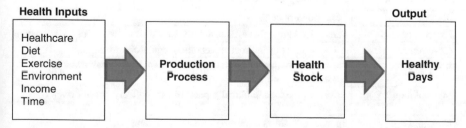

**Fig. 19.1** Diagrammatic representation of Grossman's healthcare capital [1]. Direct neurosurgical care fits primarily within the production process

## Defining the Forces Shaping Neurosurgery Healthcare Delivery Worldwide

The standard theory on how economic markets work is the model of supply and demand, in which buyers and sellers are guided by prices to an efficient allocation of resources. Not dissimilar to many other markets, the economic market of healthcare delivery in general, and neurosurgery specifically, deviates from these models in many ways as it is shaped by many forces and stakeholders. This is not surprising as healthcare often represents a major proportion of a nation's total economic output (gross domestic product, or GDP). There are many relevant *stakeholders* in the healthcare market, a term defined as individuals or groups that have an interest in the decisions or activity of the organization. Below we review the main forces that shape neurosurgery (Table 19.2).

### *Externality*

*Externality* is defined as market exchange that affects a third party who is outside of the exchange. As an example, an externality arises when a person engages in an activity that influences the well-being of a bystander but neither pays nor receives compensation for that effect. If the impact of the bystander is adverse, this is called a *negative externality*. If it is beneficial, it is called a *positive externality*. In the presence of externalities, societies interest in a market extends beyond the well-being of the buyer and seller who participate in the market to include the well-being of the bystander who are affected indirectly. This happens because buyers and sellers neglect the external effects of their action when deciding how much to demand or supply.

Take the example of vaccines. If one person vaccinates himself/herself against a disease, he/she is less likely to catch it. But because he/she is less likely to catch it, he/she is less likely to become a carrier and infect other people. Thus, getting vaccinated conveys a positive externality. If getting vaccinated has some cost either in

**Table 19.2** The neurosurgery enterprise and its market forces

| Force | Definition/effect |
|---|---|
| Externality | Market exchange that affects a third party who is outside of the exchange |
| Government | A major direct or indirect stakeholder, regulatory oversight |
| Insurance | Prevents individuals from having a financial detrimental effect by consequences of health |
| Medical industry | Advances the technological aspects of care delivery, profit driven by nature |
| Nonprofit organizations | Sponsor educational/training/research programs |
| Uncertainty | For example, COVID-19 pandemic |

money, time, or risk, too few people will choose to get themselves vaccinated because they will likely ignore the positive externalities when weighing the cost and benefits. This is a situation where an external force like the government might remedy the problem by subsidizing the development, manufacture, and distribution of vaccine or by requiring vaccination. Without the intervention from an "outsider," the externality can render the unregulated market outcome inefficient. This general conclusion is crucial to understand the healthcare market as well as the neurosurgery enterprise. Externalities are very prevalent in the healthcare market and neurosurgery. These externalities necessitate the government intervention to remedy potential market failures.

## *Government*

Market deviation caused by many factors including externalities are at the basis of government intervention in healthcare and neurosurgery worldwide. The government can be a stakeholder directly or indirectly. The government is a direct stakeholder in healthcare and neurosurgery in countries where it holds a significant percentage of the healthcare spending, in part because it is financially contributing to the health insurance coverage for their citizens. The percentage of governmental share varies from almost 100% in countries with socialized medicine to approximately 50% in the USA [2, 3], to smaller amount in countries where out-of-pocket is still the prevalent coverage.

Even in countries where the government is not the major stakeholder of healthcare and neurosurgery, it can be a major player in shaping neurosurgery by means of several broad areas that in turn have a direct financial impact on the government itself (Table 19.3).

First, the government can control commodity taxes and subsidies. For example, it can decide that in order to decrease its healthcare expense, it will tax tobacco or sugary drinks as they both have an impact on health. Second, the government can issue laws to prevent or to foster monopoly depending on how the monopoly will benefit the country/government. Combining the two concepts, we can take as example a medical innovation. In some countries, the government law is such that a discovery can be "patented." The patent process will result in income to the government and cost to the inventor, but the inventor may ultimately financially benefit from the temporary monopoly to license or manufacture the innovation. The upfront cost of

**Table 19.3** Governmental interventions on the neurosurgery enterprise

| Intervention | Example |
| --- | --- |
| Control commodity taxes and subsidies | Tax sugar drinks |
| Laws | Prevention/establishment of monopoly |
| Transfer programs | Subsidize research |
| Regulations | Food and Drug Administration |

the patent to the inventor will increase the price of the good (the invention) which may result in high prices for the consumer (and ultimately the patient). Given market dynamics, higher prices may decrease the market and drive the price even higher to recoup the initial investment. At this point the government may intervene and subsidize the item to allow lower-income patients access to it. This example was given to explain the complexity of interaction between the government and our field.

Additionally, the government can influence our field by transfer programs. Let's take the example of medical research. In some countries, the government supports medical research with a substantial budget to improve the overall health of the nation and by so doing possibly by decreasing costs related to healthcare delivery. Finally, in most countries the government has an active role on our field by means of regulating. In the USA, an example is the Food and Drug Administration (FDA), a government agency founded in 1906 responsible for the safety, efficacy, and security of human and veterinary drugs, biological products, and medical devices [4].

## Insurance

In countries where healthcare is not provided or subsidized in part by the government, health insurances exist and are stakeholders of a sizable slice of the healthcare market. Since the majority of the population tends to be risk adverse, insurances are common in many economic markets including healthcare. Let's take the example of a disease that affects 2% of the population and everyone is equally likely to be stricken. Treatment costs $30,000. In this case, the expected cost of healthcare is 2% of $30,000, which is $600. If people are risk averse, they prefer to pay $600 with certainty over a 2% chance of having to pay $30,000.

The existence of insurances in turn creates at least two forces that impact the healthcare market. The first is *moral hazard*, defined as the tendency of a person who is imperfectly monitored to engage in dishonest or otherwise undesirable behavior. As an example, if you have a car insurance, you will be less worried about parking your car on the street. In this scenario, your car may be dented, but with insurance, you may not be required to pay for the whole cost of repair. In contrast, on the insurance side, *adverse selection* (defined as exploiting asymmetric information) may occur and cause market imperfections. In this example, insurers may selectively choose to insure a healthier population in order to limit their overall payouts.

## Medical and Pharmacological Industry

The medical device and pharmacological industries are an aggregation and integration of sectors within the economic system that provides goods and services to treat patients with curative, preventive, rehabilitative, and palliative care. For the neurosurgeon, the industry segment that handles medical technology is the most impactful as very often neurosurgeons drive this segment and simultaneously are driven by it. Neurosurgeons have often been leaders in technological advances, both inventing new devices and performing clinical trials to verify the safety and efficacy of these devices and interventions. The examples of neurosurgeons as inventors and technological leader are numerous, including the introduction of the bipolar [5] and the stereotactic frame [6] that allowed our field to progress to provide safer surgeries and to broaden the scope of diseases treated and further technology invented. From the neurosurgeon's perspective, innovation allows for improved treatment of a particular disease state or improves the speed, safety, or ergonomics of a particular technique. However, the private industry's role in innovation may often be financially driven. Here, large corporations often choose pathologies with high prevalence in which to innovate, to optimize the addressable market and therefore the profit margin. Government has intervened in this realm as well, creating pathways to highlight underserved patient populations, such as the US FDA Humanitarian Device Exemption, which allows for marketing of a device used to treat a disease affected less than 8000 patients each year.

## Nonprofit and Academic Organizations

Philanthropy is a driving force worldwide. The desire to provide welfare to others is innate to human nature. The generosity of private individuals or company is often directed toward private foundations. In neurosurgery, foundations and other nonprofit organizations including academic institutions have a significant impact on our field. Private foundations play an important role in supporting the design, execution, and evaluation of innovative educational programs that will address the needs of our field globally. They can also provide a role in generating information that will better inform healthcare workforce policies. Finally, foundations can provide seed funds to execute preliminary research and/or educational programs important to start new projects.

## Uncertainty

Unpredictable factors can influence any economic market. As first remarked by Kenneth Arrow, Nobel Prize in Economics in 1972 and one the founder of healthcare economics, uncertainties affect healthcare more than other industries [7]. Not surprisingly, his paper entitled "Uncertainty and Welfare Economics of Medical Care" (1963) remains one of the most cited in economics 50 years after its publication [8].

More than ever before, the uncertainty due to the COVID-19 pandemic has influenced all market sectors globally. The COVID-19 pandemic is one of the most profound sociological phenomena in recent human history. Most likely its deep impact on every industry including healthcare will persist long after the pandemic is brought under control. Neurosurgery clearly was not spared from its effect. Many emergent and urgent neurosurgical operations proceeded as usual even during the peak of the COVID-19 crisis. Yet highly profitable elective procedures in many healthcare systems decreased dramatically, which strained institutions' bottom lines. Despite this, the pandemic also highlighted our field's resilience, in that we are able to progress and overcome difficulties to continue caring for our patients. The delivery of virtual care through tele-health, remote patient monitoring, and other tools where by necessity greatly accelerated and expanded due to the pandemic. This is not likely to return to baseline. Rather combined with payment changes and other technology, it is poised to catalyze even more transformation in the neurosurgery healthcare delivery model.

## Conclusion

Neurosurgery as a specialty is unique in the complexity both of pathologies treated and the surgical treatments available. Neurosurgeons are highly reliant on technology and institutional support to be able to provide for our patient populations. Given this, there are many complicated, interrelated stakeholders in the neurosurgery enterprise. Understanding that neurosurgical care is not simply performing the operation but also a product of the pre- and postoperative care, supply chain optimization, government regulation, and private industry innovation is key to optimizing care for our patients.

## References

1. Grossman M. On the concept of health capital and the demand for health. J Polit Econ. 1972;80(2):223–55.
2. The Federal Share of American Health Spending is Now Approaching 50%: Conover, Chris. Forbes, June 1, 2018.
3. https://www.cms.gov/research-statistics-data-and-systems/statistics-trends-and-reports/nationalhealthexpenddata/downloads/highlights.pdf.
4. https://www.fda.gov.
5. Bulsara R, Shahid S, Nimjee M. History of bipolar coagulation. Neurosurg Rev. 2006;29:93–6.
6. Rahman M, Murad G, Mocco J. Early history of the stereotactic apparatus in neurosurgery. Neurosurg Focus. 2009;27(3):E12.
7. Arrow KJ. Uncertainty and the welfare economics of medical care. Am Econ Rev. 1963;53:941–73.
8. Savedoff WD. Kenneth Arrow and the birth of health economics. Bull World Health Organ. 2004;82(2):139–40.

# Chapter 20
# Medical Technology Innovation and Entrepreneurship in Neurosurgery

Alexandre C. Carpentier and John R. Adler Jr.

## Ultrasound-Induced Blood-Brain Barrier Opening: The Neurosurgeon's SonoCloud Solution

Brain drug delivery remains a challenge due to the blood-brain barrier (BBB). Pulsed ultrasound is a new technique that is capable of safely and transiently opening the BBB. After fundamental research and conception of a new medical device for BBB opening, the CarThera entrepreneurial adventure began. Innovation transfer implies numerous challenges, especially for development of a fundamentally new technology with no precedents. The SonoCloud has further challenges as an implantable device, regulatory hurdles as it is used in combination with drugs, and since it targets a sensitive organ – the brain.

## Step 1: The Vision

*To innovate, one has to envision the ideal clinical practice several decades in the future. Present* **unmet needs** *(fundamental, surgical, organizational, or computational) have also to be precisely identified and defined. By the confrontation of*

A. C. Carpentier
Chief Neurosurgery Department, Pitie Salpetriere Hospital, Sorbonne University, Founder CarThera Inc., Paris, France

J. R. Adler Jr. (✉)
Department of Neurosurgery, Stanford University, Stanford, CA, USA
e-mail: jra@stanford.edu

© The Author(s), under exclusive license to Springer Nature Switzerland AG 2022
I. M. Germano (ed.), *Neurosurgery and Global Health*,
https://doi.org/10.1007/978-3-030-86656-3_20

*future (ideal practice) with present (unmet needs), a **vision** will be born, and the **process of innovating** will start and should not be inhibited by any immediate difficulties or apparent **technical challenges**.*

One of the major *fundamental unmet needs* in neuroscience is brain drug delivery, a constant challenge due to the blood-brain barrier (BBB). Approximately 99% of drugs can't cross the BBB. Existing approaches to circumvent the BBB are insufficient (convection enhanced delivery, local wafers) or toxic (osmotic drugs, electroporation). In the 1990s, pharmaceutical companies and start-ups developed functionalized drugs or nanoparticles to cross the BBB using receptor-mediated transcytosis such as transferrin receptors. Such approaches didn't achieve significant clinical efficacy due to acquired resistance at the endothelium and receptor downregulation/blockage. For brain tumors, only two chemotherapies have efficient brain uptake (temozolomide 25%, nitrosoureas 20%), whereas most other drugs fail to cross the BBB at levels higher than 3–5%, explaining why numerous trials have failed over the last 20 years. This *clinical unmet need for brain drug delivery also includes* numerous other brain pathologies including neurodegenerative diseases. This BBB challenge is amplified by the arrival of new molecules with higher molecular weights (antibodies, nanoparticles, etc.) which cannot cross the BBB and have only a <1% penetration from the blood to brain tissue.

Russian research in the 1960s had shown that pulsed ultrasound could open the BBB, but this high-intensity "sonoporation" also impacted brain cells, resulting in significant toxicity. In 2001, Kullervo Hynynen, PhD used a lower intensity pulsed ultrasound emission but coupled the ultrasound with intravascular ultrasound contrast agents (microbubbles) commonly used in clinical diagnostic routine [1]. These microbubbles resonate in response to the acoustic energy delivered, leading to "cavitation," causing a shear stress at the vascular endothelium inducing a transient (6 h) and reversible disruption of the BBB. Although the technique works with an external ultrasound transmitter in small animals with thin skulls, the adoption of the technique in humans has several hurdles: absorption and acoustic defocusing induced by the thickness and irregularity of the cranial bone.

Two complementary technological achievements were then born to make up for these problems: an external HIFU (high-intensity focused ultrasound) device and an implanted LIPU (low-intensity pulsed ultrasound) device.

HIFU, designed by physicists, consists of a helmet of 1000 converging ultrasound emitters (Exablate by Insightec). Installed on a shaved head, cooled and immobilized in a stereotactic frame, the ultrasound sonication procedure requires a prior acoustic burst under MRI to check the target and the treatment intensity before launching the pulsed opening sequence of the BBB. While the technique is perfectly adapted for pathologies of the deep brain, it is less efficient in the cortical region. Moreover, the procedure time (3 h) is difficult for routine clinical practice for repeated treatments, for example, at each chemotherapy treatment in the management of brain tumors.

LIPU, designed by neurosurgeons, consists of an implantable device with 1–9 emitters, convergent or not (SonoCloud by CarThera). The device is installed in the thickness of the skull, in an extradural position, during tumor removal surgery before classically closing the patient's skin, avoiding the issue of transmission through the skull bone. The acoustic pressure delivered to the brain is then perfectly controlled, without attenuation or distortion, so that MRI is no longer necessary. The aim here was to extend the applications of the BBB opening to cortical brain pathologies, brain tumors, more diffuse pathologies, and to the need for repeated treatments. The LIPU procedure to open the BBB takes 10 min, making possible repeated treatments at each chemotherapy session, with a clinical routine feasibility with low time consumption and a minimal learning curve.

## Step 2: Preclinical Research

*An innovation can result from a clinical vision (majority of medical device advances), and then preclinical research will follow to establish a **preclinical proof of concept**. Alternatively, an innovation can result from preclinical research (most drug discoveries), and then the clinical vision is established. In both cases, to accelerate future transfer to patients, preclinical research should be performed with the **final device/drug** to satisfy regulatory considerations for clinical trial authorization. The prototype/device/drug conception and production must take into account these regulatory and clinical factors very early on in development (biocompatibility, MRI compatibility, patient's feasibility, etc.), and preclinical research must be performed using **good laboratory practice (GLP) guidelines**. An early initial patent is then recommended. Then, a **multidisciplinary team** (fundamental research, physicists, engineers) and strategic collaborations can be established to proceed with additional innovation, production, and preclinical research.*

The SonoCloud (ultrasound implantable device) was developed between 2010 and 2012 in my Sorbonne research academic lab, through a close collaboration with a dedicated French public research lab specializing in therapeutic ultrasound (INSERM/LabTAU, Lyon, France). At that time, a basic prototype (Fig. 20.1), not

**Fig. 20.1** SonoCloud-1 by CarThera: ultrasound implanted medical device for 5 cm³ BBB opening

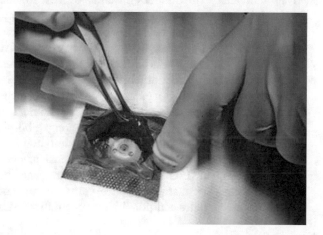

yet compatible for human use, was developed for preclinical proof of concept. After establishing the proper parameters, the LIPU technology was used to confirm that the BBB can be transiently disrupted after 2–4 min of nonfocused ultrasound emission in contact with the dura matter [2]. Mice, rabbits, dogs, and then primate experiments not only showed efficiency of the technique (using contrast agents indicating BBB disruption such as Evan's blue and contrast-enhanced MRI) but also its safety (in PET, EEG, EP, histology) even for repeated sessions every 15 days [3–6]. After each session, the BBB closes spontaneously between 6 h and 24 h after sonication (ultrasound emission), a crucial physiological repair to avoid secondary effects of long BBB opening duration. Mice models of high-grade glioma demonstrated increased survival with opened BBB during drug IV administration [7]. The preclinical proof of concept was then achieved.

## Step 3: Translation from "Proof of Concept" to Clinical Trials

*After preclinical research proof of concept was demonstrated, and after essential validation of interest by key opinion leaders (KOLs), the entrepreneurial adventure can start with **building a dedicated team consisting** of engineers, clinical, regulatory, and business experts. Top engineer and technical conception are essential for device **technical conception**, reliability, **production**, subcontractor selection, and regulatory strategy. Most of the time, big medical device companies are not willing to embrace an early stage development due to the high business risks, long development times, and liability issues that could result if any adverse safety events occur during initial clinical trials. A start-up is often the ideal solution to navigate the risks and maximize the opportunities of such an endeavor. The **business model** and **fundraising** will be strengthened by the user conviction: the neurosurgeon.*

CarThera, a university start-up, was created in 2010 to develop the SonoCloud device. *Business plan* and neurosurgeon implications allowed for fundraising among private individuals (love money), family offices, foundations, and public grants. Even if the inventor has to fund symbolically the company, he/she can keep substantial equity by valuating his in-kind assets: university patents [8] licensed to the start-up, preclinical proof of concept, personal expertise, and future implication.

Between 2012 and 2014, besides continuing fundamental research, the team focused on device production for future clinical trials. Such production had to respect the numerous state *regulatory requirements* such as risk management (EN ISO 14971), biocompatibility (ISO 10993-1), electrical and mechanical safety (EN 60601-1&2, EN 45502-1), electromagnetic compatibility (EN 60601-1-2), medical software (EN 62304), packaging and sterilization (ISO 11135 - EN ISO 11607-1&2), degradation analysis (EN 62366), good clinical practices (EN ISO 14155), and quality management (ISO 13485). Such requirements may require additional animal experiments; for example, even if composed of biocompatible materials, the final device may require additional biocompatibility testing. Additionally, a certain amount of the prototype devices will have to be analyzed by independent certification companies to prove they conform to the applicable regulatory norms.

This step was achieved in mid-2014 and cost three times the preclinical research stage. The start-up creation is not a goal in itself. It is only a means for funding such regulatory steps that are normally not financed by academic grants. As a neurosurgeon, a biologist, or an inventor, the fundamental science and clinical development are our most important input in the project, and it is important to maintain this role, keep our clinical routine activities, and decline any day-to-day management functions in the company.

## Step 4: Clinical Trials

*After completion of preclinical proof of concept, potential patients benefit evaluation, efficacy comparison with existing therapeutics, and preclinical proof of safety, the regulatory dossier can be submitted to FDA (Food and Drug Administration) or EMA (European Medical Agency). Clinical trials will have to first prove safety on humans (phase 1) and then prove efficacy (phase 2/3) with previous validation of the strategy by regulatory authorities. Randomized trials are more and more mandatory, with all their complexity in terms of control arm choice, bias, and costs. Even if FDA/EMA clearance is the ultimate goal to reach, clinical trials should never forget to first convince the scientific/clinical community, so that trial designs must be validated by external scientific board advisers prior to any of the other steps.*

At La Pitie-Salpctrière Sorbonne Hospital, we have therefore started the first clinical trial to open the BBB in 2014 in recurrent glioblastoma after patients have received standard of care treatment. Patients eligible for new tumor resection were implanted with the SonoCloud device to avoid a dedicated surgery for device implantation. Carboplatin chemotherapy was chosen to be IV injected concomitantly to BBB opening since this drug was shown to be non-neurotoxic in previous convection enhanced drug (CED) delivery trials. Several days after implantation, the first sonication was performed using a transdermal needle to provide energy to the device (no internal battery to be MRI compatible for tumor follow-up MRI). On 19 patients and 65 BBB opening sessions, not only tolerance of BBB opening was proven for the first time on humans [9] but also a trend of delayed tumor progression [10]. Another trial was performed to extend by ninefold the field of ultrasound using a newly developed SonoCloud-9 device (Fig. 20.2), inducing a large BBB opening region (Fig. 20.3), still with good tolerance. A pivotal phase 3 study is planned to prove better overall survival versus currently available therapies, the key criteria demanded by regulatory authorities. Due to its cost, usually only a single pivotal trial can be performed by a start-up, so that this decision is major in terms of technology survival.

Pilot trials are also ongoing to explore interest of the technology for other indications such as for pediatric brain tumors [11], other drug association [12], including

**Fig. 20.2** SonoCloud-9 by
CarThera: ultrasound
implanted medical device
for 45 cm³ BBB opening

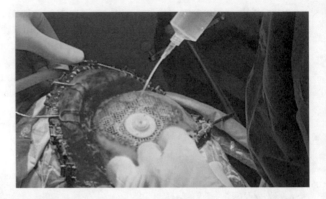

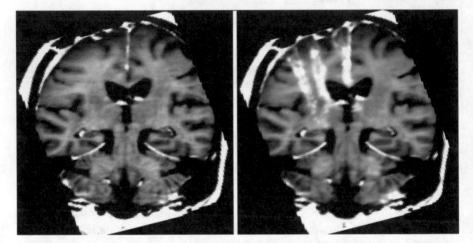

**Fig. 20.3** Contrast enhancement as a surrogate showing ultrasound-induced blood-brain barrier opening. Note the contrast enhancement in front of three ultrasound emitters

brain tumor with check point inhibitors [13], but also for Alzheimer's disease with no associated drug, which is also being pursued by others using transcranial approaches [14]. Indeed, preclinical work on Alzheimer's disease mice model showed that amyloid plaques, neurofibrillary deposits, and cognitive impairment were decreased by repetitive sonication [15, 16].

## Step 5: User Adoption

*User adoption or deployment of a technology can be envisioned if you obtain improved treatment efficacy/process or care cost diminution. To reach market access, the most difficult step is to obtain clearance from regulatory authorities. After this critical step, reimbursement is the main limitation before widespread adoption. In this latest step, the clinician is once again the best ambassador.*

A disruptive innovation is a totally new innovation or treatment approach, without existing predicates on the market. One has to be aware before developing such an innovation, because its development involves many challenging steps, with a slow progression due to the amount of proof required for regulatory authorities (e.g., a PMA through the FDA) and evidence for reimbursement. Additionally, existing treatment habits may lead clinicians to modify their practice, especially if the patient's flow is significantly altered. On the other hand, the absence of predicate devices will give significant time for proper development and at the end bring significant value to the project. The SonoCloud development is an example of such a disruptive innovation, having in addition to deal with fundamental science and drug issues.

An incremental innovation is an optimization of an existing device that does the same therapeutic effect. Such innovation, although less challenging, can progress much faster and is easier to deploy. Additionally, the technology is most often matching with existing treatment habits so that clinicians will not have to modify their practice and the learning curve and adoption is much easier. The 510 K FDA regulation procedure is also easier since it focuses on differences with existing, approved devices. On the other hand, the value of the project is limited due to the existence of competing technologies.

## Saving Lives by Other Means: Enabling Radiosurgery for Two Million Patients per Year

### Step 1: My Serendipitous Path

Who is a doctor? A simple question, yet with myriad answers. I stumbled into medicine with only the most superficial appreciation for what it means to be a physician. Coming from a small town I understood the prestige given to the immigrant town doctor as well as the economic security he enjoyed. And in school, I always liked science and embraced hard work. However, I had never given deep thought about "the profession" of medicine, and before I knew it, I was a medical student and then neurosurgical resident. Just like my fellow classmates and residents, the path into my future career was seemingly laid out for me. Little was I aware of the abrupt turn it might take [17].        Somewhat randomly my young family and I went to the Karolinska Institute in Stockholm, expecting during a year fellowship to dabble in research but, seemingly even more importantly to me then, spend significant time in the operating room doing cerebrovascular cases. But soon I would meet Lars Leksell. Before spending much time with "the man" himself, I got a furtive glimpse here and there of his very big idea, noninvasive brain surgery via "his radiosurgery." Suddenly I was asking if the long-term future of brain surgery might not involve open surgery at all? If so, did I want future neurosurgeons to think of me the way I thought of Civil War era surgeons, who were little more than amputation machines and vectors for contagium? Despite being nearly retired, Leksell's ideas permeated the entire Department of Neurosurgery at the Karolinska Institute, driving nearly all clinical innovation and, most importantly, saving lives. I was dazzled by the notion that a surgeon's ideas and not necessarily their hands might save the most lives. It should have been immediately apparent to me that turning Leksell's big ideas into reality also required a parallel ubiquitous societal structure, business. However, I was largely oblivious to that dimension of innovation because in Lars Leksell's world, his nonhospital-based sons did the heaviest lifting when it came to business.

Not long after leaving Sweden, a growing family in tow, I was finishing up my residency at Harvard and needed to find a home where I might pursue my own dreams and big ideas. Taking some vague notions about this idea for image guidance and a device that would someday become the CyberKnife, I interviewed with a handful of academic institutions looking to hire a poorly paid junior faculty member. Serendipitously I found my way to Stanford and the surrounding Silicon Valley. At Stanford I was clearly at the very bottom of the neurosurgical pecking order, largely ignored and tucked away at the local VA Hospital. Cut off from significant patient referrals, little was asked or expected from me. How truly fortunate I was.

When not covering the ER or relegated to taking night call, I had enough time on my young assistant professor hands to find my way to the Stanford School of Engineering, believing that they might help me realize my innovation for image-guided radiosurgery. However, rather quickly my dreams became too big and tangible for a university lab, even a big research institution like Stanford, so I wandered off campus and found my way into the land of big dreams: Silicon Valley. Truthfully, I had no guide, no mentor, and not even a like-minded colleague with whom I might share the adventure or, more importantly, who might provide emotional support in the world of mega-drama I was about to enter.

## Step 2: Leverage Your Environment

From the outside, the world looks at Silicon Valley and sees a collection of massive all-powerful world-renowned companies like Apple, Google, Facebook, Intuitive Surgical, etc. However, I soon learned that what really makes Silicon Valley special is a motley community of small-scale, intrepid entrepreneurs offering an unmatched collection of capabilities in just about every aspect of technology. For many of these small businesses, big time commercial success had evaded them, yet for the majority, they simply love the process of innovation more than commercial success and are not unhappy to just be "tinkerers." But not for me. I was in the early 1990s a man on a mission, determined to disrupt radiosurgery as the world knew it. Before long I had found a base of operation outside Stanford in a very small R&D shop named Schonberg Radiation that was living a virtual hand to mouth existence but which also made very small (x-band) linear accelerators. Like many Silicon Valley companies, innovation was in part an aphrodisiac for the eclectic founders of Schonberg, and my radical notion for changing therapeutic radiation certainly appealed to that side of their nature. A few small government grants were followed by rejection after rejection. NIH grant reviewers commented, "who would want to do radiosurgery outside the brain" and "why would anyone want to fractionate SRS for brain lesions"; the radiation therapy elite really saw no significant value to my dreams. In response I turned to industry for funding: GE, Siemens, and Philips. Again, rejection after rejection. Then I turned to the ever-present Silicon Valley venture capital community who are supposed to be inclined to make big bets on big ideas, especially here in "The Valley." Yet again rejection after rejection. After almost 3 years of rejections, I said "enough," I will try to do this myself. Cobbling together a grand total of $600,000, mostly from neurosurgeon friends of mine, as well as one advance order from Stanford Medical Center for a "Neurotron 1000," and teaming up with several technologist, the youngest of which was 25 years my senior, a new company was founded, and in short order it was named Accuray by my wife Marilyn.

I, who was merely a young neurosurgeon, had no idea what I was getting myself into when I founded Accuray. Without any business or engineering experience, I was oblivious to the challenges of a grossly underfunded complex and heavily regulated medical device company, and in hindsight my much more seasoned cofounders seem to have been even more clueless than me. In fact, whenever the going got tough, it was me who had to solve the problems, despite also working a full-time job as a reasonably busy neurosurgeon at Stanford and being the father of two young children. It is me who went around the USA and found five more customers for the Neurotron 1000, which would soon morph into the CyberKnife brand, each sale coming with a hefty down payment used to support company R&D and other operations. It was me who led most additional, albeit extremely modest, funding efforts, again mostly from angel investor often neurosurgeon friends of mine. A second mortgage on my house became a revolving source of cash for the business, yet with such limited funding Accuray needed to cut corners everywhere. Because the company lacked funding to build a proper radiation-shielded facility for testing inside the company, the first prototype machine was actually built inside Stanford Hospital. In comparison, Intuitive Surgery (which has become my lifelong stalking horse) was founded at almost exactly the same time as Accuray and was located only a few miles from our office, and both new technologies (Da Vinci Robot and CyberKnife) were of comparable technical complexity, yet Intuitive had serious venture capital funding and Accuray did not; the difference between the two was literally 20X! Despite always needing to bootstrap operations, a naïve but determined team of engineers and me found a way to treat the first CyberKnife patient, an elderly woman with a solitary brain metastasis (Fig. 20.4).

## Step 3: The Business Plan

At best my "frameless" CyberKnife procedure was on par with standard frame-based Linac SRS, yet the effort involved in treating that first patient was easily ten times greater. Seeing how much improvement "my" CyberKnife required to get anywhere close to my vision and, even more importantly, to meet my promises to

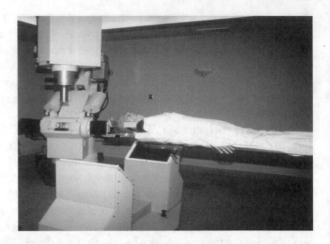

customers, left me often feeling ashamed and like a failure. I had no basis for appreciating that disruptive technologies always initially represent a practical step backwards. Sadly, no one in my world took me aside to explain how the innovation game ALWAYS works; to some extent, "You must fake it until you make it!"

Ashamed or not, I had treated my first patient which was some cause for short-term celebration. However, when my supposedly seasoned cofounders proved incapable of raising even the most modest investment, Accuray literally ran out of money only 6 months after our "first in man!" I had to sell machines, fundraise, promote, treat patients, recruit talent, help manage R&D, drive the board of directors, and more, all the while striving to be a full-time hard-charging academic neurosurgeon and also a good father. I just couldn't keep the entire enterprise together, and so the company ran out of money. The next 3 years were frankly hellish. Day after day, sleepless night after sleepless night, I would feel constant despair, uncertain how I might ever save my CyberKnife baby. I tried everything, short of making a deal with the devil. I entertained the sketchiest of characters who promised to help the company, but in hindsight "help" meant little more than help themselves. Ironically my clinical practice at Stanford was by then booming, fueled in part by the attention garnered by "my" CyberKnife, yet this only added to the incessant stress and ever-present feeling of being a fraud and a failure.

Throughout all the doom and gloom, a core group of 8 crazy zealous mostly engineering employees (having been reduced from a one-time team of 40) had the tenacity to hang in there, and slowly over time the CyberKnife technology improved. Although still living a hand to mouth existence, the team found a way to install the four other US CyberKnifes I had previously sold. Soon thereafter we got a near miraculous Japanese regulatory clearance and with that a handful of sales. Then Accuray yet again almost ran out of funds for the umpteenth time. However, on this occasion a longtime champion, neurosurgeon Jim Doty, came along and agreed to invest what was then a near unimaginable sum of 500,000 dollars, providing he was also made CEO. Experience or not, the board and I took the deal, also investing more myself over my poor wife's objections. Not much time had passed before an Asian-based venture capital firm agreed to invest 8 million dollars in Accuray, suddenly brightening the outlook for my baby appreciably. But like so much of my saga, the good times lasted about a year when a precipitous spat with the board resulted in Jim Doty walking out the door. In literally an instant I decided to take a sabbatical from Stanford and become Accuray's new CEO.

Overnight I became the leader of what by then was nearly a 100-employee business. Accuray's chaotic past leadership, and a booming 1999 Silicon Valley, poisoned upfront any grace period a new leader by all rights might have been afforded. Within days I, yet another inexperienced neurosurgeon CEO of Accuray, had a management revolt on my hands, eventually leading to the departure of several senior employees who headed out to apparently "greener pastures." In hindsight all these seemingly seasoned hands made terrible strategic blunders in their careers. The first year of my CEO tenure proved to be very tough. I was naïve and untested, and in parallel all the stars were aligned against us. Not long after, the CEO of a key supplier to Accuray, Fanuc Robots, made a summary decision to not sell their robots to us; Fanuc's CEO and all-powerful founder was frightened by the risk of seeing his robots being used in the first ever truly robotic surgery system, the CyberKnife. It was incredibly traumatic to have to turn the entire product upside down and build it around an entirely new robot, Kuka, but the company managed to do it in only 4 months led by one exceptionally talented charismatic engineer. Meanwhile 1999 was a brutal year in Silicon Valley for recruiting desperately needed engineers, who were simultaneously being courted by the richest technology companies. Stock prices in "The Valley" were soaring, everyone, even secretaries were getting million-dollar paydays, but not poor Accuray where a hand to mouth financial existence and a parsimonious CEO ruled. Although chronically short of funds, Accuray still managed to survive, finally securing its first US FDA regulatory clearance in 1999 and then even more critically another 510(k) clearance a year later.

Despite having US regulatory clearance in hand and a more stable CyberKnife technology, it proved impossible to secure more funding for Accuray, in large part because of the financial bust that followed the bursting of the technology bubble and then September 11, 2001. So needing more money, I entered back into serious sales mode in both the USA and Japan, after what had been a nearly 5-year hiatus. And then in my third year of being CEO everything finally started to click for the business. Despite customer skepticism the company was able to finally resume sales in the USA in part through my relentless sales evangelism. Meanwhile we released very cool technology (in large part my inventions) for treating spinal lesions and both lung and prostate cancer. Real revenue was starting to flow from Japanese and US sales and that in turn made it possible to ultimately raise significant venture investment. Accuray was entering this virtuous cycle of success, and it was utterly joyful, and yet, it was at this very juncture that I needed to enter into one of the most fateful decisions of my life.

## Step 3: User Adoption and Academia

The founder and CEO of a start-up is utterly critical to business success, arguably more important than product. However, for a disruptive medical device company it may be physician innovators that are even more important. Fender Musical Instruments Corporation made amazing electric guitars, but without Jimi Hendrix playing their "Stratocaster," would the world have ever known? So once the business was stabilized, I realized that Accuray and I did not have our Jimi Hendrix of new clinical applications. It dawned on me that the CyberKnife user best able by far to fill that role was me. It seemed much easier to find a "professional CEO" to manage the business than a neurosurgeon to drive clinical innovation. Unfortunately, Stanford University's obsession with conflicts of interest made it impossible to work both roles. And so I found myself needing to make what was the difficult (and ultimately fateful) choice of my career: remain the CEO or return to Stanford as a neurosurgeon and drive clinical innovation.

Following a small search by a headhunter, Accuray hired its "professional CEO," an individual with prior experience in industry and, uniquely enough, brain radiosurgery. I then returned to Stanford about 3 years after leaving. The ensuing 6 years proved to be some of the most academically productive of my career. Despite lots of handwringing by myself and colleagues, my core surgical skills quickly returned, much like riding a bicycle! Being back at Stanford and freed of management responsibilities at Accuray, I was finally able to focus entirely on developing multiple new clinical applications with the CyberKnife, most of these representing "medical firsts" which today are commonplace procedures for spine, thoracic, and urologic surgeons. I was also publishing nonstop, frequently using the many long plane trips I was taking worldwide, always to promote the CyberKnife and grow Accuray's burgeoning sales backlog; at this point my children were off to college, and I could travel without regret. Meanwhile the business was booming, and John Adler was the face of a growing and even at times celebrated brand.

Although it was great fun jetting around the world and being treated as a celebrity, albeit within only a small niche of medicine (radiosurgery), problems were brewing on the home front. While Accuray's revenues were growing very quickly, literally doubling every year, a knowledgeable insider like me could see worrisome signs. The company's new CEO convinced himself first, and then the board, that he personally was the reason for the company's recent growth. He took over all decision making around the business but even more importantly the product evolution. Inside the business I was sidelined, and sometimes even contractually handcuffed, to be the "doctor" face of the company, merely schmoozing with customers and investors alike but without any internal authority. The result was the leveling off of CyberKnife technical innovation and clinical applications, and I was powerless to intervene, with the CEO having utterly convinced the board he was the business genius behind the business' recent successes; as is so often true, revenue growth does not tell the entire story about a business's prospects. Yet from the outside, and even to many inside the company, all appeared well.. Things appeared good enough to do a listing on a public stock market, which is what happened in 2007. Yes, I celebrated this event but, from afar, needing to host a previously committed to big sales dinner on the West Coast with potential physician customers. While Dr. Adler was attending to business, the Accuray management team metaphorically whooped it up celebrating ARAY's NASDAQ IPO in New York City.

## Step 4: The Impact of Historic Financial Market Events

The problems for Accuray that I was sensing were greatly magnified later that year when organized Radiation Oncology (ASTRO) and its industry counterpart, Varian, ganged up to put this upstart in its place. The CyberKnife's accelerating success treating prostate cancer, arguably the single disease most critical to the financial success of all of radiation oncology, was a direct threat to both entities. In a hugely influential *Radiation Oncology Red Journal* editorial, it was argued that hypofractionated CyberKnife treatment for prostate should still be deemed "unproven," "experimental," and "investigational" [18]. Overnight, insurance companies stopped paying for experimental (and ironically even less expensive) prostate cancer treatment, and CyberKnife sales quickly dried up. Nevertheless, Accuray management was still too busy celebrating their IPO success and largely oblivious to this existential threat. I was worried, deeply worried, especially as the USA started to enter its "Great Recession." Meanwhile I never stopped being the public face of Accuray to customers. Sometimes that could be fun, when things were working well, but sometimes it was extremely frustrating when there were problems, and I have no control.

Responsibility without authority inevitably makes one feel powerless and is extremely stressful. Totally frightened about where "my company" was heading, I decided to lead a rear-guard revolt with selected key employees and hoping ultimately to convince the Accuray board of directors that a change in CEO was needed. Some employees who I knew to be key to the business were utterly supportive and really yearned for me to make a Steve Jobs-like return. However most senior managers were quite content, clearly aware that if the revolt failed, they would be out of a job. With whatever employee troops I could muster waiting for my order, I made a fateful presentation to the Accuray board of directors in February 2008 demanding the replacement of the CEO. It fell on utterly deaf ears. I was deemed a jealous ingrate, and bluntly informed the CEO would stay. Hearing that, I knew it was me who must leave Accuray despite giving my heart and soul to the company for almost two decades. Over the ensuing year I worked my way out of the company starting with my resignation from the board. It was a horrible time to be selling any stock during the depths of the Great Recession, but I did not have much choice needing to sell my company stock at rock bottom prices. By the end of 2008 I was out. My baby, my Accuray, was now on its own, and so was I.

While arranging my departure from Accuray, I started to give thought to what's next in my life. What hung over me was not the past success of my professional career but the failure to get radiosurgery more widely embraced. An approach to surgery, which I reckoned to be the most advanced in history, literally as important as the genetics revolution (which I believe still), was embraced only tepidly by the medical world, even by my own neurosurgical colleagues. What struck me was that this failure, my failure, stemmed not from clinical outcomes but rather stark practical realities about medicine. Science in medicine does matter, yet sadly money and power often matter more. The radiosurgical field I loved was held hostage in a political struggle between two medical specialties, in large part because very generous insurance reimbursement flowed not too physicians (neurosurgeons) but to the biggest and richest hospitals. What dawned on me was that when incentives are misaligned, patients do not get the best care no matter what medical science might argue; for ivory-tower academic types, who insist that "evidence-based medicine" must drive decision-making, this real-world experience proved an epiphany. It was this singular insight that set me off on my latest medical device start-up.

I convinced myself that just maybe I could "rescue" brain radiosurgery from a slow death stemming from growing neurosurgical disinterest. As I saw things, a major problem with "the practice" of radiosurgery stemmed from a lack of clinical innovation, and if that was to be reversed, neurosurgeons needed to reengage and be passionate; better reimbursement should also be part of a solution to incentivize neurosurgeons. The big challenge with radiosurgery as a procedural field is that it requires the most complex to operate and expensive equipment in all of healthcare. This practical reality is why SRS had become bottled up inside big institutions; at the same time I believe the world is just now starting to witness the gradual decline of big hospitals and medical schools as being the primary centers for surgical innovation. So my simple answer was "less complex, less expensive" radiosurgery by creating a specialized surgical robot.

Getting radiosurgery out of big expensive radiation therapy vaults seemed like an important step if I was to "democratize" the procedure. Brainstorming with myself, I quickly realized I would need a lower energy linear accelerator to make my new dream into a reality. With this need in mind, I approached Varian Medical Inc., which is immediately next door to Stanford and knows more about Linacs than any company in the world. However in a turn of events the CEO of Varian convinced me to join Varian and make my newest dream happen inside his company instead; multiple members of the board of directors also met with me, each explaining with the utmost sincerity that my entrepreneurial spirit would be just the shot in the arm that a stodgy Varian needed to reinvigorate it.

In no time there was a plan and financial offer that was hard to refuse, even for a well-paid chaired professor of NS. With the utmost enthusiasm, I took another leave of absence from Stanford, this time committed to making a next-generation radiosurgery device to democratize the field. What excited me the most was that this time around I had the backing of a big company, and therefore it could not possibly be so completely arduous. After what happened at Accuray, I didn't feel I had the courage or stamina for another raw start-up. Yet again, I was in for a surprise!

## *Step 5: Doing It All Over Again!*

Unfortunately, the honeymoon with Varian lasted less than 2 years. A quarterly earnings shortfall meant budget cuts, and like most old-fashioned unimaginative companies, which by then I realized Varian to be, the first thing cut is the unpredictable scary innovation stuff. Fortunately, or not, Varian invited me to find outside investors to fund what would become a technology spin out named Zap Surgical. Although never explicitly stated as such, my impression was that Varian management, knowing how challenging fundraising for medical device companies can be, truly hoped I would come up empty-handed and my pesky notions of radiosurgical innovation would ultimately just disappear; Varian senior management from the onset felt deeply ambivalent about Zap's success given their own "kludge" (my words) of a solution for brain radiosurgery and wanting to avoid competition from a more optimized neurosurgical product. Still Varian was willing to grant me a license to MY own inventions if fundraising succeeded. My ideas for a next-generation SRS device were now moving forward (Fig. 20.5).

Rather than feeling excitement, I was ironically frightened and emotionally spent. I had promised myself since Accuray that there would be no more difficult start-ups in my life, and suddenly I was late in middle age doing yet another raw start-up. And if that wasn't depressing enough, I had also "blundered" my way into creating and managing (as CEO) a "Next Gen" medical journal named *Cureus*, having initially started that company around an operations leader with lots of internet experience [19]. I naively founded *Cureus* believing the operating president would do the heavy lifting and I would just be an evangelist and the chairman filled with good ideas. However 2 years into *Cureus*, when things started getting a little tough, as they ALWAYS do, the president washed out. While I viewed *Cureus* as an exciting world changing idea and as a great business opportunity, it was very much a fresh start-up requiring lots of attention and increasingly associated with all the stereotypical start-up anguish. So, having just crossed age 60, a time when so many colleagues are thinking about slowing down, I found myself being the CEO of two raw start-ups happening in parallel.

**Fig. 20.5** Schematic of Zap-X

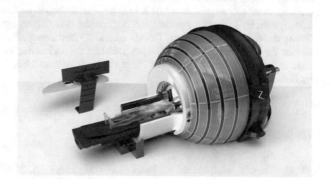

While both *Cureus* and Zap Surgical have had their ups and downs, neither one over the ensuing years remotely resembled Accuray when it comes to emotional drama. More than a decade after inception, both *Cureus* and Zap Surgical are doing well and seem poised, in time, to become big successes, maybe even colossal successes, within their respective niches [20]. Still the idea of slowing down and not giving everything I have to these two other virtual children of mine remains unthinkable. I console myself with the idea that an eternity of rest awaits me inside one's grave. Until that time, I'll stay laser focused on the millions of patients' lives at stake. Rightly or wrongly my concern is that if I as a neurosurgeon don't do this work, who will?

## Conclusions

As neurosurgeons, our biggest satisfaction resides in patients' care and postoperative results. Research performed by many neurosurgeons ultimately improves standard of care by introducing new treatments. By raising funds for research and development (R&D), regulatory clearance, and production entrepreneurship makes it possible to bring novel technologies to the bedside. Medical device start-ups are exceptionally difficult endeavors, typically requiring more than a decade to merely get serious traction. While neurosurgeons are innately innovative, it is a difficult decision to start a business given what an extreme distraction it will be from the typical clinical practice. Should a neurosurgeon choose to start an innovative medical device (or Pharma) company, it will prove to be the most difficult challenges of their professional lives. However, it will also be the most rewarding career experience of one's life. Clinicians' expertise and their clinical activities are the best ambassadors for new technology development and adoption. The road is long, but contributing to treatment optimization across the world represents an exciting mission and gives enormous motivation to overcome difficulties along the development path.

**Acknowledgments** Prof. Carpentier sincerely thanks Michael Canney, Jean-Yves Chapelon, Cyril Lafon, Dr. Kevin Beccaria, and Dr. Catherine Horodyckid for their fundamental support and co-development since the very beginning of this project. For the first clinical trial and ongoing ones, he thanks Pr Ahmed IDBAIH for his huge contribution as a neuro-oncologist and principal investigator, by including patients and performing complementary fundamental researches. He thanks Pr John deGroot, Pr Amy Heimberger, Dr. Adam Sonabend, Pr Roger Stupp, and Pr Mitch Berger for their strong belief in this program and for performing additional research and clinical trials in the USA. He also thanks CarThera's impressive team based in Paris, Lyon, and Denver, run by Frederic Sottilini.

## References

1. Hynynen K, McDannold N, Vykhodtseva N, Jolesz FA. Noninvasive MR imaging-guided focal opening of the blood-brain barrier in rabbits. Radiology. 2001;220(3):640–6.

2. Beccaria K, Canney M, Goldwirt L, Fernandez C, Adam C, Lafon C, Chapelon J-Y, Carpentier A. Opening of the blood-brain barrier with an unfocused ultrasound device in rabbits. J Neurosurg. 2013;119(4):887–98.

3. Horodyckid C, Canney M, Vignot A, Boisgard R, Adam C, Willer JC, Lafon C, Chapelon JY, Carpentier A. Safe long-term repeated disruption of the blood-brain barrier using an implantable ultrasound device: a multiparametric study in primate. J Neurosurg. 2016;10:1–11.

4. Beccaria K, Canney M, Goldwirt L, Fernandez C, Piquet J, Perier M-C, Lafon C, Chapelon J-Y, Carpentier A. Ultrasound-induced opening of the blood-brain barrier to enhance temozolomide and irinotecan delivery: an experimental study in rabbits. J Neurosurg. 2016;124(6):1602–10.

5. Goldwirt L, Canney M, Horodyckid C, Poupon J, Mourah S, Vignot A, Chapelon J-Y, Carpentier A. Enhanced brain distribution of carboplatin in a primate model after blood-brain barrier disruption using an implantable ultrasound device. Cancer Chemother Pharmacol. 2016;77(1):211–6.

6. Asquier N, Bouchoux G, Canney M, Martin C, Law-Ye B, Leclercq S, Chapelon JY, Lafon C, Idbaih A, Carpentier A. Blood-brain barrier disruption in humans using an implantable ultrasound device: quantification with MR images and correlation with local acoustic pressure. J Neurosurg. 2019;1:1–9.

7. Dréan A, Lemaire N, Bouchoux G, Goldwirt L, Canney M, Goli L, Bouzidi A, Schmitt C, Guehennec J, Verreault M, Sanson M, Delattre JY, Mokhtari K, Sottilini F, Carpentier A, Idbaih A. Temporary blood-brain barrier disruption by low intensity pulsed ultrasound increases carboplatin delivery and efficacy in preclinical models of glioblastoma. J Neuro-Oncol. 2019;144(1):33–41.

8. Carpentier A. Apparatus for the treatment of brain affections and method implementing thereof. PCT/EP2010/052206 (2010), PCT/EP2011/052611, WO2011101492 (2011), Granted EP2539021 (B), CA2789096 (A1), US20130204316 (A1), US8977361, EP2539021B, CN103002950 (A), JP2013520216 (A).

9. Carpentier A, Canney M, Vignot A, Reina V, Beccaria K, Horodyckid C, Karachi C, Leclercq D, Lafon C, Chapelon JY, Capelle L, Cornu P, Sanson M, Hoang-Xuan K, Delattre JY, Idbaih A. Clinical trial of blood-brain barrier disruption by pulsed ultrasound. Sci Trans Med. 2016;8(343):343re2.

10. Idbaih A, Canney M, Desseaux C, Vignot A, Bouchoux G, Asquier N, Law-Ye B, Leclercq D, Belin L, Bissery A, DeRycke Y, Trosch C, Capelle L, Sanson M, Hoang-Xuan K, Dehais C, Houillier C, Laigle-Donadey F, Delattre JY, Carpentier A. Safety and feasibility of repeated and transient blood brain barrier disruption by pulsed ultrasound in patients with recurrent glioblastoma. Clin Cancer Res. 2019;25(13):3793–801.

11. Beccaria K, Canney M, Bouchoux G, Puget S, Grill J, Carpentier A. Blood-brain barrier disruption with low-intensity pulsed ultrasound for the treatment of pediatric brain tumors: a review and perspectives. Neurosurg Focus. 2020;48(1):E10.

12. Zhang DY, et al. Ultrasound-mediated delivery of paclitaxel for glioma: a comparative study of distribution, toxicity, and efficacy of albumin-bound versus Cremophor formulations. Clin Cancer Res. 2020;26(2):477–86.

13. Beccaria K, Sabbagh A, de Groot J, Canney M, Carpentier A, Heimberger AB. Blood-brain barrier opening with low intensity pulsed ultrasound for immune modulation and immune therapeutic delivery to CNS tumors. J Neurooncol. 2020;151(1):65–73.

14. D'Haese P-F, et al. β-amyloid plaque reduction in the hippocampus after focused ultrasound-induced blood–brain barrier opening in Alzheimer's disease. Front Human Neurosci. 2020;14:422.

15. Jordão JF, et al. Amyloid-β plaque reduction, endogenous antibody delivery and glial activation by brain-targeted, transcranial focused ultrasound. Exp Neurol. 2013;248:16–29.

16. Karakatsani ME, et al. Unilateral focused ultrasound-induced blood-brain barrier opening reduces phosphorylated tau from the rTg4510 mouse model. Theranostics. 2019;9(18):5396.

17. Adler JR. https://www.cureus.com/articles/3-accuray-inc-a-neurosurgical-business-case-study.

18. Bentzen S, Wasserman TH. Balancing on a Knife's Edge: evidence-based medicine and the marketing of health technology. Int J Radiat Oncol Biol Phys. 2008;72(1):12–4. https://doi.org/10.1016/j.ijrobp.2008.05.044.
19. Adler JR. https://www-ncbi-nlm-nih-gov.laneproxy.stanford.edu/pmc/articles/PMC3515965/.
20. Weidlich GA, et al. https://www.cureus.com/articles/13225-characterization-of-a-novel-3-megavolt-linear-accelerator-for-dedicated-intracranial-stereotactic-radiosurgery.

# Chapter 21
# Digital Technology in Neurosurgery: A Successful Entrepreneurship Story

Federico Nicolosi, Paolo Raimondo, and Giannantonio Spena

## The Problem

Neurosurgery is, by definition, the medical discipline that deals with some of the most complicated pathologies being the brain not only a largely unexplored organ but also the one that holds the most intricate anatomy. Neurosurgical training is a long, complicated, multifaceted, and demanding path that asks the trainees to combine hard cognitive skills with 3D spatial orientation, coordination, procedural automatisms, and a vast theoretical knowledge. This process takes years. The methods to apprehend neurosurgical anatomy mainly rely upon the acquisition of theoretical concepts through lectures, textbooks, operative videos, medical images, and, of course, operating theaters. Finally, the learning process requires to translate this two-dimensional information into tridimensional mental imagery. This task is, at the same time, the most important and the most difficult to accomplish in neurosurgery, as it involves the ability to imagine the position of neural and vascular structures and to locate pathologies from different surgical perspectives and accesses (approaches). In addition, a trainee is asked to learn manual automatisms, dexterity, and psychomotor coordination in order to reduce the error rate during his/her performance. Somehow, the accuracy and rapidity to roll out these processes differentiate the experienced neurosurgeon from a younger or less experienced one.

In recent years neurosurgical training has become more difficult due to regulations in Western countries that limit the working hours of residents in neurosurgical

F. Nicolosi
Humanitas Research Hospital, Rozzano, Milan, Italy

P. Raimondo
UpSurgeOn, Milan, Italy

G. Spena (✉)
HospitalNeurosurgery, Policlinico San Matteo Foundation, Pavia, Italy

departments [1]. For this reason, worldwide, neurosurgeons have access to a limited number of surgical procedures, both during the training period and during the activity in wards. In a system where manual training coincides almost completely with live surgery experience, educators need to guarantee both training opportunities and patient's safety at once. In this scenario cadaver labs, which remains the gold standard to explore the human anatomy and train young surgeons, represent generally a very limited timeframe in the whole surgical curriculum. Among the traditional limits to the diffusion of cadaveric dissection, the most important is related, intuitively, to costs. This issue of neurosurgical training is particularly delicate for LMICs (low- to middle-income countries) are concerned. In these areas of the world, there is a severe shortage of neurosurgeons due to educational costs with a calculated volume of about five million patients who will never undergo their necessary surgical procedures [2–4].

## The Dawn of New Ideas

While coming from a similar background, the first and senior authors (FN and GN) were at different points of their career when they first got together to discuss a new idea. With hundreds of surgical cases performed and 10 years of surgical practice as consultant, GN had the ability to easily translate all the information derived from neuroimaging anatomy and pathology into the operating room. As a new practitioner in the neurosurgery residency, FN had, on the other hand, the will and the passion to explore this complicated universe and to infuse a fresh approach and contamination of 3D technologies to conceive new ways to speed up this long learning process. The mix of their two points of view was fundamental to pave the way of a new approach in teaching and learning neurosurgery.

Being versed in computational thinking, FN's very first step was to explore the world of digital segmentation and reconstruction of medical images for both normal and pathological neurosurgical anatomy. It almost immediately became clear that the comprehension of neurosurgical anatomy and, specifically, of the surgical corridors was clearly enhanced by the tridimensional digital reconstruction.

With such good premises, the collaboration of the two soon gave the desired results: a new software was developed for the evaluation of best approach to cerebello-pontine angle tumors which would later became the title of FN's final residency program thesis. However, their main focus was again the visualization of tridimensional neurosurgical anatomy, and, thanks to the intuition to apply photogrammetry (the process through which three-dimensional measurements can be extracted from two-dimensional data) to surgical scenarios and generating a virtual and explorable intraoperative surgical field [5, 6], the result was not long in coming.

At that time, there was a global interest toward the rapidly spreading 3D printing technology which gave the hint to create an in-house lab and reproduce patient-specific bony structures with operative planning purposes. Through this process, they moved to deal with the patient-specific soft tissue designing a 3D-printed mold (a negative) where a silicon mixture was dropped to obtain a very realistic and, more important, patient-specific brain surface.

The first initial self-made prototypes, with the hybridization of digital and physical products, made clear to the two "inventors" that they were on the right path: they understood that global technologies and the Internet were so advanced that also a purely scientific group could upgrade its daily educational activities without passing through medical companies and in a completely novel way. The combination of accurate and detailed tridimensional digital images, faithful physical models, and strong scientific bases would constitute the main pillar of a new vision in neurosurgery where teaching and learning would become easily available, more effective, and accurate. Thanks to the deep knowledge of the needs, they identified a learning process of mental, hybrid, and manual training and a series of technologies potentially able to cover these three stages.

## The Challenge: Creating a Team and a Developing Process

The excitement for the new idea and the perspective of new potential projects to follow soon gave way to the awareness that it was time to transform passion into a solid object that could have an impact on future generations of neurosurgeons. To do so, a working team had to be put together to manage the project in an organized process. The ambition to succeed set very strong assumptions from the very beginning: the end users – the neurosurgeons – would also be designers of the project. This was undoubtedly one of the most interesting and potentially successful aspect of the project. In fact, by leveraging their neurosurgical background, they were able to pick up-to-date and verified scientific references and to collect textbooks, anatomy lab pictures, and intraoperative videos. An enthusiastic pool of medical students and residents happily joined the project and helped in organizing the content (many of them are still members of the UpSurgeOn scientific team). On the other hand, the digital content development needed strong professional developers and 3D artists to reach the highest level of accuracy and usability. By the same logic, new tools for neurosurgical training should have been accessible globally. In other words, they needed to develop mobile-based 3D technologies to allow portability and widespread diffusion.

Given the dimension of the starting vision, they soon understood the importance of a financial support, and so they decided to self-finance the project and hire developers and digital artists. After few months the project had a name: UpSurgeOn. It comes from the fusion of "upsurge" and "surgeon," and it encompasses the whole message and spirit of the enterprise, giving the neurosurgical community a burst. The scientific team ("ST") and the developing team (DT") started immediately working together under the new name following what will be the "7-Step Scientific Modelling" process which is still at the core of all the developing processes of UpSurgeOn (see Fig. 21.1).

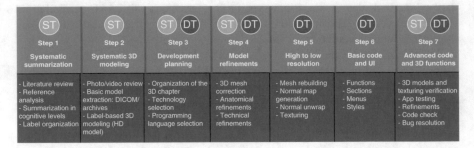

| | | | | | | |
|---|---|---|---|---|---|---|
| ST | ST | ST DT | ST DT | DT | DT | ST DT |
| Step 1 | Step 2 | Step 3 | Step 4 | Step 5 | Step 6 | Step 7 |
| Systematic summarization | Systematic 3D modeling | Development planning | Model refinements | High to low resolution | Basic code and UI | Advanced code and 3D functions |
| - Literature review<br>- Reference analysis<br>- Summarization in cognitive levels<br>- Label organization | - Photo/video review<br>- Basic model extraction: DICOM/ archives<br>- Label-based 3D modeling (HD model) | - Organization of the 3D chapter<br>- Technology selection<br>- Programming language selection | - 3D mesh correction<br>- Anatomical refinements<br>- Technical refinements | - Mesh rebuilding<br>- Normal map generation<br>- Normal unwrap<br>- Texturing | - Functions<br>- Sections<br>- Menus<br>- Styles | - 3D models and texturing verification<br>- App testing<br>- Refinements<br>- Code check<br>- Bug resolution |

**Fig. 21.1** A schematic representation of the productive and developing process named "7-Steps Process." *ST* scientific team, *DT* developing team

On January 30, 2017, the first educational app was released: 3D Skull Atlas. 3D Skull Atlas was engineered with innovative technologies to offer the most impressive 3D educational experience ever: three different visualization modes provide tools to explode, isolate, customize view, and arrange the bones. But there's more: hundreds of labels and descriptions from the scientific literature offered the widest bibliography ever seen in an anatomy app. With more than 700,000 downloads, the app in now a huge success.

## The Times and the Spaces: Evolving Toward a Company

As the project grew quickly, it was evident that to achieve its objectives, they had to level up. In their restless journey, FN and GN realized that ambitious projects do not easily find financial support in Italy which is, on the contrary, a country where imagination, creativity, and ability to act upon the problem are strongest. In this environment, they eventually met a person who radically changed their approach and their vision, allowing the necessary change. With more than 30-year experience in project management and start-up development, PR brought a pragmatic approach, and his contribution gave an extraordinary burst to the project. At this point, they all decided to ambitiously apply to Horizon 2020, the most important research and innovation program within the EU. The application selection to the grant was extremely rigorous, but, thanks to the team's hard work and dedication, they finally entered the competition. The project they presented was named UpSurgeOn Academy and was a completely new way of conceiving simulation. The foundation of the project is based on the assumption that the standard education, traditionally affected by a gap between theoretical knowledge and practice, could benefit from a hybrid educational platform provided by digital and physical hi-tech and low-cost technologies to support mental and manual training. The simulation prototype was conceived starting from the assumption that reproducing entire cranial anatomy implies high production costs and, hence, a limited accessibility. The new simulator was the first ever "hybrid simulator" (physical plus augmented reality) engineered to allow the exploration of a restricted cranial volume (approach) from the skull to the internal neuroanatomy, in an extremely detailed manner. Superficial anatomy was digitally "augmented" by 3D virtual animated models representing all the steps, from skin to bone. In this way the extracranial surgical phases were digitally represented for a visuospatial training, while the craniotomy and the intracranial contents were physically explored by the interaction with life-like materials. In other words, the user touches what he needs to touch and sees, virtually, what he only needs to see. The modular engineering with universal components (common to all the elements of the series) and specific components (specific of an element of the series) represents an additional innovation. Such organized approach enabled the switch from a surgical scenario to another by just changing only the specific components and maintaining the universal ones. This strategy reduces the costs, in line with the global need of innovative instruments capable to provide additional support to neurosurgical training even for settings with limited facilities, e.g., LMICs (low- to middle-income countries).

In July 2019 they succeeded and received a grant from the EU. From that moment on UpSurgeOn forever changed its aspect (www.upsurgeon.com).

## What Is UpSurgeOn Now and Where Is It Going to?

Since the awarding of H2020 project grant, UpSurgeOn has been expanding as a company; more than ten people have been hired to develop the 7-Step Scientific Modeling process with speed and accuracy.

In the UpSurgeOn laboratory, the scientific team continuously interact with the technical interdisciplinary team (developers, digital artists, modelers, bioengineers, and expert in materials are working) to develop the in-house process technologies for both virtual and physical simulation. Before the publication of this book, we have delivered a brand new neuroanatomy app which is the evolution of 3D Skull Atlas, this time with an ultra-detailed intracranial anatomy (from dura mater to nerves, veins, artery, and so on). Furthermore, the first hybrid Neurosimulator is available on smartphone and tablet and allows to digitally train on nine different cranial approaches (pterional, mini pterional, frontal, supraorbital, temporal, mini temporal, retrosigmoid, mini retrosigmoid, fronto-parietal). This app also interacts through AR with the physical models to help the users have a life-like experience with excellent tactile feedback and the opportunity to better visualize and explore intracranial tridimensional anatomy (Figs. 21.2 and 21.3).

Thanks to these instruments, UpSurgeOn promotes a novel cognitive and psychomotor training based on a triple categorization: anatomy (knowledge of three-dimensional anatomy); skills (knowledge of specific skills) and execution of operating techniques (craniotomy, suture, catheter insertion, etc.); and procedures (knowledge of operating procedures conceived as a logical sequence of actions and steps [e.g., patient positioning, craniotomy, approach to pathology, closure, etc.]).

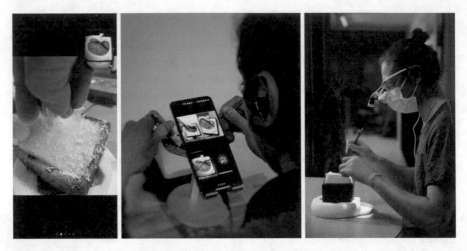

**Fig. 21.2** This picture shows the simulation box (in this case pterional approach). The model allows to perform craniotomy and explore the ultrarealistic intracranial anatomy, via a smartphone used as magnifier or a surgical loupe

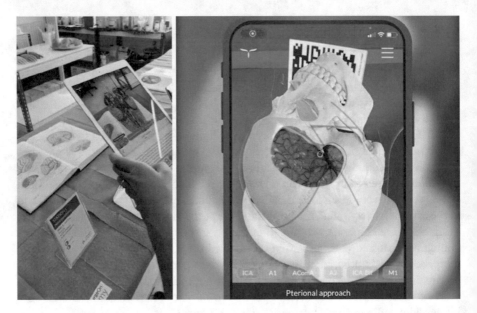

**Fig. 21.3** An example of how augmented reality app can help explore those parts of the anatomy that are not reproduced in the physical module

According to the funding principles of the absolute importance of strong scientific bases, the UpSurgeOn team continues to broaden and strengthen the endorsement by scientific institutions at global scale and to collaborate with companies interested in new surgical training methods.

For some months now we have been working with Global Neuro (globalneuro. org), the largest training institution for neurosurgery in Europe. Global Neuro, as many other companies affected by SARS-COVID-19 pandemic emergency, had to convert its classroom courses into a new way of doing distance learning. The working team, formed by the Global Neuro's scientific committee and UpSurgeOn founders, has realized that training needs, now more than ever, a revolution to distribute knowledge and to export surgical excellence skills in any socioeconomic context. By understanding and embracing the potential of the cadaver-free training revolution, Global Neuro is now developing a series of training modules (based on the UpSurgeOn platform technology) that will allow distance learning delivered by international masters who can teach neuroanatomy and neurosurgical procedures through the UpSurgeOn Academy. These learning modules are composed by a virtual part delivered through 3D apps and a physical part executed on a "cadaver-like" brainbox. This new learning methodology will be delivered directly to neurosurgery schools or to individual users, at their own homes, located anywhere in the world. This is a completely new training paradigm that has revolutionary potential and represents new hope for developing countries.

## Conclusion and Perspectives

It's a fact that, as for many other start-ups (medical and nonmedical), the difficulty to raise interest and to fight skepticism is the rule rather than the exception. Nevertheless, we had the chance to find many young people who overwhelmed us with enthusiasm and positive energy. We also injected into the project a solid vision of the future derived not only by the competencies and the expertise in neurosurgery but also by the need of a deep change in training paradigms. It is interesting to note that while struggling to find financial support in Italy, we discovered extraordinary abilities and know how available at relatively low costs.

UpSurgeOn is rapidly gaining consensus from both academic institutions and company interested in developing a brand new way to create and deliver new training procedures [7, 8]. This training model shifts the traditional paradigm that considers theory and practice as two consecutive steps with no specific path. The presence between these two cornerstones of an intensive cognitive and psychomotor simulation step represents a natural educational and cultural evolution of modern surgery.

Neurosurgery has been the starting point due to the founders' background. However, such a robust, scientifically validated, and technically sophisticated method can easily be applied to other surgical disciplines in order to expand the exploitation of such revolutionary simulation tools.

# References

1. Sedney CL, Spirou E, Voelker JL, Rosen CL. More learning in less time: optimizing the resident educational experience with limited clinical and educational work hours. World Neurosurg. 2017;107:881–7. https://doi.org/10.1016/j.wneu.2017.08.082. Epub 2017 Aug 24
2. Gnanakumar S, Abou El Ela Bourquin B, Robertson FC, Solla DJF, et al. The world Federation of Neurosurgical Societies Young Neurosurgeons Survey (part I): demographics, resources, and education. World Neurosurg X. 2020;8:100083.
3. Robertson FC, Gnanakumar S, Karekezi C, Vaughan K, Garcia RM, et al. The World Federation of Neurosurgical Societies Young Neurosurgeons Survey (Part II): barriers to professional development and service delivery in neurosurgery. World Neurosurg X. 2020;8:100084.
4. Nicolosi F, Rossini Z, Zaed I, Kolias AG, Fornari M, Servadei F. Neurosurgical digital teaching in low-middle income countries: beyond the frontiers of traditional education. Neurosurg Focus. 2018;45(4):E17.
5. Servadei F, Rossini Z, Nicolosi F, Morselli C, Park KB. The role of neurosurgery in countries with limited facilities: facts and challenges. World Neurosurg. 2018;112:315–21.
6. Nicolosi F, Spena G. Three-dimensional virtual intraoperative reconstruction: a novel method to explore a virtual neurosurgical field. World Neurosurg. 2020;137:e189–93.
7. Fontanella MM, Zanin L, Fiorindi A, Spena G, Nicolosi F, Belotti F, Panciani P, Cornali C, Doglietto F. Surgical management of brain cavernous malformations. Methods Mol Biol. 2020;2152:109–28. https://doi.org/10.1007/978-1-0716-0640-7_9.
8. Mattogno PP, Guerrini F, Nicolosi F, Panciani PP, Olivi A, Fontanella M, Spena G. Minimally invasive subfrontal approach (MISFA): how to make it safe and effective from the olfactory groove to the mesial temporal lobe. Skull Base accepted manuscript (CEN-2020-06-TN-2786).

# Chapter 22
# The Role of Nonprofit and Academic Institutions in Global Neurosurgery

Anthony T. Fuller, Miguel A. Arraez, and Michael M. Haglund

## Brief Historical Background

Before exploring the historical background, we must review the definition of global neurosurgery if we are to have any hope of creating a representative timeline. In our prior work [1, 2], and work by others [3, 4], global neurosurgery has been defined as "an area for study, research, practice, and advocacy that places priority on improving health outcomes and achieving health equity for all people worldwide who are affected by neurosurgical conditions or have a need for neurosurgical care." Using this as the definition, it is clear that global neurosurgery has been ongoing at least as long as the field of neurosurgery has existed and that essentially all neurosurgery everywhere could be encapsulated by this definition. In a series of exchanges in *World Neurosurgery* [5–7] prompted by the emergence of global neurosurgery as an emergent term in the past few years, the definition of global neurosurgery was addressed. Ultimately, the conclusion appeared to be that no matter if the term global neurosurgery is used or not, if we are to address the inequities present in neurosurgical care worldwide, we must collaborate. We wholeheartedly agree; thus, we highlight collaborative efforts throughout this chapter.

In light of the above discussion, it is nearly impossible to fully agree when nonprofit and academic institutions began contributing to global neurosurgery

A. T. Fuller
Department of Neurosurgery, Duke University, Durham, NC, USA

M. A. Arraez
Department of Neurosurgery, Malaga University, Malaga, Spain

M. M. Haglund (✉)
Duke Department of Neurosurgery, SIngHealth Duke-NUS Global Health Institute, Duke Health, Duke University, Durham, NC, USA
e-mail: michael.haglund@duke.edu

© The Author(s), under exclusive license to Springer Nature Switzerland AG 2022
I. M. Germano (ed.), *Neurosurgery and Global Health*,
https://doi.org/10.1007/978-3-030-86656-3_22

**Table 22.1** Global neurosurgery strategies and their definitions

| Strategy | Definition |
|---|---|
| Surgical camps | Collaborations with a primary focus on the delivery of neurosurgical care to populations in need |
| Education | Collaborations with a primary focus on increasing the knowledge and skills of the current neurosurgical care providers |
| Training | Collaborations with a primary focus on increasing the number of neurosurgical care providers |
| Research | Collaborations with a primary focus on using various research methods to scientifically explore neurosurgery topics |
| Health system strengthening, health policy, and advocacy | Collaborations with a primary focus on improving the health system drivers that impact the delivery of safe, affordable, accessible, and high-quality neurosurgical care |

collaborations. Our team within Duke Global Neurosurgery and Neurology (DGNN) published a scoping review of global neurosurgery collaborations which identified collaborations dating back to the 1960s [1]. This paper with a more recent publication [2] will serve as guideposts within this chapter. Much of the "Current Status" section draws heavily upon our work cited above.

For our purposes, global neurosurgery collaborations fall into five broad strategies (Table 22.1).

Our five strategies above reflect both the overarching historical timeline of global neurosurgery and the primary goals and drivers of global neurosurgery collaborations. Most of the early collaborations focused on the provision of neurosurgery to populations in need, which allows collaborators to immediately care for neurosurgical patients. Recent collaborations have focused on improving the health system infrastructure which allows neurosurgery collaborators to work holistically to meet the current burden. All five strategies are needed within global neurosurgery given the magnitude of the problem and the need for balancing short-term and long-term needs.

# Current Status

## *Surgical Camps*

Worldwide there are over five million people in need of neurosurgical care beyond the current capacity [8]. The primary driver of the inability to perform enough operations differs from country to country although a few key challenges are common to most locations. These include lack of neurosurgeons, inequitable in-country distribution of neurosurgical care facilities, a high volume of trauma cases overwhelming the ability of neurosurgeons to perform other operations, inaccessible surgical equipment needed for cases, and lack of necessary consumables to perform cases safely. Surgical camps are an expeditious way to provide care in places around the world that face the challenges outlined above.

At the most basic level, neurosurgery surgical camps provide neurosurgery to those in need wherever that need exists. The earliest method for surgical camps, one that is still used frequently today, involves a single neurosurgeon (or a small neurosurgery team) traveling and providing surgical services for a short period of time. Henry Marsh's work in Ukraine that started in 1992 is a perfect example [9, 10]. Marsh's Ukrainian efforts represent the core elements of individual surgical camps: (1) exposure to inequities drives action; (2) taking personal time, effort, and finances to travel and perform surgery; (3) repeated trips, usually on an annual basis; and (4) developing a strong partnership with the local neurosurgeon(s) and hospital. A few examples of other efforts include Alessandro Olivi and Ben Carson's trips to Ghana, Nigeria, and Kenya [11]; Alfredo Quiñones and Michael Lawton's trips to Mexico and the Philippines [12]; Paul Young and Jose Piquer's trips to Kenya and Tanzania [13]; Peter Nakaji's trips to Tanzania, Peru, Ecuador, and Nicaragua [14]; Charlie Teo's work in Peru, Indonesia, and Vietnam7 [15, 16]; and Robert Dempsey's work in Ecuador and Kenya [17]. There are many more neurosurgeons worldwide that see the current suffering that exists and decide to act by offering their surgical expertise. Some of them decide to develop new collaborations on an individual level while others seek out existing collaborations.

Individual neurosurgeons' efforts have motivated institutions to develop institutionally backed surgical camps which allow for a broader scale and the promise of sustainability. The Co-Pilot Project [18] and International Neurosurgical Children's Association [19] are two programs that currently work in Ukraine helping to provide neurosurgical care with an added emphasis on education and training of local practitioners. Another example of an institutional program is Project Shunt out of the University of Michigan, which has been going to Guatemala since 1997 and exists as a partnership between the Departments of Neurosurgery, Anesthesia, and Operating Rooms [20]. The program out of the University of Toronto is one of the larger endeavors globally with over 25 surgical camps to various hospitals in Indonesia, Ethiopia, Kenya, Zambia, Nigeria, Ukraine, Cambodia, and Ghana [21].

Adding to the diversity are neurosurgery surgical camps sponsored and supported by various NGOs/foundations, nonprofit organizations, missionary groups, and corporations. Chaine de l'Espoir (Chain of Hope- Europe) is a network of around six European NGOs that provide surgical care to populations in need across the globe, and some of their work, like in Cambodia, focuses on neurosurgery patients [22]. World Medical Missions, which is part of the larger missionary organization Samaritan's Purse, helps plan and link interested providers with medical and surgical camps around the world [23]. Some of their offerings include surgical camps for neurosurgeons, like their partnership with Tenwek Hospital in Bomet, Kenya, which has been developing their neurosurgery capacity in recent years and examining outcomes [24]. Tenwek Hospital has also set up post-residency program, which was most recently filled by William Copeland. Medical device companies have also pitched in with some, like Nuvasive, developing foundations or corporate responsibility departments that support global neurosurgical work. The Nuvasive Spine Foundation has in recent years annually supported nearly 20 trips to all parts of the world [25].

## *Education*

Surgical camps fulfill a direct medical need, and it cannot be denied that many patients that would have died otherwise are now living fulfilling lives due to these camps. This does not overshadow the variety of fundamental concerns levied at surgical camps spanning from the lack of attention to follow-up care after the camp is over to the perpetuation of colonialism due to camps promoting an image that outside neurosurgeons are "better" than the ones in the country. Many, if not all, of the surgical camps listed above have responded to these concerns by broadening their efforts to include components like the education and training of local providers.

Education is a central tenet for developing long-term, sustainable solutions to the issues faced in global neurosurgery. In defining this strategy of global neurosurgery engagement, we must differentiate education from formal training in neurosurgery. Education in this context is defined by interventions that focus on skills transfer, teaching medical students/residents/neurosurgeons about specific conditions by giving lectures, and providing educational materials like books, pamphlets, and videos. Global neurosurgery education programs seek to improve the quality of care that is provided in the country through sharing and improving knowledge. This is distinct from training, which is a formal process meant to increase the number of neurosurgeons or neurosurgery capable professionals in the country.

A common scenario faced in global neurosurgery is a hospital that has one neurosurgeon operating in less than ideal conditions, usually in an operating room shared with other specialties. The neurosurgeon likely completed their formal training outside of their home country and chose to return. In this setting, education not only for the neurosurgeons but also for the other healthcare providers and staff becomes important for a variety of reasons.

First, many of the neurosurgeons have been operating below their level of training due to resource limitations. This means that even formally trained neurosurgeons require some level of education and skills transfer when global neurosurgery efforts bring modern equipment that they haven't used in years or ever [26].

Second, education of the next generation of interested students becomes exceedingly challenging when you are the only neurosurgeon in your district, region, or country. Global neurosurgery programs allow interested students to learn and become interested in neurosurgery, and many have lecture series embedded that discuss common neurosurgical conditions and management. An example of this type of program is the Weill Cornell Medicine Neurosurgery Mission in Tanzania, founded in 2008 by Roger Härtl, which has added training components to their trips in addition to setting up a fellowship cosponsored by Fundación NED (Neurocirugia Educacion y DeSarrollo), a nonprofit organization based in Valencia, Spain, and supported by Paul Young, José Piquer, and Mubashir Mahmood Qureshi [17, 27].

Third, many LMICs have limited access to educational materials like books, operative videos, and other educational platforms so an important facet of some programs is donating and setting up access to these materials to all interested providers and students. The education of biomedical engineers and techs is also part of some programs as maintenance of donated equipment and supplies is vital to impact beyond the surgical camps [27]. Lastly, extremely complex cases and "first-ever in the country" cases are common during surgical camps; thus the education of neurosurgeons through skills transfer during the case is the only way to create competencies so that those procedures can be performed outside of surgical camps. Additionally, due to the need for complex medical management and the short-term nature of many trips, education on postoperative follow-up is imperative for successful neurosurgical outcomes.

## Training

Training more neurosurgeons and neurosurgery-capable providers is the only solution to increase the number of providers to close the gap in the neurosurgeon to population ratio. Global neurosurgery engages in training through the development of visiting residencies or fellowships, development of in-country residency or fellowship programs, and formalized neurosurgical skills transfer to other healthcare professionals to develop their ability to care for neurosurgery patients.

The University of Toronto has been training neurosurgeons from around the world as part of their Neuro-oncology and Skull Base Surgery Fellowship at the Toronto Western Hospital since 2010 [21]. This fellowship is a 1-year program that allows the visiting trainee to be exposed to and to learn the latest techniques and then return to their home country. A similar fellowship in pediatric neurosurgery has been established at the Hospital for Sick Children [28]. Brain drain is a common criticism brought against these types of programs, and while evidence implicating any one program is scarce, the phenomenon is undeniably present.

One way to address the concern of brain drain is to develop long-term, collaborative, in-country training programs. An example of such a program is the collaboration between Project Medishare and the Global Institute of the University of Miami Miller School of Medicine (UMMSM). They have developed a program in Haiti to train general surgeons to become neurosurgeons [29]. Other training programs have been developed by a neurosurgeon moving to another country and working with the local team and partners to develop training programs. Benjamin Warf in Mbale, Uganda, and A. Leland Albright in Kijabe, Kenya, are two perfect examples of neurosurgeons who decided to do just that. Benjamin Warf in partnership with CURE International helped develop a pediatric neurosurgery training program in Uganda, which now has visiting trainees from across Africa [30]. Warf's work additionally led to advancements in the care of hydrocephalus patients, which are being applied globally [31–34]. A. Leland Albright was able to accomplish a similar feat in Kijabe, Kenya, accompanied by his wife Susan Ferson, a pediatric neurosurgery nurse practitioner. They moved to Kijabe, Kenya, in 2010 and helped care for patients while developing a training program for pediatric neurosurgeons [35–38]. Both of these efforts exemplify what can be accomplished in global neurosurgery with motivated global neurosurgeons and outstanding in-country neurosurgeons and partnerships.

The Foundation for International Education in Neurological Surgery (FIENS) has been promoting the training of neurosurgeons on a global scale since 1969 [39, 40]. FIENS has made a tremendous impact in Central America, South America, Asia, and most recently in Africa, due to the past leadership of Merwyn Bagan and the current leadership of Robert Dempsey. An important distinction of the work FIENS has engaged in has been its emphasis on the development of in-country residencies/fellowships to train neurosurgeons. Providing in-country opportunities for neurosurgery training is a massive step toward decreasing the gap and creating a sustainable future for neurosurgery. The Neurosurgical Training Program of East Africa led by Moody Qureshi from Kenya and approved through the College of Surgeons of East, Central, and Southern Africa (COSECSA) has developed neurosurgery training programs in Ethiopia, Kenya, Tanzania, and Uganda [41]. Our group, Duke Global Neurosurgery and Neurology, helps support the Uganda program, which started in 2009, and to date, we have trained five Ugandans to become neurosurgeons, graduated the first woman neurosurgeon, and have ten more residents in the program [42]. In Ethiopia, the neurosurgery training program has been incredibly successful at increasing the number of neurosurgeons and the number of neurosurgery cases performed and has been supported since 2004 through a partnership between the University of Bergen, Haukeland University Hospital, the Black Lion Specialized Hospital, and a private hospital in Addis Ababa [43].

The Foundation of the World Federation of Neurosurgical Societies (WFNS) was created in 2000 by Professor Majid Sami, who made a personal donation of $10,000, and Professor Gerardo Martin Rodriguez. Its mission focuses on three goals. First, the foundation provides training and support for the postgraduate education of young neurosurgeons in developing countries. Second, it provides travel scholarships to young neurosurgeons to attend educational courses and fellowships. Third, it provides high-quality, low-cost instrument sets and equipment to neurosurgeons in developing countries. The latter is done in partnership with medical companies (Aesculap, Carl Zeiss, Storz, Xi Zhan) contributing to this efforts by providing instruments and equipment free of charge. The WFNS Foundation has partnered with academic and governmental institution to create WFNS training centers in LMIC where young neurosurgeons can be trained in the same continent where they will practice. The first of such centers was established in 2002 in Rabat (Morocco). For the past 20 years, many African neurosurgery resident from the sub-Sahara regions have been trained with full financial support by the WFNS Foundation. These trainees have successfully returned to their sub-Sahara countries after training was completed [44]. Additionally, the WFNS Foundation has established opportunities in over 30 training centers around the world where young neurosurgeons from LMIC can seek short training experiences with full room and board support, including a small stipend (https://www.wfns.org/training-centers).

Task-shifting or training an entry-level provider to do very specific tasks has been widely used throughout global health and has advocates within global surgery due to its expediency and cost implications. Faced with a neurosurgeon ratio gap that is nearly impossible to close rapidly, the length of time it takes to fully train a neurosurgeon, and the increased incidence of traumatic brain injuries requiring care, global neurosurgery strategies have included task-shifting as a necessary component. Led by Dilan Ellegala, a successful task-shifting model described as "train forward" has had great success in Tanzania through an organization called Madaktari Africa whose mission is to "advance medical expertise and care in sub-Saharan Africa through the training and education of local medical personnel." [45, 46]. While this model may not be applicable in all countries, using a "train-the-trainer" model and having neurosurgeons teach general surgeons how to perform basic trauma neurosurgery procedures is a viable solution to increase not only capacity but decentralize neurosurgical care, which is usually localized to major city centers.

## Research

There has been a rapid expansion in the number of dedicated global neurosurgery research articles in the past two decades. Article topics range from defining the current capacity and burden of neurosurgery globally to examining the impact of specific global neurosurgery interventions. The increased emphasis on research corresponds to the need to define the field and identify the most effective strategies for expanding access and improving the quality of neurosurgery care. Additionally, as the number of people interested in global neurosurgery increases in tandem with additional neurosurgeons globally, there are new opportunities for neurosurgeons to focus on academic pursuits alongside clinical work. Research collaborations help to answer important scientific questions while directly and indirectly impacting research capacity in-country.

A central research aim in any area of scientific inquiry is to understand the magnitude of the problem. For global neurosurgery, the central problem is the total number of neurosurgeons and the number of people requiring neurosurgery worldwide. There were initial efforts to define the problem regionally such as the work by El Khamlichi in 2001 defining the number of neurosurgeons in Africa [47], prior to the seminal work published by Dewan et al. [8] which highlights the problem at a global level. The initial paper by Dewan et al. has led to the establishment of a global collaboration to update the burden and workforce data regularly as well as articles exploring global trends [48]. Using the results as a starting point, global neurosurgery collaborations can begin to set specific goals for their efforts and assess their impact against these goals.

Our group, DGNN, has made research a core component of our global neurosurgery efforts in combination with our other core components: service and training [49]. In collaboration with our in-country partners, we have established a research plan that encompasses quantitative and qualitative methods with full-country projects to single-intervention assessments. Since our founding in 2014, we have published over 50 peer-reviewed manuscripts that have helped shape neurosurgery and neurology care in Uganda. Through this work, we have established ongoing neurosurgery patient registries, improved in-hospital neurosurgery outcomes, and have begun exploring innovative solutions to challenges inherent to providing neurosurgery care in Uganda. Most importantly, we have involved Ugandan neurosurgeons, neurologists, and other researchers in these efforts throughout and have trained Ugandan students in research methodologies. It is our ultimate goal to have all of the neurosurgery trainees in Uganda participate in research projects as part of their residency and fellowship experiences.

## Health System Strengthening, Health Policy, and Advocacy

The expert global opinion is shifting within global health beyond vertical projects to horizontal projects that aim to address the underlying issues within the health system [50]. This change has occurred partly because noncommunicable diseases and chronic conditions cannot be solved by the traditional global health approaches applied to infectious disease. Global neurosurgery work falls within this mind-set shift, as surgery provision in its best form requires a well-functioning health system [50]. Within the past 5–10 years, more neurosurgery groups are broadening their scope to include health system strengthening projects, examining health care policy, and advocating at national and international levels. This strategy of global neurosurgery focuses on the system of care surrounding neurosurgeons and their patients. While there are more programs domestically and abroad, we wanted to highlight the Global Neurosurgery Initiative (GNI) within the Program in Global Surgery and Social Change (PGSSC) at Harvard University.

PGSSC is a collaborative effort between the Harvard teaching hospitals, the Department of Global Health and Social Medicine at Harvard Medical School, Boston Children's Hospital, and Partners In Health [8]. PGSSC's primary objective is to advocate for universal access to safe, affordable surgical, obstetric, and anesthesia care when needed. The Global Neurosurgery Initiative (GNI) exists within PGSSC's framework and focuses on research, policy, and advocacy within global neurosurgery. Ongoing work from GNI includes pediatric neurosurgical training in Mbale, Uganda; research examining health policy and economic implications for global neurosurgery; and global surveys examining neurosurgeon perspectives and current capacity in LMICs which is being done in partnership with the World Federation of Neurosurgical Societies (WFNS) and the National Institute for Health Research (NIHR) Global Health Research Group on Neurotrauma. GNI focuses on advocacy at the global level through participation in various international conferences, World Health Organization sponsored events, country-level Ministry of Health discussions, and through the dissemination of their work through opinion articles, Twitter, podcasts, and news station interviews.

## Future Opportunities and Unmet Needs

Collaboration as mentioned at the start of this chapter is at the heart of global neurosurgery nonprofit and academic institutional efforts. Tremendous progress has been made; nevertheless, for global neurosurgery to fully realize its aims, the field remains with unmet needs and ample opportunities for improvement in each of the strategies outlined.

## Surgical Camps

Common criticisms of surgical camps are that they are not fully planned with the in-country team in mind, prioritize camp attendee's education instead of the local team, bring unnecessary and sometimes useless supplies and equipment, and lack attention to follow-up care. Each of these critics is valid in varying degrees to a majority of ongoing neurosurgical camp collaborations. An increased emphasis on pre-camp planning and sharing of best practices will help address these concerns.

Pre-camp planning should begin well in advance of the trip and if possible at least 4–6 months prior to the trip. This amount of time ensures that the in-country team has adequate time to identify the most pressing needs and the best time for the hospital to host the camp. Many surgical camps are able to provide neurosurgery to a large number of patients in a short period of time, but if not planned in advance, the local hospital may not have the opportunity to alert the other departments that a camp is happening. This can lead to the neurosurgery camp straining the local resources from anesthesia providers, oxygen and blood supplies, and intensive care unit space.

Pre-camp planning can also address not only the local needs for neurosurgical care but also the educational needs for the local healthcare providers. Identifying these needs in advance allows the camp team to select cases that aid the local neurosurgeons and residents improving their skills to manage those cases outside of camp. Additionally, this allows the visiting team to tailor educational lectures or other materials to discuss while the team is in the country. Often the education of the nursing, intensive care unit, and equipment maintenance staff is overlooked during camps despite the high correlation of good outcomes associated with these staff being well trained. With this added emphasis on in-camp education, it becomes clear that the local educational needs supersede those of the visiting team.

Many surgical camps bring with them neurosurgical equipment, supplies, and consumables most of which is in dire need to safely perform the camp operations. Unfortunately, pervasive intellectual concepts such as "anything is better than nothing" and "I'm sure they need this" cause many camps to bring equipment and supplies in excess of what is truly needed. Advanced discussions are needed to agree on the local needs, how to procure the equipment and supplies in the country, how equipment will be maintained and serviced prior to and upon arrival, and what the plan is for sustainable access to necessary consumables.

There are an abundance of other best practices that neurosurgery camps have implemented over the years leading to successful camps and long-term collaborations. Within our field, we must create a central location to learn about the workings of different neurosurgery camps as well as use this location to share best practices and other helpful materials. Currently, it is an arduous task to find the specifics or even know where to find details if you are planning your own neurosurgical camp or hoping to improve your existing camp. Apart from scrapping small clues from journal articles and online descriptions, neurosurgeons interested in surgical camps are left with contacting the key people involved and hoping for a response. We must also develop a standardized approach for monitoring and evaluating our efforts to identify areas in need of improvement. A helpful resource to begin this effort would be for all current neurosurgery camp programs to either use The Framework for the Assessment of InteRNational Surgical Success (FAIRNeSS) to evaluate their programs [51] or for current programs to work collaboratively to develop a neurosurgery-tailored, standardized assessment tool. These evaluations could then be submitted and undergo peer review prior to becoming accessible in a central location online.

## *Education*

In addition to the educational initiatives during surgical camps outlined above, education of the current neurosurgical workforce has additional needs. These needs include full access to the most current books, articles, videos, and online platforms; attention to the educational needs beyond the neurosurgeons; and developing an environment that promotes learning.

Access to the most up-to-date and innovative learning resources is taken as a given in many parts of the world that have academic and other institutions that pay exorbitant institutional licensing fees for educational materials. This cost-influenced divide leads individuals in many countries to either deal with subpar, outdated educational materials or rely upon alternative means of access, typically collaborators providing them access. While it may not be possible overnight to change licensing agreements, global neurosurgery collaborators should make it a priority to advocate at their institutions for full access to the same educational materials for all of their in-country partners.

Neurosurgery is supported by a host of other important healthcare providers and hospital staff. Their education is essential to effective preoperative, in-hospital, postoperative, and post-hospital management of patients to achieve the best outcomes for our patients. Thus, increased attention, beyond surgical camps, is needed for these other key contributors. An excellent starting place is the nursing staff on the wards, in the operating theaters, and in the intensive care unit. Improving the education of these nurses will allow for a substantial portion of the improved outcomes mentioned earlier to be achieved.

One of the many things that the COVID-19 global pandemic exposed for those that were unaware was that your learning environment matters. For many neurosurgery trainees, their learning environment is inadequate due to limited space for uninterrupted studying, unreliable Internet access, and strenuous clinical loads that do not take into account study time. Global neurosurgery collaborators must work together to develop innovative approaches to set up space for trainees to study, provide them reliable access to the Internet and the means and devices to connect, and work to carve out educational time into the clinical schedules for trainees.

## Training

The massive shortage of neurosurgeons worldwide is critical, especially in light of the rapidly increasing populations in some countries. Many countries may not even have a fully trained neurosurgeon capable of training the next generation. In order to start a program, the needed requirements include trainers whether in country or from outside academic institutions. Besides the program leadership, there is a great need for institutional support, appropriate equipment, supply chains, and intensive care, step-down, and floor nursing and allied professional care such as occupational and physical therapy, and placement abilities.

Tailored curricular development is important, and the foundational learning opportunities are available through the World Federation of Neurological Surgeons (WFNS) and the FIENS. Also, many societies such as the Congress of Neurological Surgeons, Senior Society of Neurological Surgeons, and the American Association of Neurological provide significant online learning opportunities. The ACGME Milestones and Residency Review in Neurological Surgery as part of the ACGME in the United States have specific milestones of progression that should occur throughout training. Live online learning experiences for surgical training are growing with Aaron Cohen-Gadol's Virtual Neurosurgery Atlas (https://www.neurosurgicalatlas.com) which provides live OR demonstrations that would be important for the trainees to view and learn about more complex procedures.

Paid positions must also be available for graduates upon training completion or programs run the risk of their graduates leaving the country. Graduates unable to find a position in their home country may leave to neighboring countries or to the USA or the UK. Successful placement of neurosurgeons depends on the Ministry of Health and other governmental agencies being willing to fund the positions. Training programs must develop and cultivate relationships with the Ministry of Health during the early stages to avoid brain drain.

## Research

Research is a valuable aspect of global neurosurgery for its ability to define the size of the problem, its contributions to knowledge, and for the advancement of innovative ideas that can be tested prior to implementation. Advanced research methods and techniques are only recently beginning to take hold in global neurosurgery collaborations. We still need to create central data repositories, develop research opportunities for local trainees and interested collaborators, and promote grant funding mechanisms that do not require a US or European collaborator to access.

Standardized data repositories hold incredible promise because they allow researchers to utilize the most recent advances in computational efficiency and statistical methods to answer previously unanswerable questions. In global neurosurgery, there are current ongoing efforts to develop a global system to track the number of neurosurgeons and burden along with efforts to establish standardized metrics for tracking traumatic brain injury outcomes. These are important first steps and help set the stage for global neurosurgery researchers to think big and develop methods that help us to securely share data to answer questions that one center or one country is unable to answer.

Neurosurgery training programs need to include opportunities for trainees to learn research skills and time for them to explore a specific research question. Understandably, this may not be possible in all circumstances given resource constraints and the need for clinical management of excessive caseloads can be done by allotting dedicated research time within the current training paradigm or expanding the length of training for interested trainees. Providing training in neurosurgery research is an incredibly important step to help address the often-cited problem that many global neurosurgery articles are published with US or European first and/or senior authors. Building the local research capacity allows for research questions to better align with local needs and for the local researchers to position themselves better for academic posts. This added attention to research skill development, which would need to include grant writing, would allow for local researchers to be better positioned for grant funding. As the local research capacity increases, a concordant increase should occur in the number of grants offered that do not require US or European collaborators. This point cannot be overemphasized given that many high-quality researchers are unable to access grant funding unless they have a US or European collaborator.

## Health System Strengthening, Health Policy, and Advocacy

Health system strengthening must be central to our discussions about global neurosurgery if we are to have any hope of achieving our lofty goals. It is impossible to deliver accessible, safe, affordable, and high-quality neurosurgical care to all those in need without a well-functioning health system. Neurosurgery patients rely on surgeons to work closely with radiologists, anesthesiologists, nurses, rehabilitation professionals, and many others in the health system to decrease morbidity and improve their chance of survival. All of this then additionally needs to be delivered in a way that doesn't cause patients and their families catastrophic healthcare expenditures. When the problem is positioned in this way, it is clear that the only hope is that global neurosurgery efforts begin to collaborate with each other as well as with other global surgery and broader global health efforts. Some of this work has already begun with multiple conferences dedicated to global neurosurgery and global neurosurgery dedicated sessions at international neurosurgery and global health conferences.

Healthcare delivery is inextricably linked to policy at the national and international levels. With this in mind, global neurosurgery goals must begin to be integrated into policy that impacts the delivery of neurosurgical care. The World Health Organization plays a key role internationally in informing policy, and having individuals like neurosurgeon Dr. Walter Johnson, who leads the WHO's Emergency & Essential Surgical Care Programme, is important for bringing global neurosurgery into these conversations. Another avenue is through the development of National Surgical, Obstetric and Anesthesia Plans (NSOAPs), an idea that was first pitched by the Lancet Commission of Global Surgery and has been pushed forward by partnerships with Ministries of Health and PGSSC. Another policy topic that is important for global neurosurgery to work on is helping curb the impact of road traffic accidents through improved road infrastructure and helmet laws.

Beyond policy work, there is a need for advocacy efforts within global neurosurgery aligned with the current decolonization of global health movement. As already mentioned in this chapter, there is a need for our field to advocate for full, open access to educational materials, increase equity in the grant process, and consider equity in all of our efforts. There are a few things that we should be able to implement immediately. With our conferences, we should shift their locations to be positioned with equitable accessibility in mind, we should ensure that every panel discussion promotes the voices of the local collaborators, and we should provide free access to conference presentations and materials for those unable to attend. During the COVID-19 pandemic, we have seen virtual conferences and new ways of engagement setup for international conferences. These innovations must remain a key pillar for planning conferences even as restrictions ease internationally. With our research publications, we should position local collaborators to be first and senior authors, we should work closely with our collaborators before developing intervention ideas, and we should ensure that local trainees can participate in research projects to build up their research skills. These ideas are already being implemented, in part, around the world; however, we must never forget that we must keep the concepts of equity and decolonization at the forefront of our decision-making and iterative evaluation processes.

## Conclusion

In summary, collaboration is the central theme for the development of impactful and sustainable global neurosurgery academic and nonprofit partnerships. The passion to bring this to fruition needs all sides to be dedicated to seeing it through and for open and honest communication about goals. There are many difficult roadblocks to overcome, but we believe that the many examples in this chapter serve as templates to accomplishing the extraordinary goal of decreasing the global neurosurgery inequity that exists.

## References

1. Fuller AT, et al. Global neurosurgery: a scoping review detailing the current state of international neurosurgical outreach. J. Neurosurg. 2020;134(3):1316–24. https://doi.org/10.3171/2020.2.JNS192517.

2. Haglund MM, Fuller AT. Global neurosurgery: innovators, strategies, and the way forward: JNSPG 75th Anniversary Invited Review Article. J Neurosurg. 2019;131:993–9.
3. Dare AJ, et al. Global surgery: defining an emerging global health field. Lancet. 2014;384:2245–7.
4. Park KB, Johnson WD, Dempsey RJ. Global neurosurgery: the unmet need. World Neurosurg. 2016;88:32–5.
5. Andrews RJ. What's in a name? 'Global neurosurgery' in the 21st century. World Neurosurg. 2020;143:336–8.
6. Agrawal A, Shrivastava A, Mishra R, Raj S, Chouksey P. Letter to the editor regarding 'what's in a name? "Global neurosurgery" in the 21st century'. World Neurosurg. 2020;143:644–5.
7. Andrews RJ. In reply to the letter to the editor regarding 'what's in a name? "Global neurosurgery" in the 21st century'. World Neurosurg. 2020;143:646.
8. Dewan MC, et al. Global neurosurgery: the current capacity and deficit in the provision of essential neurosurgical care. Executive Summary of the Global Neurosurgery Initiative at the Program in Global Surgery and Social Change. J Neurosurg. 2018; https://doi.org/10.3171/2017.11.JNS171500.
9. March H. Do no harm: stories of life, death and brain surgery. Weidenfeld & Nicolson; United Kingdom. 2014.
10. Smith G. The English Surgeon. Eyeline Films and Bungalow Town Productions; England. 2010.
11. NeuroNow. Mission to Africa. Johns Hopkins Hospital. 2011. https://www.hopkinsmedicine.org/news/publications/neuronow/neuronow_spring_2011/mission_to_africa.
12. Our History. Mission: Brain Foundation. 2020. https://www.missionbrain.org/history.html.
13. Qureshi MM, Oluoch-Olunya D. History of neurosurgery in Kenya, East Africa. World Neurosurg. 2010;73:261–3.
14. Meeusen, A. J. Barrow Beyond Borders. 2013. http://barrowbeyondborders.weebly.com/.
15. 40th Annual Meeting of the International Society for Pediatric Neurosurgery, Sydney, Australia, September 9–13, 2012. Childs Nerv Syst. 2012;28:1589–669.
16. Lee VJ, Low E, Ng YY, Teo C. Disaster relief and initial response to the earthquake and tsunami in Meulaboh, Indonesia. Ann Acad Med Singapore. 2005;34:586–90.
17. Piquer J, Qureshi MM, Young PH, Dempsey RJ. Neurosurgery Education and Development program to treat hydrocephalus and to develop neurosurgery in Africa using mobile neuroendoscopic training. J Neurosurg Pediatr. 2015;15:552–9.
18. The Co-Pilot Project. Razom for Ukraine. 2020. https://razomforukraine.org/projects/cpp/#:~:text=The%20Co%2DPilot%20Project%20(CPP,million%20people%20in%20eastern%20Europe.
19. All children deserve modern brain surgery. International Neurosurgical Children's Association. 2018. http://www.incachildren.org/.
20. Project Shunt. University of Michigan Neurosurgery. 2020. https://medicine.umich.edu/dept/neurosurgery/project-shunt.
21. Almeida JP, et al. Global neurosurgery: models for international surgical education and collaboration at one university. Neurosurg Focus. 2018;45:E5.
22. Chain of Hope. Chain of Hope-Europe. 2020. https://www.chainofhopeeurope.eu/.
23. World Medical Missions. Samaritan's Purse. 2020. https://www.samaritanspurse.org/medical/world-medical-mission/.
24. Kanyi JK, Ogada TV, Oloo MJ, Parker RK. Burr-Hole Craniostomy for chronic subdural hematomas by general surgeons in Rural Kenya. World J Surg. 2018;42:40–5.
25. Giving Back. NuVasive Spine Foundation. 2020. https://www.nuvasive.com/about/nuvasive-spine-foundation/.

26. Kahamba JF, Assey AB, Dempsey RJ, Qureshi MM, Härtl R. The second African Federation of Neurological Surgeons course in the East, Central, and Southern Africa region held in Dar es Salaam, Tanzania, January 2011. World Neurosurg. 2013;80:255–9.
27. NED Foundation. NED Foundation. 2020. https://nedfundacion.org/.
28. Fellowship in Clinical Pediatric Neurosurgery. University of Toronto. 2020. https://surgery.utoronto.ca/fellowship-clinical-pediatric-neurosurgery.
29. Shah AH, et al. Bridging the gap: creating a self-sustaining neurosurgical residency program in Haiti. Neurosurg Focus. 2018;45:E4.
30. Dewan MC, et al. Subspecialty pediatric neurosurgery training: a skill-based training model for neurosurgeons in low-resourced health systems. Neurosurg Focus. 2018;45:E2. Warf BC. Combined endoscopic third ventriculostomy and choroid plexus cauterization for treatment of infant hydrocephalus. Pediatric Hydrocephalus. 2018. https://doi.org/10.1007/978-3-319-31889-9_79-1
31. Kulkarni AV, et al. Endoscopic treatment versus shunting for infant hydrocephalus in Uganda. N Engl J Med. 2017;377:2456–64.
32. Kulkarni AV, et al. Endoscopic third ventriculostomy and choroid plexus cauterization in infants with hydrocephalus: a retrospective Hydrocephalus Clinical Research Network study. J Neurosurg Pediatr. 2014;14:224–9.
33. Cairo SB, Agyei J, Nyavandu K, Rothstein DH, Kalisya LM. Neurosurgical management of hydrocephalus by a general surgeon in an extremely low resource setting: initial experience in North Kivu province of Eastern Democratic Republic of Congo. Pediatr Surg Int. 2018;34:467–73.
34. Albright AL, Ferson SS. Developing pediatric neurosurgery in a developing country. J Child Neurol. 2012;27:1559–64.
35. Munyi N, Poenaru D, Bransford R, Albright L. Encephalocele–a single institution African experience. East Afr Med J. 2009;86:51–4.
36. Githuku JN, et al. Assessing the prevalence of spina bifida and encephalocele in a Kenyan hospital from 2005-2010: implications for a neural tube defects surveillance system. Pan Afr Med J. 2014;18:60.
37. The Kenya Initiative. The Kenya Initiative. 2018. https://kenyainitiative.weebly.com/about.html.
38. Bagan M. The foundation for international education in neurological surgery. World Neurosurg. 2010;73:289.
39. Dempsey RJ, Nakaji P. Foundation for International Education in Neurological Surgery (FIENS) global health and neurosurgical volunteerism. Neurosurgery. 2013;73:1070–1.
40. Budohoski KP, et al. Neurosurgery in East Africa: innovations. World Neurosurg. 2018;113:436–52.
41. Haglund MM, et al. Past, present, and future of neurosurgery in Uganda. Neurosurgery. 2017;80:656–61.
42. Lund-Johansen M, Dahl JW, Eilertsen GM, Wester K. Establishment of neurosurgery training in Ethiopia. Tidsskrift for Den norske legeforening. 2017; https://doi.org/10.4045/tidsskr.17.0282.
43. Forrester JD. Unlikely surgeons. Health Aff. 2017;36:2026–7.
44. Karekezi C, El Khamlichi A, El Ouahabi A, El Abbadi N, Ahokpossi SA, Ahanogbe KMH, Berete I, Bouya SM, Coulibaly O, Dao I, Djoubairou BO, Doleagbenou AAK, Egu KP, Ekouele Mbaki HB, Kinata-Bambino SB, Habibou LM, Mousse AN, Ngamasata T, Ntalaja J, Onen J, Quenum K, Seylan D, Sogoba Y, Servadei F, Germano IM. Impact of African-trained neurosurgeon on Sub-Sahara Africa. JNS Neurosurg Focus. 2020;48(3):E6. PMID: 32114560
45. Madaktari Africa. Madaktari Africa. 2020. https://madaktari.jimdo.com/home/our-mission/.
46. El Khamlichi A. African neurosurgery: current situation, priorities, and needs. Neurosurgery. 2001;48:1344–7.

47. Kanmounye US, et al. Emerging trends in the neurosurgical workforce of low- and middle-income countries: a cross-sectional study. World Neurosurg. 2020;142:e420–33.
48. Frenk J. The global health system: strengthening national health systems as the next step for global progress. PLoS Med. 2010;7:e1000089.
49. Fuller A, Tran T, Muhumuza M, Haglund MM. Building neurosurgical capacity in low and middle income countries. eNeurologicalSci. 2016;3:1–6.
50. Meara JG, et al. Global Surgery 2030: evidence and solutions for achieving health, welfare, and economic development. Lancet. 2015;386:569–624.
51. Ibrahim GM, Cadotte DW, Bernstein M. A framework for the monitoring and evaluation of international surgical initiatives in low- and middle-income countries. PLoS One. 2015;10:e0120368.

# Chapter 23
# The World Health Organization and Neurosurgery

Walter D. Johnson, Emmanuel M. Makasa, S. William A. Gunn, and Meena N. Cherian

## Historical Background

In the immediate aftermath of the Second World War, diplomats met to establish the United Nations (UN), which officially came into existence on October 24, 1945. This organization was founded by 51 countries "committed to maintaining international peace and security, developing friendly relations among nations and promoting social progress, better living standards and human rights" [1].

That same year, the UN Conference on International Organizations was held in San Francisco, California, resolved to establish a new international health organization, and the International Health Conference in New York crafted and

W. D. Johnson (✉)
Department of Neurosurgery and School of Public Health, Loma Linda, CA, USA

Center for Global Surgery, Loma Linda University, Loma Linda, CA, USA

Emergency and Essential Surgical Care Programme, World Health Organization, Geneva, Switzerland

E. M. Makasa
University Hospitals, Lusaka, Zambia

Wits-SADC Regional Collaboration Centre for Surgical Healthcare, University of the Witwatersrand, Johannesburg, Republic of South Africa

Former Health Counsellor at the Permanent Mission of the Republic of Zambia to the United Nations in Geneva and Vienna, Johannesburg, Republic of South Africa

S. W. A. Gunn
Emergency Humanitarian Operations, World Health Organization, Rolle, Switzerland

International Association for Humanitarian Medicine, Rolle, Switzerland

M. N. Cherian
Emergency & Surgical Care Program, Geneva Foundation for Medical Education & Research (GFMER), Geneva, Switzerland

© The Author(s), under exclusive license to Springer Nature Switzerland AG 2022
I. M. Germano (ed.), *Neurosurgery and Global Health*,
https://doi.org/10.1007/978-3-030-86656-3_23

approved the Constitution of the World Health Organization (WHO). Between 1946 and 1948 an Interim Commission, comprised of 18 states, took over the work of L'Office International d'Hygiene Publique (European Health Commission), the original Health Organization of the League of Nations in Geneva, Switzerland, and the Health Division of the UN Relief and Rehabilitation Administration. Enough signatures were obtained, and the WHO Constitution came into force on 7 April 1948 – a date we now celebrate each year as World Health Day [2].

The first World Health Assembly (WHA) was held in Geneva in 1948 (Fig. 23.1), establishing as priorities the following: malaria, tuberculosis, venereal diseases, maternal and child health, sanitary engineering, and nutrition, as well as wide-ranging disease prevention and control efforts against yaws, endemic syphilis, leprosy, and trachoma. The original annual budget was US$5 million.

The WHO is the health technical arm of the UN, with core functions that include providing leadership on crucial health matters, setting the research agenda for generating and disseminating valuable knowledge, creating standards and guidelines, articulating ethical and evidence-based policies, providing technical support to build sustainable health system capacity, and monitoring health situations and assessing health trends [3]. The WHA, currently comprised of 194 health ministers representing all Member States (countries) of the UN, is the governing body of WHO, which sets the global health agenda, creates mandates for WHO's work, and elects the director-general (D-G). This body sets the what, how, how long, and with what means programs are conducted by WHO through resolutions and decisions. To facilitate activities of the WHA, an executive board (EB), made up of 36 Member States, creates a more nimble executive function, sets the WHA agenda, including proposed resolutions and decisions. While WHA meets each May, the EB meets twice yearly [4].

The EB prepares the provisional agenda of each regular session of the WHA after consideration of proposals submitted by Member States and the D-G. The EB then includes on this provisional agenda (among other things): (a) the annual report of the D-G on the ongoing work of WHO; (b) all items that the WHA has, in a previous

## WHO EESC Timeline

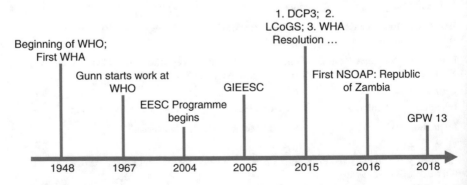

**Fig. 23.1** World Health Organization (WHO) Emergency and Essential Surgical Care (EESC) schematic historical timeline

session, ordered to be included; (c) any items pertaining to the budget for the next financial period and to reports on the accounts for the preceding year or period; (d) any item proposed by a Member State or by an Associate Member; (e) subject to such preliminary consultation as may be necessary between the D-G and the secretary-general of the UN, any item proposed by the UN; and (f) any item proposed by any other organization of the UN system with which WHO has entered into effective relations. The EB may recommend to the WHA the deferral of any item under (d), (e), or (f) above. Member States can, under exceptional circumstances, introduce a new item for consideration by the WHA prior to or during its seating [5].

An agenda item that is considered by the EB and WHA is traditionally accompanied by a WHO Secretariat report and can be proposed for (i) notation only, (ii) consideration with an associated resolution, or (iii) consideration with an associated decision. The text of the resolution is drafted through negotiated consensus by Member States under the principle of "Nothing is agreed until everything is agreed." During these negotiations, the WHO Secretariat prepares an associated agenda item report for consideration by the EB or WHA but only supports this process with editing and recording of ongoing progress. While voting is a legal option, WHA resolutions are traditionally adopted by consensus during the WHA. Non-state actors in official relations with WHO are invited to comment on the record and register their positions on any agenda item under consideration during the EB and WHA, after WHO and Member States have made their statements.

Resolutions are proposals that are brought forward and championed by a Member State or group of Member States and are formal expressions of the opinion or will of the WHA, bearing operative mandates for both Member States and WHO Secretariat through the D-G. WHA resolutions also reflect the views of the Member States, provide policy recommendations, assign mandates to the WHO Secretariat, and decide on all questions regarding the WHO budget. Decisions are another type of formal action taken by WHA bodies and often concern procedural matters such as elections, appointments, time, and place of future sessions. Decisions bear mandates for the WHO Secretariat through the director-general only, but none for Member States as is the case with resolutions. Decisions may also be used to record the adoption of a text representing the consensus a given scientific committee or technical working group. WHA resolutions and decisions have the same legal status. Except for decisions regarding payments to the regular WHO budgets, resolutions and decisions are not binding on Member States. However, the implementation of all policy recommendations contained in resolutions and decisions is the responsibility of each Member State.

The WHO headquarters is located in Geneva, Switzerland; the work is divided between six world regions and implemented through regional offices, namely, Africa (Brazzaville, Congo), Americas (Washington, DC, USA, originally the Pan American Health Organization (PAHO), established in 1902), Eastern Mediterranean (Cairo, Egypt), European (Copenhagen, Denmark), Southeast Asia (Delhi, India), and Western Pacific (Manila, Philippines). Each Regional Office is primarily responsive to the country offices within that region; there are over 150 country offices in total [4].

The first surgeon to serve at WHO was Dr S William A Gunn (author), a Canadian surgeon who began the WHO global disaster care program in 1967. Dr Gunn is credited with coining the term "essential surgery" to identify those procedures that covered the basic surgical needs of most global populations. During his tenure at WHO, Dr Gunn greatly influenced his friend and third D-G, Dr Halfdan T Mahler, as to the importance of essential surgical care within the primary care framework of Alma Ata. Gunn is also recognized as significantly contributing to Mahler's oft-quoted speech *Surgery and Health for All*, given at the 1980 International College of Surgeons meeting in Mexico City [6].

The WHO Emergency and Essential Surgical Care (EESC) Programme was initiated in 2004 under the direction of Dr Meena N Cherian (author) [7]. Early accomplishments included publication of the manual *Surgical Care at the District Hospital*, followed by various publications leading to a better understanding of the importance of strengthening essential surgical and anesthesia services in district and subdistrict levels of care in low- and middle-income countries (LMICs) [8]. The WHO *Global Initiative for Emergency and Essential Surgical Care*, a global forum of multidisciplinary stakeholders, was established in 2005 for collaborations on knowledge and resources for evidence-based policies and practices to reduce the burden of death and disability through access to safe and timely surgical care and anesthesia, particularly within more vulnerable populations [9]. Furthermore, two global databases were created: WHO global database of surgical and anesthesia care service delivery at various levels of health facilities in LMICs through a combination facility and service delivery assessment tool and a WHO global database on surgical workforce. These databases have been utilized into many significant manuscripts establishing a baseline of care in many LMICs [10–12].

Additionally, key collaborative projects with various WHO programs and other UN agencies involved access to safe surgical care within a wide range of disease burdens and the development of safety checklists (including the WHO Surgical Safety Checklist, 2008), priority medical devices, essential medicines, health workforce, quality health service in universal health coverage (UHC), neglected tropical diseases, and the best practices in the care of children, women, and adults [13].

Historically, WHO has been primarily focused on the prevention, treatment, and reduction of morbidity and mortality of communicable diseases, maternal and childhood diseases, and those incurred during humanitarian emergencies and crises. Celebrated among these is the massively successful effort to entirely eradicate smallpox in 1980. However, over the past decade, the global epidemiological profile has rapidly changed to where communicable diseases are being eclipsed by noncommunicable diseases (NCDs), primarily cancer, heart and cerebrovascular diseases, diabetes, chronic respiratory illnesses, mental illness, and injuries. Current global cancer deaths of around 10 million (2018) are predicted to triple to 13 million by 2030, with 75% occurring in LMICs. This has necessitated a protracted change in WHO priorities and budgets and occasioned a major paradigm shift which is ongoing. This dramatic trend conveys a rapid and parallel increased demand for surgical care globally [14, 15].

For the first time, WHO's World Health Report 2008: Primary Health Care (Now More Than Ever) included surgical care as a critical component of the primary care hub of coordination and networking within the community to ensure comprehensive responsibility for that population [16].

Since that time, the importance of surgical care (and notably neurosurgical care) within the context of UHC has been increasingly highlighted within WHO's agenda in response to worldwide demands on how surgical care issues impact global health and place a huge strain on health systems, particularly by the urgent needs of the communities during disasters and emergencies.

## Modern History

In January 2015, the UN introduced the Sustainable Development Goals (SDGs), with expectations of at least partial fulfillment by 2030. Within Goal 3, *to ensure healthy lives and promote wellbeing for all at all ages*, includes at least four targets which will never be achieved without safe, timely, and affordable surgical care and anesthesia: SDG 3.1, reduce maternal mortality rate; SDG 3.2, reduce preventable newborn and under 5 years of age mortality; SDG 3.4, reduce by one third premature deaths from NCDs; and SDG 3.6, reduce by one half deaths and injuries from road traffic accidents (mandated to be fulfilled by 2020) [17].

Later in 2015, three timely events occurred in rapid succession: (1) the Lancet Commission on Global Surgery (LCoGS) [18]; (2) Disease Control Priorities 3rd Edition, Volume 1 Essential Surgery, which laid out the economic case for surgical care [19]; and (3) WHA resolution 68.15 on strengthening emergency and essential surgical care as a component of universal health coverage, endorsed unanimously by *every* Member State and provided the political impetus toward making this a global priority [20]. This resolution, the first specifically to focus on surgical care and anesthesia care, incorporated several specific initiatives: (1) advocacy and resource development; (2) service delivery – access to care and service integration; (3) information management – data acquisition, analysis, and ongoing monitoring; (4) essential medicines; (5) health workforce – training, credentialing, competence, and oversight; and (6) report back to the WHA on progress of the resolution in 2 years. For first time surgical indicators were included in the WHO Global Reference List of 100 Core Health Indicators, 2015 [21].

The LCoGS created immense global awareness and impact with five key messages (Table 23.1). This publication fundamentally transformed the understanding and working paradigm of global surgical care, highlighting the needs, particularly in the poorest and most vulnerable populations, of drastically improving surgical healthcare service delivery [18].

In 2018, for the first time, surgical care was mentioned in the WHO Global Programme of Work 13, the WHO stated list of agenda priorities for a 5-year interval [22].

**Table 23.1** The Lancet Commission on global surgery's five key messages [18]

| |
|---|
| 5 billion people on this planet do not have access to safe, timely and affordable surgical care and anesthesia |
| Of 313 million surgeries performed each year, only 6.5% occur in the world's poorest one third of countries; 143 million additional surgeries are needed each year above current capacity to adequately avert death and disability |
| 33 million individuals suffer catastrophic financial burden following surgical care and anesthesia, which rises to 81 million when including indirect costs |
| Investing in surgical care and anesthesia is affordable, reduces mortality, and stimulates national economic growth |
| Surgical care and anesthesia are integral components of UHC |

## Current Status

### *Partnerships with WHO Surgery*

Partnerships are critically important in global efforts to promote health, sustainability, and development. In fact, the final goal incorporated into both the UN's Millennium Development Goals and their replacement, the SDGs, is partnerships where joint action is needed: economic, technology, capacity building, trade, and system development.

Currently, there is one full-time position within the WHO EESC Programme. Considering that surgical care and anesthesia involve some aspect of virtually all other WHO departments, that roughly 30% of the global burden of disease includes surgical care, and the sheer magnitude of all global aspects this care encompasses, necessitates that WHO EESC Programme maintain strong partnerships with health ministries, professional societies, academia, and the nongovernment sectors. These critical partnerships provide not only human resources but project assistance, political influence, and much needed input on local/regional priorities and contexts.

Within WHO, there were few departments that did not connect in some manner with the EESC Programme. However, several stand out as close partners on specific projects, and practically all have some bearing on neurosurgical conditions [23]. These are summarized in Table 23.2.

**Maternal, Newborn, Child, and Adolescent Health** This large department partnered on key obstetric surgical issues, such as C-sections and obstructed labor, postpartum hemorrhage, safe abortions, obstetric fistula, and sterilization, among other topics. All aspects of children's surgery, including all subspecialty areas, regarding congenital malformations, injuries, and other common surgical conditions of childhood.

**Violence and Injury Prevention** This group had the strongest ties with surgeons through trauma surgery networks and working groups. Of particular interest were trauma systems, guidelines, checklists, and protocols. This is of critical importance to low-resource settings as poorer countries have higher injury death rates than

**Table 23.2** Summary of major WHO departments partnered with the Emergency and Essential Surgical Care (EESC) Programme. See text for details

| WHO EESC Programme major internal partners |
| --- |
| Maternal, newborn, child, and adolescent health |
| Violence and injury prevention |
| Disability and rehabilitation |
| HIV/AIDS and neglected tropical diseases |
| Noncommunicable diseases, including surgical oncology |
| Primary care, including integrated patient-centered health services |
| Health workforce |
| Health economics and health policy |

higher-income countries. Additionally, 90% of the world's fatalities occur in LMICs, even though these countries have only about half of the world's vehicles. Estimates from DCP-3 project that 68% of the burden of avertable deaths in LMICs are due to injury and could be prevented by scaling up basic surgical care delivery at the first-referral hospital.

This group, in partnership with US Centre for Disease Control and Prevention (CDC), published *Standards for the Surveillance of Neurotrauma* (1995), as well as developed the WHO Helmet Initiative.

**Disability and Rehabilitation**   Although this group is small, rehabilitation is virtually nonexistent for the majority of populations in the global south but is being increasingly viewed as a critical need, especially for recovery from injury, stroke, and surgical care. Within this group are also those working in blindness and deafness prevention, treatment, and recovery.

## HIV/AIDS and Neglected Tropical Diseases

The main topics of overlap were the following:

- HIV/AIDS: evidence has grown that male circumcision reduces the heterosexual transmission of HIV by 60%. Male circumcision is now a common procedure in much of the world and is emphasized in this preventive capacity. Surgical techniques and guidelines were developed and implemented.
- Lymphatic filariasis: within the "filariasis belt" there remain millions of individuals that suffer from the obstructive lymphedema resulting from this parasite. Clinical manifestations include elephantiasis or lymphedema of the lower extremity and lymphedema of the scrotum.
- Ebola/Marburg viral disease: with each outbreak of Ebola virus disease (EVD), surgical teams have been among those most seriously affected. One positive EVD surgical patient has been witnessed to infect up to eight members of a surgical team in which most or all die. The use of personal protective equipment cannot be overemphasized and every precaution undertaken.

**Noncommunicable Diseases** Surgical Oncology: within cancer care for solid tumors, surgical excision has been shown to contribute most to overall survival and at the lowest cost when compared with adjunctive chemotherapy or radiation. These latter two modalities are often completely unavailable in the LMICs due to out-of-pocket expenses and the lack of relevant medication or equipment.

Stroke in the developing world: this group were strong partners in global stroke work and will be discussed further below.

Surgical care of diabetic patients: although diabetes mellitus is not considered a surgical disease, the secondary manifestations frequently require surgical care. Given the large global numbers of diabetic patients, this creates overwhelming demand on surgical services.

**Primary Care** This group has official relations with *WONCA*, the *World Organization of National Colleges, Academies and Academic Associations of General Practitioners/Family Physicians.* In partnership with WONCA, surgical care models were developed within the primary care framework, attempting to conform to Alma Ata Declaration of 1978 and the more recent Declaration of Astana [24]. In rural areas of Australia, Canada, and the USA, some primary care/family medicine doctors undergo an additional specialty training for 1 year, allowing them to practice higher-level surgical, obstetric, or anesthesia care, thus greatly reducing the need for long-distance transfers for relatively routine care. Developing similar skills training into primary care/family medicine curriculum in LMICs is one method of building healthcare workforce for surgical services. Highlighted in primary care is the concept of *integrated people-centered health services.*

**Health Workforce** This department partnered to quantify the surgical, anesthesia, and obstetric workforce worldwide and placing this information on the WHO Global Health Observatory.

**Health Economics and Policy** These individuals worked to uncover out-of-pocket expenses and greatly assisted in the development of National Surgical, Obstetric, and Anesthesia Plans.

Official partnerships with WHO fall under two main categories: WHO collaborating centers (CCs) and non-state actors (NSA) in official relations with WHO [25]. WHO CCs assist WHO in particular niches of expertise and providing crucial technical guidance within those areas. Current WHO CCs on surgical and anesthesia care include:

1. Ulaanbaatar, Mongolia: National Health Sciences University of Mongolia, Department of Surgery, expertise in distance learning and quality initiatives
2. Ontario, Canada: University of Western Ontario (Western University), Department of Anesthesia's *M*edical *E*vidence, *D*ecision *I*ntegrity, *C*linical *I*mpact (MEDICI) Center, expertise in perioperative care and outcomes
3. Mumbai, India: Bhabha Atomic Research Center (BARC) Hospital, Surgical Services, expertise in access to surgical oncology service delivery in remote areas

4. Lund, Sweden: Lund University, Department of Paediatrics (Surgery), expertise in global surgical workforce data collection and evaluation

5. Boston, MA, USA: Harvard University, Program in Global Surgery and Social Change, expertise in national surgical health policy, implementation, and outcomes; and 6. Bogotá, Colombia, Universidad El Bosque, expertise in traumatic brain injury.

Non-state actors in official relations with WHO are nongovernmental organizations that allow a certain number of individuals in that organization access to the WHA and EB meetings [25]. These individuals may make comments on the floor of the assembly in support or against legislation that is under discussion but cannot vote. It also allows access to key individuals that may be able to assist the NSA in their worldwide endeavors, through influence, politics, or resource development. Examples of NSA supported by WHO EESC (with headquarters):

1. World Federation of Neurosurgical Societies (WFNS) (Nyon, Switzerland)
2. World Federation of Societies of Anesthesiologists (London, UK)
3. International Society of Orthopaedic Surgery and Traumatology (SICOT) (Brussels, Belgium)
4. International Federation of Surgical Colleges (London, UK)
5. International College of Surgeons (Chicago, IL, USA)

Lastly, professional societies were strong partners worldwide. Each region has surgical societies that were deeply involved with professional advancement, credentialing, training programs, and quality initiatives. While not with specific official relations with WHO, these organizations contributed greatly to the WHO EESC Programme, especially through north-south collaborative efforts, such as twinning programs and training exercises. Examples of these organizations include the American Association of Neurological Surgeons, College of Surgeons of East, Central and Southern Africa, Pan-African Association of Neurosurgical Societies, and The Foundation for International Education in Neurological Surgery.

Most recent accomplishments of the WHO EESC Programme include completion of:

1. WHO Global Guidelines for the Prevention of Transmission of Ebola or Marburg Virus During Surgery and Invasive Procedures, with a decision-making algorithm to advise policy and all personnel involved with any procedures (awaiting final approval)
2. WHO surgical approaches to the urogenital manifestations of lymphatic filariasis: report from an informal consultation among experts [26]
3. Optimal Resources for Children's Surgery [27]
4. World Health Organization World Federation of Societies of Anesthesiologists (WHO-WFSA) International Standards for a Safe Practice of Anesthesia [28]
5. WHO Guideline on Voluntary Medical Male Circumcision for HIV Prevention [29]
6. WHO consultation to define priority medical devices for cardiovascular disease, diabetes and stroke management targeting low- and middle-income settings [30]

## WHO and Neurosurgery

The overwhelming neurosurgical issues at WHO are traumatic brain and spine injuries and stroke. Traumatic Brain Injury (TBI) is among the most lethal injury in every country on the globe. Many of these injuries are low-velocity injuries that could be easily and successfully treated with excellent outcomes if there were capable local healthcare facilities and trained neurosurgical workforce. Most frequently, however, facilities are long distances away, transportation is limited, imaging is unavailable, out-of-pocket expenses high, and neurosurgeons are nonexistent, not to mention lack of integrated health services, ICUs, and ventilators. These necessities of basic neurosurgical care can also be applied to all other uniquely neurosurgical pathologies, such as hydrocephalus, tumors, degenerative spine disorders, and children's neurosurgery.

WHO has long been involved in reducing the global injuries through programs and publications such as WHO Helmet Initiative, Trauma Checklist, Standards for Surveillance in Neurotrauma, Guidelines for Essential Trauma Care, and Strengthening Care for the Injured, among many others [31].

Several aspects of neurosurgical care are included within the scope of WHO's mandates of work. However, building a service delivery platform that can deliver over several diagnoses and specialties is preferable and more sustainable than working within the silos of a single diagnosis or a single entity such as surgery. Building healthcare system capacity is predicated on several factors, which will be highlighted individually.

Stroke is rapidly becoming one of the most common causes of death, particularly in LMICs. The current available data shows that 75% strokes occur in LMICs and that 87% of the burden of disability and death is borne by LMICs. In LMICs, stroke incidence has more than doubled in the past four decades while being reduced by 42% in high-income countries. On average, strokes in LMICs occur 15 years of age younger, generally at times ages of peak productivity. Furthermore, there is a higher incidence of hemorrhage, at least 34% in LMICs vs 9% in the USA. Stroke is now one of top three causes of death in almost every country, a glaring reality that primary prevention has failed. In LMICs there is largely no rehabilitation to successfully reintegrate patients back into daily life. Stroke also creates economic catastrophe for individual and families, as well as having a huge impact on a country's socioeconomic development. As stroke is no respecter of rank or person, stroke can have a devastating toll on leadership within institutions and create political instability [32].

### Children's Neurosurgery

The unique challenges of operating on children are several, including (1) higher risks due to smaller body size and blood volume, (2) distinctive pathologies (congenital malformations, etc.), (3) children inability to afford surgery, and (4) in democratic societies children do not vote and therefore remain a "silent" population. For these reasons (and likely others), surgeons not specifically trained in pediatric surgical specialties are often reluctant to operate on children. However, in sub-Saharan

Africa (SSA), currently on average, 43% of the populations are under the age of 15; in many of these countries the numbers approach 50% or higher. Children are a highly vulnerable population for surgical issues, particularly injuries such as road traffic accidents as passengers or pedestrians, burns, falls, drownings, or violence. It is estimated that 85% of children require some type of surgical intervention by the age of 15 years; thus the gap in surgical care delivery to this population is enormous.

Pediatric neurosurgery is massively engulfed within the vortex of this trend. In many countries, there are no trained pediatric neurosurgeons (PNS); in SSA, the average in LICs is 1 PNS/30 million population, with a global need for approximately 4680 additional PNSs [33].

## Health Facilities

In many countries, local, first-level hospitals may lack 24-h electricity and running water. Furthermore, these facilities are most often staffed by young non-specialist doctors that have only completed an internship and are not in these remote areas by choice; without adequate backup or experience, many are reluctant to be very bold in their treatments. Referral hospitals are some distant away, and transportation is unavailable or too costly for almost all patients. Typically, these hospitals do not provide food or laundry services to patients in attempts at reducing costs, and family members are counted on to provide some basic-level bedside care for the patient.

Access to even basic healthcare is often lacking due to lack of local facilities and services, paucity of skilled healthcare providers, high out-of-pocket expenses, and/ or lack of trust in the local hospital.

## Health Systems

Integrated health systems that cover the majority of populations are often lacking in LMICs. First-level referral hospitals (district hospitals) frequently do not have the trust of the local population so many patients opt first to seek care at the tertiary care hospitals, creating severe backlog in cases and dramatic delays in care. If a patient is seen at a district or regional hospital, but requires advanced level surgical care, timely access to higher levels of care is problematic due to costs, case backlog, and lack of transportation. Integrated care for cancer, cardiac, and cerebrovascular events (among many others) are problematic in both preoperative and postoperative care, including rehabilitation.

## Medical Equipment

Imaging capabilities are sparse and generally unaffordable. Recent evidence shows that there are, on average, 0.32 CT scanners per 1 million population in LIC as compared with 42 CT scanners per 1 million in high-income countries (HIC). Disparity is apparent in that MRI/CT scanners per million population in HICs such as Japan 55/111, US 38/17, and Switzerland 23/14 (2019). In low-income countries, MRI/CT scanners per million population range from 0.04/0.63 to 0/0. In these areas, sonography is becoming the imaging modality of choice due to low cost of purchase and relative low maintenance requirements [34].

Intraoperative and postoperative monitoring are a major issue globally. Disparity in monitoring devices translates directly to higher mortality and morbidity rates [35]. Pulse oximetry is a significance advance as it is becoming standard of care worldwide [25].

Neurosurgical operative equipment, such as drills, instruments, and microscopes, are severely lacking in LMICs and can hamper those trained neurosurgeons in their surgical capacity [36].

## Essential Medicines

Every 2 years since its origin in 1977, WHO updates a Model List of Essential Medicines; current versions are the 21st WHO Essential Medicines List and the 7th WHO Essential Medicines List for Children updated in June 2019. The current volume includes an additional 28 drugs for adults and 23 for children as either core or complementary drugs, with the removal of 9 drugs. Additionally, indications and formulations for listed drugs are updated. These updates are based on the recommendations of the relevant expert committee. Of importance to neurosurgeons, in this volume includes the addition of Alteplase for thrombolytic therapy [37].

Worldwide, there is an enormous lack of availability of antiepileptic medications, antibiotics, adjuvant therapy for cancer, thrombolytic therapy, and adequate analgesia. Much of this is due to poverty but also to counterfeit drugs, inefficient supply chains, and fraud.

## Health Workforce/Training Programs

The global neurosurgical workforce is very limited in LMICs. Estimates for unmet neurosurgical capacity worldwide are that more than 23,000 additional neurosurgeons are needed to provide more than 5 million essential neurosurgical cases occurring in low- and middle-income countries, particularly in Africa and Southeast Asia. Academic, university-based, primarily north-south twinning programs (dyads) aimed at improving knowledge transfer between providers and institutions are becoming more common, as are residency and fellowship programs within LMICs and those offered by WFNS. Concerns regarding finished trainees immigrating to high-income countries remains, for the most part, unfounded, as those training in LMICs tend to stay where they trained or return to their home country [36].

## Catastrophic Expenditures

Out-of-pocket expenses cause massive amounts of catastrophic financial situations for millions each year. From the LCoGS, estimates point to 36 million individuals experiencing catastrophic health expenditures due to surgical care and anesthesia, with this number increasing to 81 million if indirect costs are included, such as food and travel, lost wages, etc. [18]. In many countries, any discussion of surgery will include a list of supplies which is given to the family to purchase prior to surgery: items such as gloves, antibiotics, dressings, anesthetics and analgesics, and even surgical hardware. This is due to these supplies simply being unavailable at the hospital. Frequently, this necessitates purchase on the black market.

## National Health Policy

The LCoGS first suggested the incorporation of National Surgical, Obstetric, and Anesthesia Plans (NSOAP) as an embedded component of each country's national health policy, strategy, or plan, to address capacity building of surgical care service delivery platforms. Without a formal policy, strategy, or plan, governments are ill-equipped to improve healthcare, as they are left without a suitable roadmap and political impetus for these changes.

The NSOAP pillars include (1) service delivery; (2) infrastructure, products, and technology; (3) health workforce; (4) information management; (5) finances; and (6) governance and leadership. Although each pillar is rather broad, each NSOAP attempts to define this in more focused terms based on local contexts, so that each NSOAP is specifically tailored to that Member State's priorities and resources. It is also highly dependent on local champions.

Several NSOAPs have been developed at country level, and planning workshops on NSOAP development have been carried out. However, implementation is an even greater challenge than developing an NSOAP, even with appropriate government commitments and resources. This process is ongoing in several Member States. Along with strong partnerships, WHO has been actively involved in this process [38, 39].

## *Future Opportunities/Unmet Needs*

Given the increasing emphasis on and the demand for surgical services within national governments, WHO, and the WHO regional offices, there are opportunities to develop surgical healthcare policies, develop significantly more training opportunities, and strengthen healthcare systems, including adequate infrastructure, information management, financing, governance, and partnerships.

There is especially increasing interest in forming north-south or south-south partnerships (dyads) between academic programs for both technical skills training and for research opportunities. While current trends are rightly demanding decolonization reforms for all global health work, the demand exists for forming partnerships that value equity, cultural humility, and protect the two-way dynamic that should exist in these scenarios (among other issues) [40–42].

The constant challenge at WHO is chronic and persistent underfunding. The annual base budget of WHO is less than many US state's Departments of Health budget and is approximately one-fourth of the annual base budget of the US CDC [43, 44]. This lack of sufficient funding dramatically reduces the effectiveness of WHO technical programs and limits the effective of in-country work that is necessary to achieve WHO's stated global health mandates [3].

Further challenges to neurosurgical care specifically remain the ongoing challenges of access to safe, timely, and affordable care for much of the world's populations and the development of an adequate, skilled, and available neurosurgical workforce. One stated goal of WHO under the leadership of the current D-G, Dr Tedros Adhanom Ghebreyesus, has been bringing 1 billion individuals under the umbrella of UHC, which includes the provisions for financial risk protection for all patients, including surgical patients and their families [45].

Finally, there are many issues related to WHO that are uniquely challenging. It is a political organization that delivers technical products; sadly, at times, technical output is heavily influenced by political forces. Also, any WHO recommendations are simply that, as WHO has no facility for enforcement, either of policy or Member State pledged contributions.

However, given the significant challenges, even failures of WHO at times, there are also overwhelming successes. Retaining a global health body that convenes all Member States, fulfills its stated core functions, and provides global leadership during health crises is critical to promoting and ensuring global health. No other body or Member State is capable of providing this coordinated leadership and commands global respect; no other body will bring together all 194 ministers of health into an international forum to set global health priorities and agendas. With the few exceptions of some high-income Member States, most LMICs look to WHO specifically for those core functions and rely on WHO at all levels of the organization, but particularly the country office, which is viewed as an essential ally of the local health ministry. WHO provides critical and essential resources for global health, and this world would be far less healthy or stable without it.

# References

1. https://www.un.org/un70/en/content/history/index.html. Accessed 25 Aug 2020.
2. McCarthy M. A brief history of the WHO. Lancet. 2002;360:1111–2. https://doi.org/10.1016/S0140-6736(02)11244-X.

3. https://www.who.int/about/what-we-do. Accessed 20 Sept 2020.
4. www.who.int/about. Accessed 28 Sept 2020.
5. https://apps.who.int/gb/bd/pdf_files/BD_49th-en.pdf#page=179. Accessed 7 Oct 2020.
6. https://www.who.int/surgery/strategies/Mahler1980speech.pdf?ua=1. Accessed 20 Sept 2020.
7. https://who.int/surgery. Accessed 20 Sept 2020.
8. https://www.who.int/surgery/publications/en/SCDH.pdf?ua=1. Accessed 28 Sept 2020.
9. https://www.who.int/surgery/globalinitiative/en/. Accessed 28 Sept 2020.
10. https://who.int/publications/en. Accessed 28 Sept 2020.
11. O'Neill KM, Greenberg SLM, Cherian MN, Gillies RD, Daniels KM, Roy N, et al. Bellwether procedures for monitoring and planning essential surgical care in low- and middle-income countries: caesarean delivery, laparotomy, and treatment of open fractures. World J Surg. 2016;40:2611–9. https://doi.org/10.1007/s00268-016-3614-y.
12. Spiegel DA, Droti B, Relan P, Hobson S, Cherian MN, O'Neill KM. Retrospective review of surgical availability and readiness in 8 African countries. BMJ Open. 2017;7:e014496.
13. https://www.who.int/patientsafety/topics/safe-surgery/checklist/en/
14. https://gco.iarc.fr/today/home. Accessed 25 Sept 2020.
15. Bennett JE, Stevens GA, Mathers CD, Bonita R, Rehm J, Kruk ME, Riley LM, Dain K, Kengne AP, Chalkidou K, Beagley J. NCD Countdown 2030: worldwide trends in non-communicable disease mortality and progress towards Sustainable Development Goal target 3.4. Lancet. 392(10152):1072–88. https://doi.org/10.1016/S0140-6736(18)31992-5.
16. https://www.who.int/whr/2008/en/. Accessed 25 Sept 2020.
17. https://sdgs.un.org/goals. Accessed 25 Sept 2020.
18. https://www.lancetglobalsurgery.org/. Accessed 25 Sept 2020.
19. http://dcp-3.org/surgery. Accessed 25 Sept 2020.
20. https://apps.who.int/gb/ebwha/pdf_files/WHA68/A68_R15-en.pdf?ua=1.        Accessed        28 Sept 2020.
21. https://www.who.int/healthinfo/indicators/2015/en/. Accessed 14 Aug 2020.
22. https://www.who.int/publications/m/item/thirteenth-general-programme-of-work-(gpw13)-methods-for-impact-measurement. Accessed 25 Sept 2020.
23. https://www.who.int/. (Look under health topics for specific programs). Accessed 25 Sept 2020.
24. Declaration of Astana: WHO global conference on primary health care. 25–26 October 2018, Astana, Kazakhstan. https://www.who.int/docs/default-source/primary-health/declaration/gcphc-declaration.pdf
25. https://www.who.int/surgery/collaborations/en/. Accessed 25 Sept 2020.
26. WHO. Surgical approaches to the urogenital manifestations of lymphatic filariasis. Geneva: World Health Organization; 2019. https://www.who.int/publications/i/item/WHO-CDS-NTD-PCT-2019.04. Accessed 25 Sept 2020.
27. Global Initiative for Children's Surgery. Optimal resources for children's surgical care: executive summary. World J Surg. 2019;43(4):978–80. https://doi.org/10.1007/s00268-018-04888-7.
28. Gelb AW, Morriss WW, Johnson WD, Merry AF. World health organization-world federation of societies of anaesthesiologists (WHO-WFSA) international standards for a safe practice of anesthesia. Can J Anesth. 2018;65:698–708. https://doi.org/10.1007/s12630-018-1111-5.
29. https://www.who.int/publications/i/item/978-92-4-000854-0. Accessed 25 Sept 2020.
30. https://www.who.int/medical_devices/priority/cvds/en/. Accessed 25 Sept 2020.
31. https://www.who.int/health-topics/emergency-care#tab=tab_1. These materials may be accessed and downloaded at this site. Accessed 7 Oct 2020.
32. Johnson WD, Onuma O, Owolabi M, Sachdev S. Stroke: a global response is needed. Bull World Health Organ. 2016;94:634 634A. https://doi.org/10.2471/BLT.16.181636.
33. Dewan MC, Baticulon RE, Rattani A, Johnston JM, Warf BC, Harkness W. Pediatric neurosurgical workforce, access to care, equipment and training needs worldwide. Neurosurg Focus. 2018;45(4):E13. https://doi.org/10.3171/2018.7.FOCUS18272.

34. Medical equipment data per country; WHO global health observatory. https://apps.who.int/gho/data/view.main.302010. Accessed 30 Aug 2020.
35. Biccard BM, Madiba TE, Kluyts H-L, Munlemvo DM, Madzimbamuto FD, Basenero A, et al. Perioperative patient outcomes in the African surgical outcomes study: a 7-day prospective observational cohort study. Lancet. 2018;391(10130):1589–98. https://doi.org/10.1016/S0140-6736(18)30001-1.
36. Dewan MC, Rattani A, Fieggen G, Arraez MA, Servadei F, Boop FA, Johnson WD, et al. Global neurosurgery: the current capacity and deficit in the provision of essential neurosurgical care. Executive Summary of the Global Neurosurgery Initiative at the Program in Global Surgery and Social Change. J Neurosurg. 2019;130:1055–64. https://doi.org/10.3171/2017.11.JNS171500.
37. https://www.who.int/medicines/publications/essentialmedicines/en/. Accessed 25 Sept 2020.
38. WHO. Surgical care system strengthening: developing national surgical, obstetric and anaesthesia plans. Geneva: World Health Organization; 2017. https://apps.who.int/iris/bitstream/handle/10665/255566/9789241512244-eng.pdf;jsessionid=14B57D35088746C5CD303ECF818964A7?sequence=1
39. UNITAR. National surgical, obstetric and anaesthesia planning. Geneva: United Nations Institute for Training and Research (UNITAR); 2020. https://www.globalsurgeryfoundation.org/nsoap-manual
40. Büyüm AM, Kenney C, Koris A, et al. Decolonising global health: if not now, when? BMJ Glob Health. 2020;5:e003394. https://doi.org/10.1136/bmjgh-2020-003394.
41. Affun-Adegbulu C, Adegbulu O. Decolonising global (public) health: from Western universalism to global pluriversalities. BMJ Glob Health. 2020;5:e002947. https://doi.org/10.1136/bmjgh-2020-002947.
42. Scheiner A, Rickard JL, Nwomeh B, Jawa RS, Ginzburg E, Fitzgerald TN, Charles A, Bekele A. Global surgery ProeCon debate: a pathway to bilateral academic success or the bold new face of colonialism? J Surg Res. 2020;252:272–80. https://doi.org/10.1016/j.jss.2020.01.032.
43. https://www.cdc.gov/budget/documents/fy2020/fy-2020-detail-table.pdf. Accessed 7 Oct 2020.
44. https://www.who.int/about/finances-accountability/budget/WHOPB-PRP-19.pdf?ua=1. Page 22. Accessed 7 Oct 2020.
45. https://www.who.int/data/stories/the-triple-billion-targets-a-visual-summary-of-methods-to-deliver-impact. Accessed 8 Oct 2020.

# Chapter 24
# The Impact of the COVID-19 Pandemic on Neurosurgery Worldwide

**Aristotelis Kalyvas, Mark Bernstein, Ronnie E. Baticulon, Marike L. D. Broekman, and Faith C. Robertson**

## COVID-19 Impact on Clinical Neurosurgery

The advent of COVID-19 is dramatically changing how the world practices medicine. An abundance of patients requiring hospitalization for acute respiratory management has strained the healthcare system, forcing all specialties, including neurosurgery, to combat an unprecedented shift in patient prioritization, operative risk management, workforce redistribution, and financial challenges.

A. Kalyvas · M. Bernstein
Division of Neurosurgery, Toronto Western Hospital, University of Toronto, Toronto, ON, Canada

R. E. Baticulon
Division of Neurosurgery, University of the Philippines – Philippine General Hospital, Manila, Philippines

M. L. D. Broekman
Department of Neurosurgery, Leiden University Medical Center, Leiden, The Netherlands

Department of Neurosurgery, Haaglanden Medical Center, The Hague, The Netherlands

F. C. Robertson (✉)
Department of Neurosurgery, Leiden University Medical Center, Leiden, The Netherlands

Department of Neurosurgery, Massachusetts General Hospital and Harvard Medical School, Boston, MA, USA
e-mail: frobertson@partners.org

© The Author(s), under exclusive license to Springer Nature Switzerland AG 2022
I. M. Germano (ed.), *Neurosurgery and Global Health*,
https://doi.org/10.1007/978-3-030-86656-3_24

## *Prioritization*

At the pandemic's onset, hospitals around the globe mobilized strategic plans to reduce non-COVID-related care in order to preserve resources for those with infection and to flatten the curve by decreasing contagion within the hospital [1–4]. The surge of COVID-related acute respiratory distress syndrome and consequent need for mechanical ventilation made hospital ventilator capacity a critical resource. Given that operative interventions account for the majority of ventilator use within the hospital, there were concerted efforts to reduce surgical volume. Consequently, the neurosurgical community strived to establish important principles and guidelines for prioritization of neurosurgical operations [5, 6]. These discussions incorporated ethics, biology, health systems, and lessons learned from previous epidemics like SARS [7]. The foundational question to be answered was if surgery could be deferred without significant neurological deterioration or disease progression [5]. As elective operative time was restricted, hospital committees became responsible for transparent decision-making processes regarding operative urgency, accounting for factors such as disease pathology, patient symptomatology, and the possibility of an equally effective alternative treatment. Under normal circumstances, physician rationale for treatment approach typically follows Kantian or deontological ethical theory, which favors the best possible treatment for the individual patient, regardless of the ramifications to others. However, utilitarianism or consequentialist ethical theory, which centers on treatment of many as opposed to individuals, often dictates medical practice in global health crises like the current pandemic [5, 8].

During 2020, life-threatening conditions deemed to be neurosurgical emergencies proceeded as usual across neurosurgical departments [9–11]. This included cerebral hemorrhages (epidural, subdural, subarachnoid, and intraparenchymal), acute hydrocephalus, spinal cord compression with neurological deficit, and cranial and spinal trauma emergencies. The timing of surgical management of other less urgent conditions varied. According to a recent US-based survey of leaders of 40 large academic neurosurgical programs, 62% had cancelled all nonurgent cases, 80% of respondents still preferred operating within 1–2 weeks for newly diagnosed high-grade gliomas, whereas for presumed low-grade gliomas, half of respondents monitored patients with imaging and symptoms [12]. Groups from Italy (Lombardy) [8] and the USA (New York and Detroit) [16] attempted to categorize common procedures and pathologies by urgency to facilitate clinical decisions. The Italian group classified oncological procedures in three categories: Class A++ comprised intracranial or spinal tumors that require emergency treatment (severe intracranial hypertension with declining level of consciousness, acute hydrocephalus, spinal cord compression with evolving quadri or paraparesis); Class A+ comprised tumors that need treatment within 1 week (intracranial tumors exerting mass effect with progressive neurological deficit, without declining level of consciousness); and Class A comprised conditions needing treatment within a month (tumors with imaging suspicion of malignancy) [11]. An American group prioritized the relative urgency of 86 common neurosurgical scenarios from every subspecialty into 6 tiers and respective time frames, after a consensus that was achieved among 22 neurosurgeons (14 from the New York and 8 from the Detroit metropolitan areas) using the Delphi method [13]. As more time passed, the European Association of Neurosurgical Societies put forth a unified guideline for triaging, which offered a three-tiered triaging approach but importantly noted that different countries and regions would be facing conditions that may differ greatly from one another and from day to day. Thus, they advocated for assessments using contemporary knowledge of the evolving local, regional, and national conditions, which could result in significant differences in decision-making between regions [14].

As intended, hospital prioritization of COVID management and emergency cases translated to dramatic decreases in neurosurgical case volume. For instance, at the Toronto Western Hospital, neurosurgical cases decreased from 230 in January 2020 to 146 in March and 57 in April 2020, a reduction of 36% and 75%, respectively. The subspecialties most affected were functional and spine with 80% and 73% reduction, respectively, while oncology and vascular experienced fewer cancellations, 50% and 40%, respectively. Triage schema for University of Toronto are presented in Fig. 24.1 [16]. Analogous case reduction was described in other large

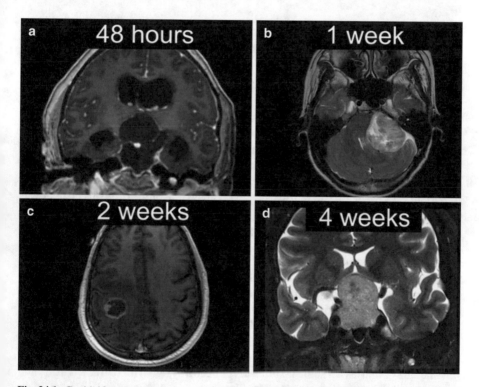

**Fig. 24.1** Covid-19 neurosurgery case triage schema at the University of Toronto. Here, classified according to the prioritization scheme published by Thomas et al. [13]. (**a**) Tier 2, intra-axial tumor with neurological decline; treatment within 48 h. (**b**) Tier 3, cerebellopontine angle tumor with hydro and/or brainstem compression; treatment within 1 week. (**c**) Tier 4, intra-axial tumor without shift; treatment within 2 weeks. (**d**) Tier 5, transsphenoidal approach for skull base lesion with optic compression; treatment within 4 weeks

North American and European institutes [6–8]. While nonurgent case cancellation produced an intentional decrease in case volume, there were significant reductions in the number of patients seeking neurosurgical care in the emergency department, noted by University of Toronto as well as Mass General Hospital [11, 12]. Furthermore, there have been significant global increases in delayed neurosurgical admissions during lockdowns and quarantine periods, as noted in Morocco [15]. Comparable declines occurred in in-person clinic visits across most neurosurgery departments [7, 10]. This is suspected to result from fear of seeking care given risk of inoculation onsite at the hospital. In contrast, telephone consultations and video clinic visits gradually increased in number to cover patient care needs, discussed further below [7]. Overall, prioritization during the pandemic forced neurosurgeons to delay nonurgent and some urgent cases with hopes that it would help optimize care delivery for COVID patients and reduce the risk of contagion in the hospital. After the first wave of the virus passed, it has left a backlog of cases to address, but a newfound appreciation for the possibility and ease of telehealth, which will likely remain a core component of care going forward.

## Preoperative Measures and Transformation of the OR

In addition to intentional decreasing of surgeries, the workflow and perioperative systems also had to transform to apply measures aiming to mitigate the perioperative spread of COVID-19 [16]. Once testing was more readily available, institutional policies began dictating that all patients undergoing surgery had to be tested for COVID-19 preoperatively. However, other institutions suggested that preoperative COVID-19 testing of asymptomatic patients should be examined according the local epidemiology and availability of testing resources [17]. This was particularly important for low-income countries; however, given that at the time this chapter was written 17.9% of infected individuals were believed to be asymptomatic carriers [18], testing everyone if feasible could potentially decrease the spread.

The use of full personal protective equipment (PPE), such as N95 masks, gowns, and gloves, by every health worker involved in neurosurgical operations was deemed mandatory at many institutions, due to the aerosol-generating potential of most neurosurgical operations (e.g., drilling; access to paranasal sinuses). Other groups have suggested that for low-risk patients (tested negative and asymptomatic with no recent travel history or contact with COVID positive patient), surgical masks and droplet precautions should suffice [16]. Having a risk-stratified PPE approach could safeguard PPE reserve in the context of worldwide shortages and particularly for low-income countries. In some institutions or health systems there were "clean" and "contaminated" patient pathways. In Toronto, specific operating rooms were reserved for confirmed or suspicious COVID-19 patients, ideally with negative pressure ventilation. Additionally, different nursing teams were assigned outside the room for circulating and providing equipment as needed. They believed the number of OR personnel and movement of personnel in and out of the OR should be kept at minimum. Paper charts were kept outside the OR, and monitors/machines were covered in plastic wrap. A rigorous decontamination after COVID-19 cases was also essential [16]. At Massachusetts General Hospital, all procedural consents became verbal as opposed to written to avoid cross-contamination with pen and paper handling. In Switzerland, Morocco, and other nations, certain buildings were designated as "green zones" to allow for COVID-negative patient and provider care to resume [15]. For each of these approaches, rigorous traffic control and attention to infection status were required.

## Intraoperative Considerations in Neurosurgery

Modifications of operative practice also took place in order to moderate the effect of high-risk settings encountered in the neurosurgical OR. Local anesthesia or conscious sedation was increasingly preferred to general anesthesia, when feasible, in order to avoid endotracheal intubation and extubation to limit aerosolization. Awake fiberoptic intubation was avoided when possible. All nonessential staff were often asked to exit the room during intubation and extubation [19]. At some institutions, ORs were also closed to entry for 30 min after intubation and extubation to allow for aerosolized particles to clear.

Operations implicating the respiratory tract, due to the high viral load [20], carry significant risk of transmission. In neurosurgery, such procedures include endoscopic endonasal, transoral, and translabyrinthine approaches, as well as any craniotomy transgressing the frontal sinuses. Equally effective and safe alternative approaches (e.g., pterional instead of endoscopic endonasal; retrosigmoid instead of translabyrinthine) could be favored, or the surgery could be deferred to a later time, when feasible.

A hypothetical and controversial risk in neurosurgery is the airborne transmission of COVID-19 following the use of aerosol-generating instruments such as drills, monopolar cautery, lasers, and ultrasonic aspirators [17]. However, the infectious potential of aerosolized particles is based on the hypothesis that they include virions. Although this is proven for the respiratory and digestive tracts [20], this is no longer believed to be the case for cerebrospinal fluid, central nervous system (CNS) tissue, or bone. As such, the recommendation to avoid or restrict the utilization of the aforementioned instruments was deemed unnecessary by many [17].

## Redeployment

As the influx of COVID-19 patients rose at each institution, hospital personnel had to adapt to a new reality, and trainees and staff from both medical and surgical specialties worldwide had to be redeployed [9]. The reassignment of staff is a common, often temporary, response to expand coverage in a crisis. With COVID-19, not only was there potential for discomfort from working in a foreign role but also susceptibility to and fear of infection. In such challenging times, strategic health systems approaches can facilitate timely access to safe and affordable care and provide reassurance that there is an element of control.

Task shifting and task sharing are workforce strategies that involve duty redistribution [21]. Task shifting is transference of clinical autonomy from highly qualified healthcare workers to those with shorter training and fewer qualifications. In contrast, task sharing uses tiered staffing models with collaborative teams of specialists and less qualified groups who share clinical responsibility and rely on iterative communication and training to preserve high-quality outcome. Ideally, hospitals requiring redeployment of workers would use a task sharing approach that invokes a three-phase model of training, practice, and maintenance (Fig. 24.2) [22, 23]. A principal step in task reassignment is strategic identification of providers and redistributing in a manner that minimizes "things to be learned" in order to satisfy the "job to be done." Once assigned, individuals should have a dedicated preparation period and ideally a competency-based evaluation of readiness. Subsequently, the practice phase should involve team-based care with tiered oversight to ensure individuals know who and when to ask for guidance when appropriate. Many neurosurgery residents were redeployed to work in COVID intensive care units, and responsibilities ranged from assisting medical teams as a responding clinician to facilitating procedures such as central lines and prone positioning. Others filled shifts in testing clinics, and some were redeployed to work on medicine triage floors or in the emergency ward. In institutions with a lower demand for workforce distribution, plans for redeployment were developed but were not required. Still, many residents took on new roles within their teams. Many hospitals developed systems in which neurosurgical non-COVID-19 patients in the wards and intensive care unit

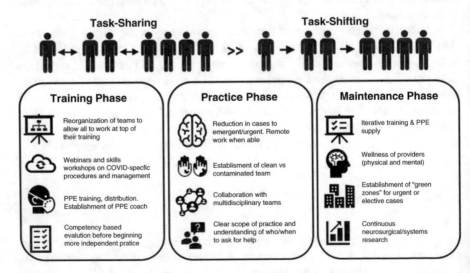

**Fig. 24.2** A strategic plan for task sharing during the COVID-19 pandemic. (Previously published by Robertson et al. [22])

(ICU) were managed with two available teams – one working in hospital and one working from home. Where redeployment plans were not enacted, hospitals have been encouraged to adequately train personnel in case of a second surge of COVID-19.

## The Rise in Telehealth for Outpatient Assessment and Postoperative Follow-Up

While digital or telehealth services existed prior to the pandemic, uptake and integration into regular clinical practice had been slow, predominantly due to learning curves, lower demand, and barriers in financial reimbursement [24]. However, the need to deliver care while reducing the use of PPE and risk of viral transmission with personal contact served as a catalyst for the exponential increases in telehealth. Benefits for the patients include less cost and time of commuting, and no need for missing work, while it can help neurosurgeons optimize their schedules [25]. A recent systematic review of 52 neurosurgical studies (25 prospective and 27 retrospective; 13 in the USA, 39 in other countries) with 45,801 patients demonstrated that 99.6% of visits were completed successfully [26]. Of the 0.4% of visits that required subsequent appointments, 81.5% were due to technology failure, and 18.5% required further face-to-face evaluation or treatment. Regarding reimbursement, 94.3% of telemedicine visits were billed using face-to-face procedural codes. Overall, both patients and providers have seemed to enjoy this transition. In a study of 596 neurosurgical patients who had telehealth visits at Michigan State University, patients reported high satisfaction with the experience, providing an average rating of 6.32 ± 1.27 out of 7 [27]. Furthermore, telehealth visits have the potential to be financially advantageous for patients. A study from Mayo Clinic on video telemedicine rather than face-to-face clinic visits for postoperative follow-up showed that patients saved an average of $888 per visit [28]. In-hospital telehealth options are also being explored. In Kuala Lumpur, Malaysia, virtual and physical ward rounds on neurocritical patients were conducted using smart glasses for an individual to broadcast rounds to the team for 103 neurocritical care patients with high overall inter-rater reliability [29].

More importantly, the potential of digital health for system improvement greatly exceeds video phone calls, and COVID-19 emphasizes the need to invest in this arena. Wearables and digital phenotyping can facilitate both active and passive data collection for remote screening and monitoring of early symptoms to indicate when a patient may need to seek higher levels of care. This technology has already been tested in neurosurgical populations, such as monitoring for physical activity rates and pain control with postoperative spine patients [30]. As such technology becomes more prevalent in home monitoring for COVID symptoms, we as a neurosurgical community should continue exploring remote management of our patients as well and advocate for appropriate reimbursement for these efforts that account for the value added to patient care.

## *Future Directions: Lessons Learned*

At the present time, healthcare protocols and national quarantine regulations have enabled countries around the globe to flatten the curve and begin resuming clinical neurosurgery activity. The next steps of health policy will focus on dealing with the backlog of the cancelled neurosurgical cases while maintaining a level of responsiveness in case of a new COVID-19 surge. The strategy should first accomplish the return to "normal" neurosurgical practice with the overarching goal of reaching full capacity. Some possible solutions would be to extend everyday operative hours and running elective ORs during weekends. Resources should be appropriately allocated – additional OR and ICU nurses should be employed, and additional ICU beds should be created. These measures put a financial strain on health systems, especially in low-income countries; however, they can help boost surgical capacity as well as create a well-prepared system for a future COVID-19 outbreak. Additionally, widespread application of telemedicine is essential to reduce viral exposure. The achieved improvements in digital health infrastructure and platforms can facilitate more timely and cost-effective outpatient care that enhances value, particularly for the patient. Even if we return to a COVID-free planet, these modes of practice will likely persist.

## COVID-19 Impact on Neurosurgery Education and Training

Similar to other medical and surgical specialties, the consequences of the COVID-19 pandemic on neurosurgery education and training cannot be understated. The experiences of the neurosurgery residents, registrars, and fellows during the acute phase of the pandemic have spurred multiple opinion pieces, letters to the editor, and survey studies conducted around the world [31–35]. Although the structure of the neurosurgery training programs varies significantly among different countries and regions, almost all neurosurgery departments have uniformly reported loss of training opportunities for young neurosurgeons. In a short span of time, adjustments had to be made in order to sustain neurosurgery education while ensuring trainee safety under challenging circumstances.

## *Loss of Training Opportunities*

The foremost concern was the significant decrease in the operative experiences of neurosurgery trainees. This was primarily due to the cancellation or postponement of elective procedures in most, if not all, neurosurgical centers, as described above. Several other factors contributed to the steep decline in surgeon logs. For instance, in Singapore and the UK, a senior surgeon was assigned to perform procedures that would have ordinarily been given to a junior trainee [36, 37]. Doing so reduced the number of people inside the operating room to limit virus exposure risk but also minimized operating time and presumably lowered the risk of perioperative complications during a period when hospital resources such as ICU beds and mechanical ventilators were being conserved for COVID-19 services. Thus, it was more challenging for trainees to gain autonomy and practice skills that were at or above their level.

There had also been a reported decline in neurosurgery consults. In the case of neurotrauma, this had been attributed to restricted mobility from mandated lockdowns and quarantines. In developing countries, limited transportation had hampered the ability of patients to reach medical care. Patients had also delayed seeking medical opinion, even for urgent neurosurgical conditions such as aneurysmal subarachnoid hemorrhage. The closure of outpatient clinics and reduction of staff during ward rounds and other patient care activities also meant that opportunities to sharpen clinical skills essential for decision-making had likewise been markedly reduced.

More often than not, trainees had to be withdrawn from their elective and research rotations. Neurosurgery trainees have also been redeployed to areas of need during the peak of the pandemic in their respective countries. Among 192 neurosurgery trainees in Italy, 30% were directly involved in the clinical management of COVID-19 patients [31]. Between 17% and 54% of trainees in Indonesia, Malaysia, the Philippines, Singapore, and Thailand reported working in COVID wards or ICUs and acute respiratory infection clinics [33].

Because of lack of hands-on experience during this period, a significant proportion of trainees around the world were worried that the pandemic would have a negative impact on their training overall: about one-third of trainees surveyed in North America [34] and as high as 74% of those in Southeast Asia [33]. In a highly technical specialty such as neurosurgery, it is essential that this concern is addressed and measures are taken to ensure that training programs continue to produce highly skilled and competent neurosurgeons.

## Adaptations Under Fire

In centers where trainees are unable to meet requirements in cases numbers set by their respective neurosurgery boards or councils, the length of the training may have to be extended to compensate for the surgical volume loss. Other strategies included increasing the exposure of the trainees to private cases performed by consultants, increasing the surgical capacity of designated non-COVID hospitals, and subsequently diverting elective neurosurgical procedures to these centers.

To maintain and develop surgical skills among trainees, neurosurgery departments have developed pandemic curricula, usually consisting of online didactics with practical, hands-on exercises on microsurgery and microanastomosis using tabletop microscopes or, when available, in dedicated simulation laboratories. Plans to develop realistic surgical simulators accelerated (e.g., https://upsurgeon.com), including the utilization of virtual and augmented reality [38, 39]. Face-to-face departmental teaching activities such as grand rounds, morbidity and mortality conferences, and subspecialty meetings were easily transitioned to the online environment using various meeting software and applications. In fact, many groups have reported an improvement in attendance during these interdisciplinary discussions, likely because of the decrease in clinical workload and ease of joining these activities, even at home. Trainees had to rapidly acquire communication and evaluation skills required for telemedicine, traditionally not taught in most training programs. Although less than ideal for getting a comprehensive clinical evaluation of patients, this replaced the learning experience from outpatient consults and follow-ups, for both trainees and medical students aspiring to get into neurosurgery.

While the pandemic introduced an abrupt barrier and negative effect on the ability to train neurosurgeons, especially in LMICs, the increased use of social media and virtual platforms is markedly improving the interactions between institutions for shared learning between neurosurgeons at an international scale. Neurosurgical societies and organizations worldwide regularly conducted online webinars on myriad topics, often focusing on clinical evaluation of neurosurgical diseases and pearls and pitfalls of neurosurgical approaches. Although the advantages of these online learning experiences are many, these have to be weighed against "Zoom fatigue," wherein long hours spent in front of a screen may lead to decreased attention span and, ultimately, loss of interest in these educational activities.

## Other Concerns of Trainees

Lack of adequate personal protective equipment was a concern for many trainees, especially in areas hardest hit by the pandemic early on [31, 33]. This was crucial, not just for trainees redeployed to COVID-19 units of their hospitals but also for those who had to perform emergency neurosurgical procedures on confirmed COVID-19 patients. Testing was likewise an issue, especially at the start when RT-PCR was not readily available in most centers and the turnaround time for tests took several days. Because of these issues, many trainees were understandably worried about their personal safety and that of their families. In a global survey of neurosurgery trainees, 90% said that the pandemic had affected their mental health [32].

A delay in career advancement is looming for many neurosurgical trainees around the world. In the USA, the Accreditation Council for Graduate Medical Education (ACGME) published multiple policies to address questions regarding how the pandemic impacted training. Ultimately, the determination of whether or not a resident or fellow can graduate as previously scheduled is the responsibility of the program director with case review by the Clinical Competency Committee [40]. The American Board of Neurological Surgery has postponed both primary and oral examinations. Similarly, in the Philippines, the Philippine Board of Neurological

Surgery has decided not to allow final-year residents to sit their exams. Because of travel, work, and visa restrictions, many trainees – especially in low- and middle-income countries – are concerned about international fellowship positions or observership slots that they have previously applied for or have already secured.

## COVID-19's Impact on Neurosurgery Research

The COVID-19 pandemic has differentially impacted scientists and researchers around the world [41]. When cases began to rise in different countries, it became necessary for academic and research institutions to reduce activity in their physical laboratories to a minimum. By conducting only essential experiments and operations, the risk of COVID-19 transmission among laboratory personnel was mitigated, and the need for PPE in these less critical areas similarly reduced. As a direct consequence of the pandemic, health researchers anticipated a decline in patient recruitment for ongoing trials, difficulty in procuring needed equipment and supplies, and subsequent delays in project completion and publication [42]. Studies that had the potential to have an impact on the prevention, diagnosis, and treatment of COVID-19 were prioritized. Others were postponed indefinitely, potentially delaying scientific productivity [38, 43]. Ultimately, those rooted in basic sciences (e.g., biochemistry, biology, chemistry, and chemical engineering) had a greater reduction in research time compared with their colleagues whose work were less dependent on physical laboratories and experiments (e.g., mathematics, statistics, computer science, and economics). In contrast, the reduction in clinical volume provided additional time for research that was able to be conducted remotely, such as outcomes, computational, and health science research. Furthermore, it has sparked an unprecedented rate of transnational collaboration on research. The short- and long-term implications of this are discussed herein.

In a global survey conducted in March 2020, out of 187 neurosurgeons, 27% reported cessation of research [44]. Women and those with young children were disproportionately affected – likely because of increased responsibilities at home – and the decline in publications authored by women has been documented [45]. Declines in research were more pronounced in low-income countries and those that had a greater COVID-19 caseload; 36% of respondents said that their research activities had decreased. In India, the researches of academic neurosurgeons were more affected than that of neurosurgeons with nonteaching positions [46]. For many neurosurgical trainees, time away from clinical responsibilities translated to more time for research; they used this period to finish pending manuscripts or revise previously rejected submissions. Out of 192 trainees in Italy, 56% said that their production of scientific manuscripts had increased [31]. In North America, 65% of residents devoted more time to clinical research [34]. These figures are in contrast to Southeast Asia, where 33–60% of residents in Indonesia, Malaysia, the Philippines, and Singapore had a decrease in their research activities [33]. Neurosurgery residents in Thailand were least affected, with 54% saying that their research work proceeded on schedule. Furthermore, 20–47% of trainees in the region reported that they would miss a research presentation at a neurosurgical conference due to travel restrictions and cancellation of international meetings. Consequently, during the spring of 2020, academic journals faced a massive surge in COVID-related manuscripts submitted to and published in scientific journals across major disciplines [47, 48]. For instance, from February to June 2020, the *Journal of Neurosurgery* recorded a 55% increase in manuscript submissions compared with the same time period in 2019 [49]. For *Journal of Neurosurgery: Spine* and *Journal of Neurosurgery: Pediatrics*, the increases were 77% and 78%, respectively.

Neurosurgical departments implemented several adaptations to maintain their research activities. Whenever possible, researchers were advised to work on the parts of their projects that could be accomplished at home, such as writing grant applications, literature review, remote data extraction, and data analysis [50]. Academic work that did not require patient contact were encouraged. These included conducting systematic reviews and meta-analyses, writing book chapters, and developing simulation models. Journal clubs were converted to virtual meetings [51]. Often, residents on their research rotation served as backup for those who rendered inpatient care and performed essential neurosurgical operations [9]. When faculty had concomitant research and clinical roles, they were only allowed to perform their research duties if they had no symptoms [52].

Other recommendations included streamlining related projects, dividing researchers into cohorts, limiting people working in the same room, and frequently decontaminating shared resources such as microscopes [50]. Over time, as scientists became more aware of the mechanics of viral transmission, it became necessary to renovate physical facilities to ensure adequate ventilation and social distance between personnel, a complete turnaround from the coworking spaces that were encouraged prior to the pandemic.

To accelerate the gathering of data and generation of recommendations in COVID-related studies, many institutions revised their protocols to expedite research processes, particularly those concerning ethics review by institutional research boards. Collaborative work among departments, organizations, and institutions were encouraged, facilitated by online networks. This was best exemplified by the COVIDSurg study [53, 54]. By rapidly recruiting international collaborators, the investigators were able to analyze the 30-day mortality and pulmonary complication rates of over 1100 patients with COVID-19 from 24 countries, concluding that the threshold for surgery in this group of patients must be raised, especially among the elderly.

To cope with the surge in manuscript submissions, major journals have had to make adaptations in their editorial and peer-review processes [48, 49]. In journals with limited human and technical resources, authors have had to contend with longer turnaround times. While there was a great need to disseminate evidence rapidly, there remained a strong responsibility to critically examine submissions for methodological flaws or scientific misconduct, especially those that had a potential impact on treatment algorithms and public health policies. In JAMA, readers were allowed to leave online comments on COVID-related content to obtain immediate feedback instead of relying on traditional letters to the editor [48]. Social media networks such as Twitter were also instrumental in swift dissemination of study findings and getting real-time peer review from the greater scientific community. More significantly, the majority of scientific journals published their COVID-related articles open access. Among the neurosurgery journals, the *Journal of Neurosurgery* released a special issue that tackled COVID-19 and its impact on all aspects of neurosurgery, while *Neurosurgery*, *World Neurosurgery*, *Acta Neurochirurgica*, and *British Journal of Neurosurgery* have all expedited the publication of experiences of neurosurgeons, trainees, and neurosurgical departments from around the world, as they grappled and coped with the COVID-19 situation in their respective countries. These articles highlighted strengths and best practices to continue providing essential neurosurgical care in both high-income and developing countries. *Neurosurgical Focus* put out a call for papers on preparedness and guidelines for neurosurgical practice during a pandemic, and the special issue is expected to be published in December 2020.

## Conclusion

The COVID-19 pandemic rapidly swept the globe in 2020 and placed an unprecedented strain on healthcare systems around the world. At the time this chapter is being written, the full impact of the pandemic on global neurosurgery research remains unknown. However, we do know that it has both caused negative and positive change. COVID adaptations decreased case volume and interrupted training in the short term but also guided neurosurgeons to reflect on protocols for case prioritization, workforce redistribution, pre- and intraoperative safety, telemedicine, and more. Regarding research, it interrupted many in-person basic science experiments but also introduced new ways of carrying out global partnerships for big data collection, such as COVIDSurg. Journals have seen surges in manuscript submissions during this time and reformatted their processes to allow for more rapid publication. Education has transformed into more broad access of shared information with online webinars and live operation teaching sessions. Overall, the time span of the virus as an acute threat for humanity is unclear, but we as a neurosurgical community should continue analyzing the positive changes which have manifested in 2020 as we prepare together for a second wave, another pandemic, or simply negotiating our "new normal."

## References

1. World Health Organization. WHO director-general's opening remarks at the media briefing on COVID-19—11 March 2020. https://www.who.int/dg/speeches/detail/who-director-general-s-opening-remarks-at-the-media-briefing-on-covid-19%2D%2D-11-march-2020. Accessed 2020.

2. Center for Systems Science and Engineering – Johns Hopkins Coronavirus Resource Center: COVID-19 Dashboard by the Center for Systems Science and Engineering (CSSE) at Johns Hopkins University. https://coronavirus.jhu.edu/map.html. Accessed 2020.
3. Remuzzi A, Remuzzi G. COVID-19 and Italy: what next? Lancet. 2020;395(10231):1225–8. https://doi.org/10.1016/S0140-6736(20)30627-9.
4. Calderwood MS, Deloney VM, Anderson DJ, Cheng VC, Gohil S, Kwon JH, et al. Policies and practices of SHEA research network hospitals during the COVID-19 pandemic. Infect Control Hosp Epidemiol. 2020:1–9. https://doi.org/10.1017/ice.2020.303.
5. Bernstein M. Editorial. Neurosurgical priority setting during a pandemic: COVID-19. J Neurosurg. 2020:1–2. https://doi.org/10.3171/2020.4.JNS201031.
6. Ramakrishna R, Zadeh G, Sheehan JP, Aghi MK. Inpatient and outpatient case prioritization for patients with neuro-oncologic disease amid the COVID-19 pandemic: general guidance for neuro-oncology practitioners from the AANS/CNS Tumor Section and Society for Neuro-oncology. J Neuro-Oncol. 2020;147(3):525–9. https://doi.org/10.1007/s11060-020-03488-7.
7. Bell JA, Hyland S, DePellegrin T, Upshur RE, Bernstein M, Martin DK. SARS and hospital priority setting: a qualitative case study and evaluation. BMC Health Serv Res. 2004;4(1):36. https://doi.org/10.1186/1472-6963-4-36.
8. Emanuel EJ, Persad G, Upshur R, Thome B, Parker M, Glickman A, et al. Fair allocation of scarce medical resources in the time of Covid-19. N Engl J Med. 2020;382(21):2049–55. https://doi.org/10.1056/NEJMsb2005114.
9. Khalafallah AM, Jimenez AE, Lee RP, Weingart JD, Theodore N, Cohen AR, et al. Impact of COVID-19 on an academic neurosurgery department: the Johns Hopkins experience. World Neurosurg. 2020;139:e877–e84. https://doi.org/10.1016/j.wneu.2020.05.167.
10. Marini A, Iacoangeli M, Dobran M. Letter to the Editor regarding "coronavirus disease 2019 (COVID-19) and neurosurgery: literature and neurosurgical societies recommendations update". World Neurosurg. 2020; https://doi.org/10.1016/j.wneu.2020.05.160.
11. Zoia C, Bongetta D, Veiceschi P, Cenzato M, Di Meco F, Locatelli D, et al. Neurosurgery during the COVID-19 pandemic: update from Lombardy, northern Italy. Acta Neurochir. 2020;162(6):1221–2. https://doi.org/10.1007/s00701-020-04305-w.
12. Goyal A, Kerezoudis P, Yolcu YU, Chaichana KL, Abode-Iyamah K, Quinones-Hinojosa A, et al. Letter to the Editor: survey of academic U.S. programs regarding the impact of the COVID-19 pandemic on clinical practice, education, and research in neurosurgery. World Neurosurg. 2020; https://doi.org/10.1016/j.wneu.2020.06.028.
13. Thomas JG, Gandhi S, White TG, Jocelyn C, Soo TM, Eisenberg M, et al. Letter: a guide to the prioritization of neurosurgical cases after the COVID-19 pandemic. Neurosurgery. 2020; https://doi.org/10.1093/neuros/nyaa251.
14. EANS. EANS advice: triaging non-emergent neurosurgical procedures during the COVID-19 outbreak. EANS; 2020.
15. Abboud H, Kharbouch H, Arkha Y. Letter to the Editor: "COVID-19 pandemic in developing countries: effects on urgent neurosurgical consultation and patients' care: experience from North Africa". World Neurosurg. 2020;141:576. https://doi.org/10.1016/j.wneu.2020.06.204.
16. Wong J, Goh QY, Tan Z, Lie SA, Tay YC, Ng SY, et al. Preparing for a COVID-19 pandemic: a review of operating room outbreak response measures in a large tertiary hospital in Singapore. Can J Anaesth. 2020;67(6):732–45. https://doi.org/10.1007/s12630-020-01620-9.
17. Iorio-Morin C, Hodaie M, Sarica C, Dea N, Westwick HJ, Christie SD, et al. Letter: the risk of COVID-19 infection during neurosurgical procedures: a review of severe acute respiratory distress syndrome coronavirus 2 (SARS-CoV-2) modes of transmission and proposed neurosurgery-specific measures for mitigation. Neurosurgery. 2020;87(2):E178–E85. https://doi.org/10.1093/neuros/nyaa157.
18. Mizumoto K, Kagaya K, Zarebski A, Chowell G. Estimating the asymptomatic proportion of coronavirus disease 2019 (COVID-19) cases on board the diamond princess cruise ship, Yokohama, Japan, 2020. Euro Surveill. 2020;25(10) https://doi.org/10.2807/1560-7917.ES.2020.25.10.2000180.

19. Cook TM, El-Boghdadly K, McGuire B, McNarry AF, Patel A, Higgs A. Consensus guidelines for managing the airway in patients with COVID-19: guidelines from the Difficult Airway Society, the Association of Anaesthetists the Intensive Care Society, the Faculty of Intensive Care Medicine and the Royal College of Anaesthetists. Anaesthesia. 2020;75(6):785–99. https://doi.org/10.1111/anae.15054.

20. Zou L, Ruan F, Huang M, Liang L, Huang H, Hong Z, et al. SARS-CoV-2 viral load in upper respiratory specimens of infected patients. N Engl J Med. 2020;382(12):1177–9. https://doi.org/10.1056/NEJMc2001737.

21. WHO. Task shifting: global recommendations and guidelines. WHO; 2008.

22. Robertson FC, Lippa L, Broekman MLD. Editorial. Task shifting and task sharing for neurosurgeons amidst the COVID-19 pandemic. J Neurosurg. 2020:1–3. https://doi.org/10.3171/2020.4.Jns201056.

23. Robertson FC, Esene IN, Kolias AG, Khan T, Rosseau G, Gormley WB, et al. Global perspectives on task shifting and task sharing in neurosurgery. World Neurosurg. 2019; https://doi.org/10.1016/j.wnsx.2019.100060.

24. Tuckson RV, Edmunds M, Hodgkins ML. Telehealth. N Engl J Med. 2017;377(16):1585–92. https://doi.org/10.1056/NEJMsr1503323.

25. Mouchtouris N, Lavergne P, Montenegro TS, Gonzalez G, Baldassari M, Sharan A, et al. Telemedicine in neurosurgery: lessons learned and transformation of care during the COVID-19 pandemic. World Neurosurg. 2020; https://doi.org/10.1016/j.wneu.2020.05.251.

26. Eichberg DG, Basil GW, Di L, Shah AH, Luther EM, Lu VM, et al. Telemedicine in neurosurgery: lessons learned from a systematic review of the literature for the COVID-19 era and beyond. Neurosurgery. 2020; https://doi.org/10.1093/neuros/nyaa306.

27. Yoon EJ, Tong D, Anton GM, Jasinski JM, Claus CF, Soo TM, et al. Patient satisfaction with neurosurgery telemedicine visits during the COVID-19 pandemic: a prospective cohort study. World Neurosurg. 2020; https://doi.org/10.1016/j.wneu.2020.09.170.

28. Demaerschalk BM, Cassivi SD, Blegen RN, Borah B, Moriarty J, Gullerud R, et al. Health economic analysis of postoperative video telemedicine visits to Patients' homes. Telemed J E Health. 2020; https://doi.org/10.1089/tmj.2020.0257.

29. Munusamy T, Karuppiah R, Faizal ABN, Sockalingam S, Cham CY, Waran V. Telemedicine via smart glasses in critical care of the neurosurgical patient – a COVID-19 pandemic preparedness and response in neurosurgery. World Neurosurg. 2020; https://doi.org/10.1016/j.wneu.2020.09.076.

30. Cote DJ, Barnett I, Onnela JP, Smith TR. Digital phenotyping in patients with spine disease: a novel approach to quantifying mobility and quality of life. World Neurosurg. 2019;126:e241–e9. https://doi.org/10.1016/j.wneu.2019.01.297.

31. Zoia C, Raffa G, Somma T, Della Pepa GM, La Rocca G, Zoli M, et al. COVID-19 and neurosurgical training and education: an Italian perspective. Acta Neurochir. 2020;162(8):1789–94. https://doi.org/10.1007/s00701-020-04460-0.

32. Alhaj AK, Al-Saadi T, Mohammad F, Alabri S. Neurosurgery residents' perspective on COVID-19: knowledge, readiness, and impact of this pandemic. World Neurosurg. 2020;139:e848–e58. https://doi.org/10.1016/j.wneu.2020.05.087.

33. Wittayanakorn N, Nga VDW, Sobana M, Bahuri NFA, Baticulon RE. Impact of COVID-19 on neurosurgical training in Southeast Asia. World Neurosurg. 2020; https://doi.org/10.1016/j.wneu.2020.08.073.

34. Pelargos PE, Chakraborty A, Zhao YD, Smith ZA, Dunn IF, Bauer AM. An evaluation of neurosurgical resident education and sentiment during the coronavirus disease 2019 pandemic: a north American survey. World Neurosurg. 2020;140:e381–e6. https://doi.org/10.1016/j.wneu.2020.05.263.

35. Kanmounye US, Esene IN. Letter to the editor "COVID-19 and neurosurgical education in Africa: making lemonade from lemons". World Neurosurg. 2020;139:732–3. https://doi.org/10.1016/j.wneu.2020.05.126.

36. Leong AZ, Lim JX, Tan CH, Teo K, Nga VDW, Lwin S, et al. COVID-19 response measures – a Singapore neurosurgical academic medical Centre experience segregated team model to maintain tertiary level neurosurgical care during the COVID-19 outbreak. Br J Neurosurg. 2020:1–6. https://doi.org/10.1080/02688697.2020.1758629.

37. Low JCM, Visagan R, Perera A. Neurosurgical training during COVID-19 pandemic: British perspective. World Neurosurg. 2020;142:520–2. https://doi.org/10.1016/j.wneu.2020.04.178.

38. Tomlinson SB, Hendricks BK, Cohen-Gadol AA. Editorial. Innovations in neurosurgical education during the COVID-19 pandemic: is it time to reexamine our neurosurgical training models? J Neurosurg. 2020:1–2. https://doi.org/10.3171/2020.4.Jns201012.

39. Zaed I, Tinterri B. Letter to the editor: how is COVID-19 going to affect education in neurosurgery? A step toward a new era of educational training. World Neurosurg. 2020;140:481–3. https://doi.org/10.1016/j.wneu.2020.06.032.

40. ACGME: Frequently Asked Questions. Accreditation Council for Graduate Medical Education. https://acgme.org/COVID-19/Frequently-Asked-Questions. Accessed Oct 2020.

41. Myers KR, Tham WY, Yin Y, Cohodes N, Thursby JG, Thursby MC, et al. Unequal effects of the COVID-19 pandemic on scientists. Nat Hum Behav. 2020;4(9):880–3. https://doi.org/10.1038/s41562-020-0921-y.

42. Peeters A, Mullins G, Becker D, Orellana L, Livingston P. COVID-19's impact on Australia's health research workforce. Lancet. 2020;396(10249):461. https://doi.org/10.1016/S0140-6736(20)31533-6.

43. Kissler SM, Tedijanto C, Lipsitch M, Grad Y. Social distancing strategies for curbing the COVID-19 epidemic. medRxiv. 2020;2020 https://doi.org/10.1101/2020.03.22.20041079.

44. El-Ghandour NMF, Elsebaie EH, Salem AA, Alkhamees AF, Zaazoue MA, Fouda MA, et al. Letter: the impact of the coronavirus (COVID-19) pandemic on neurosurgeons worldwide. Neurosurgery. 2020;87(2):E250–e7. https://doi.org/10.1093/neuros/nyaa212.

45. Kibbe MR. Consequences of the COVID-19 pandemic on manuscript submissions by women. JAMA Surg. 2020;155(9):803–4. https://doi.org/10.1001/jamasurg.2020.3917.

46. Venkataram T, Goyal N, Dash C, Chandra PP, Chaturvedi J, Raheja A, et al. Impact of the COVID-19 pandemic on neurosurgical practice in India: results of an anonymized National Survey. Neurol India. 2020;68(3):595–602. https://doi.org/10.4103/0028-3886.289004.

47. Lee JE, Mohanty A, Albuquerque FC, Couldwell WT, Levy EI, Benzel EC, et al. Trends in academic productivity in the COVID-19 era: analysis of neurosurgical, stroke neurology, and neurointerventional literature. J Neurointerv Surg. 2020; https://doi.org/10.1136/neurintsurg-2020-016710.

48. Bauchner H, Fontanarosa PB, Golub RM. Editorial evaluation and peer review during a pandemic: how journals maintain standards. JAMA. 2020;324(5):453–4. https://doi.org/10.1001/jama.2020.11764.

49. Kondziolka D, Couldwell WT, Rutka JT. Editorial. Putting pen to paper during a pandemic: increased manuscript submissions to the JNS publishing group. J Neurosurg. 2020:1–3. https://doi.org/10.3171/2020.7.JNS202691.

50. Clark VE. Editorial. Impact of COVID-19 on neurosurgery resident research training. J Neurosurg. 2020:1–2. https://doi.org/10.3171/2020.4.JNS201034.

51. Bray DP, Stricsek GP, Malcolm J, Gutierrez J, Greven A, Barrow DL, et al. Letter: maintaining neurosurgical resident education and safety during the COVID-19 pandemic. Neurosurgery. 2020;87(2):E189–E91. https://doi.org/10.1093/neuros/nyaa164.

52. Burke JF, Chan AK, Mummaneni V, Chou D, Lobo EP, Berger MS, et al. Letter: the coronavirus disease 2019 global pandemic: a neurosurgical treatment algorithm. Neurosurgery. 2020;87(1):E50–E6. https://doi.org/10.1093/neuros/nyaa116.

53. COVIDSurg Collaborative. Global guidance for surgical care during the COVID-19 pandemic. Br J Surg. 2020; https://doi.org/10.1002/bjs.11646.

54. Nepogodiev D, Bhangu A, Glasbey JC, Li E, Omar OM, Simoes JFF, et al. Mortality and pulmonary complications in patients undergoing surgery with perioperative SARS-CoV-2 infection: an international cohort study. Lancet. 2020;396(10243):27–38. https://doi.org/10.1016/S0140-6736(20)31182-X.

# Index

Printed in the United States
by Baker & Taylor Publisher Services